THIRD EDITION

THE ART OF NUTRITIONAL COOKING

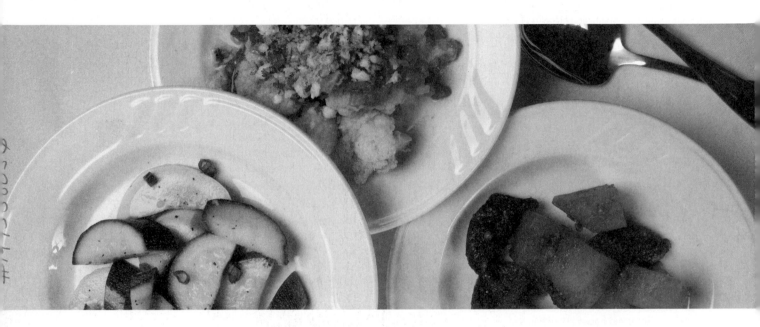

Michael Baskette, CEC, CCA, AAC

James Painter, PhD, RD

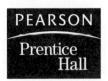

PEARSON

Prentice
Hall

Upper Saddle River, New Jersey
Columbus, Ohio

Library of Congress Cataloging-in-Publication Data

Baskette, Michael.
 The art of nutritional cooking / Michael Baskette, James Painter.—3rd ed.
  p. cm.
 Includes bibliographical references and index.
 ISBN-13: 978-0-13-045701-1
 ISBN-10: 0-13-045701-9
 1. Cookery. 2. Nutrition. I. Painter, James, PhD. II. Title.
 TX714.B373 2009
 G41.5—dc22

                                          2008030145

Editor in Chief: Vernon R. Anthony
Aquisitions Editor: William Lawrensen
Editorial Assistant: Lara Dimmick
Project Manager: Kris Roach
Production Coordination: Janet Bolton, Milford Publishing Services
Art Director: Diane Y. Ernsberger
Cover Designer: Candace Rowley
Operations Specialist: Deidra Schwartz
Director of Marketing: David Gesell
Campaign Marketing Manager: Leigh Ann Sims
Curriculum Marketing Manager: Thomas Hayward
Marketing Assistant: Les Roberts
Chapter Opening Images: Jim Smith Photography
Director, Image Resource Center: Melinda Patelli
Manager, Rights and Permissions: Zina Arabia
Manager, Visual Research: Beth Brenzel
Manager, Cover Visual Research & Permissions: Karen Sanatar
Image Permission Coordinator: Fran Toepfer

This book was set in TradeGothic Light by Aptara®, Inc. It was printed and bound by R.R. Donnelley & Sons Company. The cover was printed by Phoenix Color Corp.

Pearson Education Ltd.
Pearson Education Singapore Pte. Ltd.
Pearson Education Canada, Ltd.
Pearson Education—Japan

Pearson Education Australia Pty. Limited
Pearson Education North Asia Ltd.
Pearson Educación de Mexico, S.A. de C.V.
Pearson Education Malaysia Pte. Ltd.

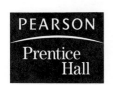

PEARSON
Prentice
Hall

10 9 8 7 6 5 4 3 2 1
ISBN 13: 978-0-13-045701-1
ISBN 10:   0-13-045701-9

CONTENTS

CHAPTER 1

Discovering Food and Nutrition   1

When Food Was Necessary   2

When Food Became Fashionable   4

The Birth of World Cuisine   5

When Food Became Convenient: The Fast-Food Generation   6

The Beginning of Nutritional Science   8

Can Good Nutrition Wait?   9

CHAPTER 2

Nutritional Guidelines   13

Nutrition in the United States Today   15

Dietary Reference Intakes   16

Dietary Guidelines for Americans   20

My Pyramid: The New Food Guide Pyramid   21

Food Labeling   24

International Dietary Guidelines   39

CHAPTER 3

Carbohydrates   43

Classification of Carbohydrates   45

Carbohydrate-Related Disorders   53

Carbohydrate Loading for Sports   55

Fiber   56

CHAPTER 4

Proteins   69

Why Do We Need Proteins?   70

Protein Discovery and Function   71

Amino Acids: The Structure of Protein   72

Protein Quality   73

Protein Requirement   75

Choosing Ideal Protein Foods   77

Food is More than Protein   77

Digestion and Absorption of Protein   79

Consequences of Insufficient Dietary Protein   80

Protein Cookery   81

Vegetarianism   81

CHAPTER 5

Lipids: Fats and Oils   87

Classification of Dietary Lipids, Fats, and Oils   89

Digestion of Fat   93

Metabolism of Lipids   94

Functions of Dietary Fat in Maintaining Health   95

Dietary Recommendations   95

Hydrogenation   96

Oxidation   97

Tips About Fatty Acids   97

Fat Replacers   98

CHAPTER 6

Vitamins   103

Fat-Soluble Vitamins   105

Water-Soluble Vitamins   115

Pseudovitamins   131

Phytochemicals   131

A Problem with Vitamin Supplements   132

CHAPTER 7

Minerals   137

Major Minerals (Macrominerals)   138

Trace Minerals (Microminerals)   150

Other Micronutrients   160

CHAPTER 8

Health and Diet   165

Diet and Aging   166

Osteoporosis   167

Diabetes 168

Heart Disease 169

Cancer 170

Arthritis 171

High Blood Pressure (Hypertension) 172

Diet and Skin Care 174

CHAPTER 9
Weight Control 177

Prevalence of Obesity 178

Causes of Obesity 180

Ill Effects of Obesity 181

Treatment for Obesity 182

Comparing Weight-Loss Diets 182

Balancing Energy Intake and Expenditure 185

Determining Calorie Need 187

Making Healthy Food Choices and Substitutions 187

Modifying Behavior 188

Environmental Factors 188

Exercise and Weight Control 191

More than Just Aerobics 192

Appetite Suppressants 193

CHAPTER 10
Serve Nutritionally Rich Foods through Proper Selection, Handling, and Cooking 197

Nutrient Sensitivity in Foods 199

Buying Nutrient-Rich Foods 202

Storing Foods to Preserve Nutrients 207

Processing Foods to Preserve Nutrients 209

Cooking Foods to Preserve Nutrients 211

CHAPTER 11
The Mechanics of Taste 217

The Components of Taste 218

Five Basic Tastes 220

Primary Odors 222

Flavor Construction 224

Sweating versus Browning to Create Flavors 225

Searing Meats for Better Flavor 226

CHAPTER 12
The Natural Flavor of Foods 229

Historical Use of Spices 230

Historical Use of Herbs 232

Flavoring with Herbs and Spices 233

Proper Handling 233

Whole versus Ground 234

Culinary Adventure 234

Olfactory Impact 235

Flavoring Vegetables 235

A Changing Palate 236

The Onion Family 237

Flavoring Stalk, Root, and Tuber Vegetables 238

Peppers for Flavor 240

Mushrooms for Flavor 240

Oils: Healthy and Flavorful 242

Responsible Butter Use 243

Acidic Flavorings 243

Alcoholic Beverages 244

CHAPTER 13
Building Recipes for Healthier Meals 251

The Challenge 252

Recipe Transformations 255

Substituting Meats and Poultry for Healthier Cooking 258

Substituting Protein Alternatives for Meats, Seafood, and Poultry 261

The Whole Plate Concept 263

Nutritional Sauces 265

Substituting Fats for Healthier Cooking 267

Portioning 271

Create New Healthier Recipes 272

Staff Development 274

CHAPTER 14
Menu Planning: Adding Nutritional Choices   **277**

Healthy Menu Construction   279

Choosing Alternative Breakfast Items   280

Creating Healthy Appetizers   281

Nutrient-Rich, Low-Fat Soups   282

Making Healthy Salads and Entremets   284

Developing Healthy Meat Entrees   288

Developing Healthy Poultry Entrees   291

Developing Healthy Seafood Entrees   292

Offering Healthy Desserts   294

Vegetarian Menus   296

APPENDIX I
Wines for Cooking   **301**

APPENDIX II
An Anthology of the Most Generally Used Herbs and Spices   **305**

APPENDIX III
Food Weights and Measures   **313**

Glossary   **319**

Index   **321**

FOREWORD

Meals are often eaten away from the home—at fast-food establishments, in workplace cafeterias, and in an endless variety of restaurants, clubs, hotels, and diners. The convenient accessibility and growing options of foods and drinks often take priority over nutrition and balance, making wise choices more difficult.

Increased nutritional knowledge, and subsequent awareness on the part of conscientious consumers, however, is fueling a growing demand for healthier food choices in all types of establishments. People still frequent steak houses in large numbers, where large portions are the industry standard. Yet some diners might be looking for low-calorie options or healthier choices than the 12-ounce prime rib or 16-ounce T-bone. Other diners will seek out the spa restaurants, vegetarian establishments, and specialty food stores for nutritious choices. These places, however, are hard to come by and often offer menus too restrictive for people who want to eat more healthful foods but not give up the dishes they are used to having.

Some consumers hear the word "nutrition" and instantly withdraw to the nearest exit. Why? Well, certainly, nutritious foods have an ill-deserved reputation of being boring and tasteless. After all, people choose food to satisfy their hunger first and their palate second. Health and nutrition are the furthest things from a hungry diner's mind. Picture yourself ordering a particular food or entree from a restaurant's menu. Do you want the large succulent steak, or the petite dry fillet of fish? Do your taste buds prefer fried chicken with garlic-buttered mashed potatoes or boiled chicken cubes over a plain lettuce salad?

It's easy to see why taste is often the primary consideration. But not all nutritious food has to be tasteless. Nutrition has a "bum reputation" because consumers hear so many conflicting, negative, vague, and boring messages about what to eat and what not to eat that they don't know what to believe. In the kitchen, cooks and chefs are asked to deliver high-quality nutritious choices, but they generally have lacked the knowledge and experience to do so. And while some chefs championed the cause of, learned, and practiced nutritional cooking early on, others still debate whether nutritional cooking is just a fad or, rather, a long-term trend.

But the demand for healthier foods is growing so large in the United States that diet-conscious customers now appear in every neighborhood. They frequent every type of dining facility and search for healthier menu choices but, at the same time, demand high-quality food and service.

Thus food service operators are constantly being challenged to offer at least some nutritious menu choices as the demand for quality nutritious foods increases. Many operations provide their traditional (i.e., daily) menus along with foods that follow strict nutritional guidelines to appease their regular clients and attract new ones. Some operators approach their cooking holistically, making everything they serve more nutritious and healthful than their standard fare would have been. In both cases it is the cooks and chefs who make this achievement possible.

The perception that foods must contain fats and salts for flavor is based on centuries of tradition and lore and common personal experiences and practice. Changing diet and culinary traditions will continue to be difficult, especially since these practices have endured the passage of time. Both diet and cooking are linked with the evolution of human civilization, which means they are woven into the fabric of the human psyche.

Abundant empirical evidence exists that poor nutrition affects everyone's overall quality of life. This fact by itself, however, isn't enough to change centuries of dining habits. Change will come slowly, and only after the foods that American dining facilities prepare and serve can meet nutritional guidelines and still satisfy hunger and appeal to customers' palates. Consumers will accept nutritionally prepared and properly balanced meals when they are constructed with the same level of detail in taste construction, eye appeal, and textural points as the traditional foods to which they are accustomed.

Heart-healthy and "light" menu items in restaurants around the country continue to gain market share every day. Consumer advocates, after winning the battle for nutrition labels on convenience foods in grocery stores, then succeeded in having similar rules applied to commercial food service operations through the Nutrition Labeling Education Act in 1997.

Consumers who are aware of the health and life benefits of good nutrition are placing the burden on restaurants and food manufacturers to present good nutritional choices. Consumers feel that they don't have time to plan and cook in a nutritional way, so it becomes the chef's challenge and the restaurant's responsibility to offer good-tasting balanced foods prepared nutritionally.

Food service in this millennium increasingly will be based on menus that combine taste and good nutrition, provide convenience and ease of preparation, and present a wide variety of healthful choices to consumers. Nutrition is fast becoming a concern for all types of people—young, old, active, and sedentary.

In television, movies, and advertisements, "thin" is portrayed as beautiful and sexy, "overweight" as unhealthy, and "obese" as unnatural. But obesity has become so commonplace in the United States that some are calling it an epidemic that affects all age groups.

The positive news about oatmeal's ability to reduce cholesterol and the health benefits of seafood's omega-3 fatty acids has made a lot of people become interested in following dietary advice. Other news about cutting dietary fat for good health fuels a growing demand for low-fat food products like turkey luncheon meats and skim and 2% milk products. What should the food service industry do in response to this demand?

Many people today want to live healthier, longer lives. This has spurred on the trend for better fad diets, exercise DVDs, and in-home exercise equipment. Spa clubs and health clubs have never been more popular. But where else could one go to find healthier food? Where could people carry on healthy traditions outside of the health clubs and spas, through everyday living and dining?

Thus an outcry for nutritional food choices and healthier alternatives to traditional menu items is under way in most types of dining environments. Consequently, cooks and chefs need to become more knowledgeable and more practiced in the art of nutritional cooking.

PREFACE

The science of nutrition, born out of our need to survive and our humanistic thirst for knowledge, has finally arrived in the modern American kitchen. Whether food is professionally prepared or prepared for home use, the pairing of good cuisine with good nutritional value is a growing concept.

This edition of *The Art of Nutritional Cooking* is both a guide and a tool for those interested in preparing healthy food. It is more than a cookbook and much more than a nutrition text. It combines the science of nutrition with the art of cooking to illustrate the infinite possibilities for healthy foods that satisfy hunger, taste, and eye appeal. We have taken the tenets of nutrition, combined them with the theories of cooking, and built a model for modern cuisine.

Good nutrition is not just something that helps heal the sick, protect the aged, and build the young. It is what we should all strive to achieve in our quest for long and healthy lives. This text does not deal solely with restrictive diets or stringent nutritional guidelines; rather, it proposes a change in the philosophy of cooking for all kitchens everywhere. The focus is on the natural flavors and textures of foods; the recipes rely on simple preparations and flavoring ingredients from around the world to heighten natural flavors and comply with nutritional guidelines.

We would like to acknowledge the support of the entire Prentice Hall staff for making this text a reality. In particular, we thank Vernon Anthony, Bill Lawrensen, and Judy Casillo, who guided us through the lengthy writing process. Special thanks to Mary Connor for her graphical design and to Nikki Mercer, Traci Frieling, and Jill North Craft for their research assistance and editorial support.

We would also like to acknowledge the following reviewers for their insightful comments: Toby Amidor, The Art Insitiute of New York City; Joan Aronson, The Art Institute of New York City; and John Hudoc, Robert Morris College.

MIKE BASKETTE   JAMES PAINTER

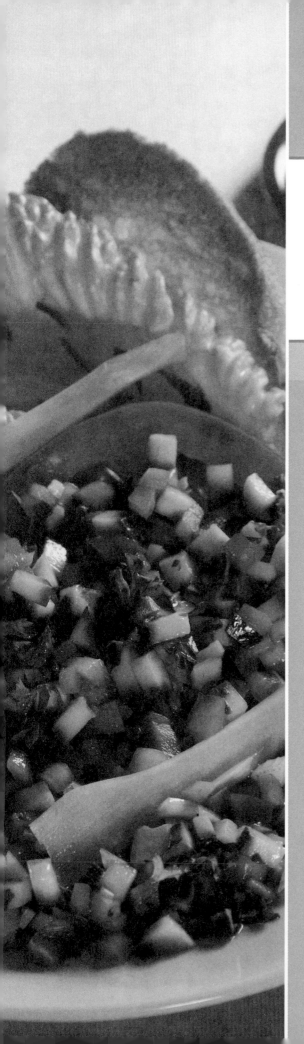

1

Discovering Food and Nutrition

KEY CONCEPTS

- Human eating habits, including our dependence on fat and salt for survival, have evolved over millions of years.
- During the Middle Ages and the European Renaissance, exotic foods became a status symbol for the wealthy and powerful, and overeating became a symbol of opulence.
- By the middle of the twentieth century, food had become a convenience item, and the fast-food generation was born.
- The science of nutrition is still relatively young. Many years of experimental studies are required to formulate and validate theories.
- The major tenets of nutritional dieting have been confirmed: Control fat intake, use salt sparingly, and eat a balanced diet.

After experimenting for thousands of years with foods, potions, and beverages, we have learned that what we choose to consume directly influences our general health, weight, and overall quality of life. **Nutritional science**, which measures relationships between the physical and chemical properties of food and drink and human metabolism, affirms this basic tenet: Moderation and balance are necessary for good health. Yet the overabundance of food in the Western world, combined with increasingly hectic lifestyles, has set the stage for overconsumption, obesity, and **malnutrition** in the United States.

Consumers have become confused about what constitutes a healthy diet, which foods they should eat, and how much they should consume. At the same time, cooks are trying to redesign traditional

NUTRITIONAL SCIENCE The study of food and nutrients and their application to health.

MALNUTRITION A condition resulting from dietary consumption that was either inadequate or excessive.

recipes to meet the strict low-fat, low-sodium, and high-fiber guidelines of nutritional cooking. What we have now is a growing uneasiness about choosing nutritious foods. In addition, the foods that we all knew and enjoyed are now being offered in less flavorful versions, smaller portion sizes, and boring plate presentations. If the notion of nutritious foods scares us, it is because we have made it that way.

THINK ABOUT IT

You may have heard chefs say that fat is what provides a lot of flavor to many different styles of foods, including savory and sweet dishes. Simply put, chefs say, fat is flavor. Likewise you may have heard that salt brings out the taste in foods. The salt bowl has never been closer to the cook's station than it is today. But is flavor something people learn to appreciate, as in the flavor of chocolate ice cream or salted pretzels, or is flavor defined by a physiological dependence on fat and salt for survival?

CASE STUDY

Is It Snack Time Yet?

John's parents both work and often come home late after a hard day at their jobs. John, on the other hand, comes home from school around 2:30 in the afternoon and rummages through the refrigerator for something to eat.

Given that he lives in the twenty-first century in a somewhat affluent family, what might John's choices be for a late afternoon snack? He doesn't want to take the time to cook anything; he just wants to grab something quick so he can run back outside to play. What items are in your own refrigerator and kitchen cabinets right now that make it easy to eat unhealthy foods? *The resolution for this case study is presented at the end of the chapter.*

WHEN FOOD WAS NECESSARY

Imagine early humans scouring the earth in search of food, always looking for their next meal. Berries, tree bark, fungi, roots, birds, snakes, and insects would all come under scrutiny through the hungry eyes of men, women, and children. Sustenance was achieved by filling their bellies with just about anything they could find that was not poisonous or otherwise unsafe to eat.

Humans learned through observation and experimentation what to eat and how to survive. No doubt, many experiments led to a better way of life or to new food sources, but some led to illness and death. Humans lived, experimented, remembered, and shared their findings on safe and dangerous foods over hundreds of thousands of years, long before written records.

Dependence on Fat for Survival

Humans recognized the need for fat in their diets from practically the beginning of their evolution. Fat is indeed necessary for life, but how did ancient humans know that or come to search for and covet fats without knowing their overall value to good health?

It did not take long, relative to over 4 million years of human evolution, for early humans to recognize the advantages of eating animals high in fat for energy and warmth. Perhaps it started at the end of the Paleolithic period (also known as the Stone

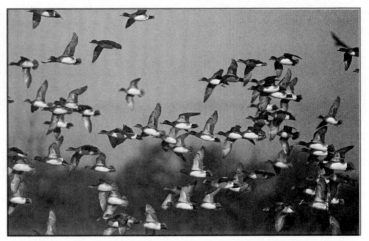
Ducks are an excellent food source, rich in protein and fat.
Nature Picture Library

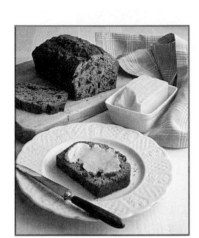
Sliced bread spread thick with butter is tempting to eat but full of fat calories.
Martin Brigdale © Dorling Kindersley

PHYSIOLOGICAL PROPERTY A property related to the functioning of the human body.

MOUTH FEEL The sensory evaluation of food in the mouth.

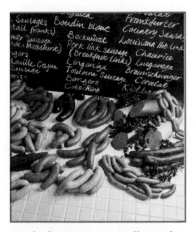
Smoked sausages are still popular today, combining smoke and fat for flavor and preservation.
Getty Images, Inc.—PhotoDisc

Age), when humans first learned to use stones and chipped bone for knives and spear tips. This enabled them to hunt a wide range of animals and birds from a distance, thus increasing their choices for each meal. Those choices began to include duck, goose, buffalo, bear, seal, and walrus meat, depending on where they lived. In addition to food, such animals supplied clothing, shoes, and other goods—all from a single source.

Fat is highly palatable and therefore very enjoyable to eat, causing both early and modern humans to crave its flavor. How many times have you heard the statement "Fat is flavor"? Well, it all boils down to the molecular structure of fat and how our bodies deal with it.

Scientists at Monell Chemical Senses Center in Philadelphia claim that the palatability of fat is partly due to its **physiological properties**. Fats, which contain twice as many calories as proteins and carbohydrates, provide the richest energy source for the human body and are therefore relished every time they are consumed.

Fat also has a certain feel or sensation in the mouth that contributes flavor to foods. **Mouth feel**, which describes the effect of textures and moisture on flavor, is an important aspect of fat. Since fats do not completely melt at body temperature, they tend to stay on the tongue longer than other foods, releasing their flavors over a longer period of time. The heavier the fat, or the more saturated it is, the longer it stays on the tongue. Together, the length of exposure to flavor coupled with fat's innate property of supplying energy and warmth made fatty foods valuable for health, energy, and protection against the cold.

Fat was also used in the early development of processed foods to give moisture to dried meats and seafood, sausages, and meat puddings. The combination of drying, salting, and smoking ground meats preserved them and gave them new flavors; fat made these foods palatable. Sausages, hot dogs, bologna, pepperoni, and thousands of other types of fresh, smoked, and dried meats are still popular menu items today.

Early Dependence on Salt

Using salt as a preservative and a seasoning also dates back many thousands of years. Early Egyptians, for example, employed salt in mummifying their pharaohs to preserve the flesh for the body's resurrection. They were already practiced in the salting of fish as a means of preservation; adapting the same method to the preservation of human flesh was a natural progression.

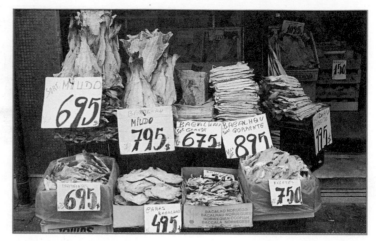

Salted cod (*bacalhau*) is still popular today, as seen at this Portuguese market.
Linda Whitwam (c) Dorling Kindersley

Another religious practice fostered the prevalence of salted foods beginning in the seventh and eighth centuries. The tradition of Christian Lent required, under penalty of death, that followers eat only fish during the 40 days of Lent, culminating with the Passion of Christ at Easter. Because fresh fish was available only to people living near water, salted fish became a source of nourishment to many inland Christians.

By the seventh century, not only salted fish but salted pork, beef, and game became a steady food supply in the absence of fresh meat.

WHEN FOOD BECAME FASHIONABLE

By AD 40, when the Roman Empire covered most of Europe, North Africa, and the Far East, agriculture and the domestication of animals and birds had advanced far enough that well-organized civilizations could grow and harvest enough food even for the commoners. Grain filled government coffers, and cooking and baking **guilds** began to flourish. The ready availability of food changed the way many people thought about food, especially wealthy and influential people. No longer forced to eat whatever could be found, they could instead plant fields (by scattering seeds), raise livestock, and import foods from foreign lands, and all this made people more adventurous in their eating habits. What a convenience it must have been to suddenly be able to eat anytime you were hungry.

This was also during the time of Marcus Apicius, the great Roman epicure whose treatise on Roman cooking still exists today, *De re coquinaria* (On Roman Cooking). It is full of complicated combinations of worldly ingredients and exotic seasonings into a series of recipes. At least for the noble Roman generals, the ability to purchase and prepare magnificent feasts was a sign of power and influence.

By the time of the European Renaissance, experimenting with food became a new trend. Members of royalty and others with wealth were willing to explore different flavor combinations and ingredients for the sake of creation rather than for mere sustenance. Food was no longer scarce, and exotic foods, which came from all over the known world for a substantial price, made their way into wealthy homes.

The availability of foods throughout the year led to overeating and obesity among wealthy Europeans. But rather than being seen as a health issue, the ability to over-

GUILD A group of professional tradesmen engaged in the same craft.

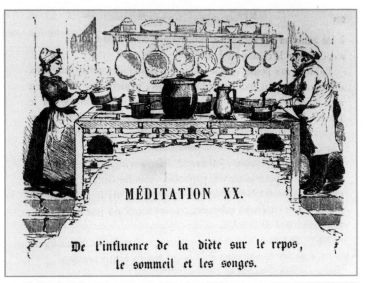

indulge was prized; eating and pleasure had become nearly synonymous to a lot of people.

This attitude was expressed by the eighteenth-century French epicure Jean Anthelme Brillat-Savarin who wrote, "And yet of all our senses, taste, such as Nature has created it, remains one which, on the whole, gives us the maximum of delight. It invites us, by means of pleasure, to make good the losses which we suffer through the action of life" (1984, p. 45)".

The taste of foods encourages us to eat when we're hungry and satisfies us when we're full. Taste combines the chemical elements and physical attributes of food and beverage with emotion to create individual boundaries of discrimination and appreciation.

We frequently use the pleasure of taste to escape from the many ups and downs of life. We eat when we are happy and overeat when we are depressed (or vice versa, depending on the individual). There are many reasons to eat for the sake of self-comforting: in anticipation of a hard day's work we allow ourselves an extra portion of this or that to fuel our physical machines; at the end of the day or week, chiffon pie becomes a prize for hard work and peach cobbler a reward for honesty.

Chefs over the centuries worked very hard to create new dishes that not only satisfied a patron's hunger but also stimulated their imaginations. Based on the foods that were available at the time and the advancements in cooking and baking technologies, the chef could experiment with and create great foods. Such foods became so admired by Brillat-Savarin that he proclaimed, "The discovery of a new dish does more for human happiness than the discovery of a new star" (1984, p. 62).

THE BIRTH OF WORLD CUISINE

As different cuisines developed around the world, indigenous game, seasonings, and other food ingredients played a critical role in early diets. Long before ships crossed the seas to gather exotic foods and caravans trekked across the deserts in search of Asian spices, necessity forced people to eat whatever they could easily put their hands on. This practice meant that food preferences were luxuries only a few could enjoy.

Foods cooked and consumed by Europeans, for example, were completely different than those cooked and enjoyed by the Asian cultures. Indigenous food ingredients were unique to their Asian and European homes, and the available herbs and spices were worlds apart.

Cooking techniques also varied around the world due to different sources of cooking fuels and different types of utensils. Where wood was plentiful for fires, large fire pits were constructed, and meats were hung over the licking flames. Later, brick ovens would be constructed to retain the heat and somewhat control the burning of the wood. Ovens led to pots, pans, and a whole array of cooking utensils. Where wood was scarce, people invented woks and steamers, which could cook foods quickly if they were cut into small enough pieces.

For thousands of years, segregated groups of people gathered, grew, cooked, and ate foods that were readily available to them. All this helped shape the cultural evolution of food preferences that are known today as *world cuisine*.

Of course, the average person did not have much of a choice of foods to eat. Only the rich and powerful people could discriminate against certain foods or discard what they considered to be inedible parts of animals and birds. To the common person, all parts of the animal were edible, and there was not a vegetable, fruit, nut, or seed that they would not consume.

WHEN FOOD BECAME CONVENIENT: THE FAST-FOOD GENERATION

People today, especially in the United States, have grown accustomed to getting food quickly. Hamburger shops, hot dog stands, and convenience stores adorn practically every street in America with their flashy signs and bargain prices. Even table-service restaurants cater to the demand for fast food with guaranteed service times, lunches in 15 minutes or less, and take-out ordering.

However, dining out is not the only place that convenience food, better known as *fast food*, has had an impact. Many of the food innovations of the past century first appeared in grocery stores for everyone to take advantage of.

Here are eight specific events in the brief history of modern convenience foods that may have contributed significantly to America's unhealthy eating habits:

1920: The refrigerator became a household appliance, providing access to all sorts of foods throughout the day or night and making snacking an easy, calorie-rich habit.

1922: The first White Castle hamburger restaurant opened, launching a revolution in fast food.

1925: Pasteurized milk became available, allowing Americans to drink more milk and to consume more dairy fat.

1930: Sliced white bread began to appear in retail bakeries, creating a convenient departure from hearth-baked, crusty breads and igniting a revolution in white bread sandwiches.

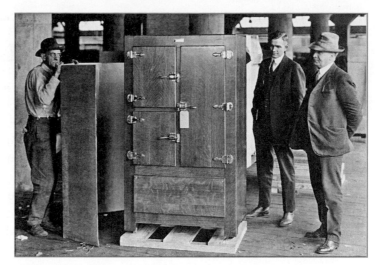

The first Frigidaire refrigerator became available around 1920 and changed the way people ate all over the world.
Corbis/Bettmann

1937: The McDonald brothers opened their first fast-food hamburger restaurant with a focus on speed and convenience.

1937: Vernon Rudolf, founder of Krispy Kreme Doughnuts, began selling his hot glazed doughnuts in grocery stores in Old Salem, North Carolina.

1945: Frozen food aisles appeared in neighborhood grocery stores, offering convenient frozen food ingredients and entire meals.

1953: Sugar-free soft drinks using saccharin as a sugar substitute hit the market.

Because of these and other convenience foods that were developed over the last hundred years, Americans today have a choice as to what type of foods to eat: convenient and fast or fresh and wholesome. Unfortunately, the hectic schedules of today's busy families, many of which have two working parents, tend to support the consumption of fast foods.

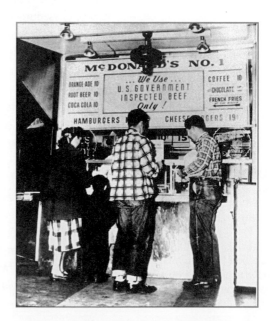

Dick and Maurice McDonald opened their first restaurant in 1948.
AP Wide World Photos

THE BEGINNING OF NUTRITIONAL SCIENCE

During the same time that the human race was evolving and the foods that we eat were cultivated and domesticated, people accorded certain healthful properties to food without really knowing how it happened or what was involved. Their reasoning was usually based on guesswork that was often laced with legend and superstition. Miracle cures abounded, but what actually caused the miracles to happen: divine intervention or nutritional science?

Garlic, for example, had been used to ward off demons since the time of the Roman Empire. There was already growing evidence that garlic and other herbs relieved people of common ailments, which were once thought to be caused by demonic possession. Then there is the old wife's tale about eating an apple a day to keep the doctor away. Is this truth or fiction? Now the evidence suggests more truth than fiction to much of what was first believed to be pure conjecture about the beneficial properties of foods. Garlic does seem to have a direct effect on human health, and the flavonoids found recently in apples have been shown to be the perfect form of antioxidant.

By the turn of the seventeenth century, sea captains learned that sailors would be less likely to contract **scurvy** if they drank citrus juice as part of their daily food allotment. Scurvy is a disease caused by a lack of vitamin C and is manifested by swollen, bleeding gums and open sores, yet nothing about **vitamins** was known back then. All that the experienced captains knew was that a daily supply of lemon, lime, or orange juice would keep their sailors healthy.

In 1846, Justus von Liebig was the first scientist to describe human and animal tissue, including food, as being composed of carbohydrates, fats, and "albuminoids," which were later called *proteins*. He hypothesized that these, together with liquids, would be the "parts of foods" needed to sustain human life. Along with other nineteenth-century theorists, von Liebig linked the mechanisms of the human body to the principles of fuel-burning engines. He conjectured that a precise connection existed between the specific types of foods consumed and good health. These initial discoveries lent support to the benefits of eating meats, fats, and starches. Fruits and vegetables were still considered supplemental foods.

It was during the same period that Louis Pasteur was perfecting his theories on the existence of **microorganisms**. Pasteur believed that it was the "high" smell of rotten foods that identified them as unfit for consumption. He sought out ways to determine what properties those smells actually contained.

The process of fermentation also intrigued Pasteur. Evidence of **fermentation** was thousands of years old, but no one could explain the process. Pasteur theorized that something came from the air itself that triggered the transformation of **malt** grains and grape juice into ale, beer, and wine, and thus he discovered wild yeast and other airborne organisms.

Thus began the search for living particles too small to be seen with the human eye. Pasteur identified and studied these microorganisms. He raised theories that would later be used to perfect the process of canning and would lead to the discovery of **pasteurization** and the use of controlled fermentation.

In 1882, a physician named Kanehiro Takaki cured deadly **beriberi** among Japanese naval crews by adding meat and vegetables to their diet, which had consisted mostly of rice. It was becoming clear there were direct connections between what humans ate and how healthy they were. A few years later, the Dutch scientist Christiaan

SCURVY A deficiency disease that results from inadequate vitamin C intake and is characterized by bleeding gums.

VITAMIN An organic substance that the body requires in very small amounts to maintain life. Vitamin C and niacin are examples.

MICROORGANISM A tiny life form that can only be seen under a microscope.

FERMENTATION A chemical reaction converting carbohydrate into its constituents, specifically carbon dioxide and alcohol.

MALT A grain, usually barley, that has been soaked in water and has begun to germinate.

PASTEURIZATION The process of heating a liquid to a high enough temperature to destroy disease-causing microorganisms.

BERIBERI A disease caused by a deficiency of thiamin, a B vitamin, and characterized by weakness, poor appetite, nerve damage, and fluid retention.

Louis Pasteur discovered tiny organisms that contributed to things like raised breads and spoiled milk.
Library of Congress

Eijkman found a direct link between polished rice and beriberi. What he found, lurking in the bran of the rice kernel, were micronutrients that were not found in the polished white rice that was the main diet of infected sailors. He then conjectured that it was these tiny substances that were needed to combat beriberi and perhaps other diseases as well.

In 1922, the Polish biochemist Casimir Funk took the study even farther and finally named these elusive compounds *vitamine* (meaning "amine essential to life"). He was convinced that there were many similar substances, yet to be discovered, in other foods that were also necessary for good health.

Thus the science of nutrition, which is the precise discrimination of the composition of foods and their effect on human health, was born.

CAN GOOD NUTRITION WAIT?

Scientific knowledge, based on the study of nutrition and health, strengthens the arguments of dietitians who lead the cause for nutritional awareness. It can take many years, however, to validate theories with measurable observations. Furthermore, the average person sees a dietitian only when sick or hospitalized. When someone is in the hospital, his or her main concern is getting well, not developing nutritional awareness.

Many patients have already accepted that hospital food tastes bad because of bad publicity or preconceived notions, and they often solicit visitors to smuggle in ice cream or potato chips. It's only when patients are hospitalized for health problems caused by diet that they begin to accept the nutritional guidance of hospital-based dietitians and nutritionally selected and prepared foods as medicine. Bland, low-fat, and no-salt foods may then become necessary parts of their diets to recover good health. But their good eating habits last only as long as it takes to get well; poor eating habits are harder to change.

Consumers are expected to sift through the multitude of nutritional and health claims that food manufacturers and their marketers make and to balance that information with what dietitians claim is important for good health. When is a product claim nothing more than a marketing tool by a promotions company? When is it a true conclusion based on years of empirical study? Are eggs high in cholesterol? What is the difference between

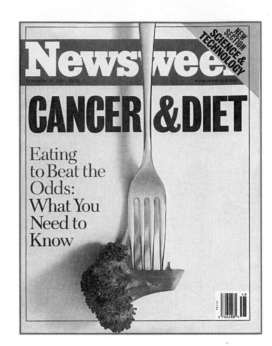

Newsweek magazine addressed nutritional claims in November 1985.
PhotoEdit Inc.

"good" and "bad" cholesterol anyway? How can cholesterol be bad if our own bodies generate cholesterol through other foods that we eat? What makes chocolate bad for you one day and good the next? What are the real concerns about salt? How can salt be bad and necessary for human health at the same time? How do you measure what is good and what is bad? Which "experts" do you believe?

One reason why Americans tend to ignore dietary recommendations from **nutritionists** and **dietitians** is because the effects of poor nutrition often do not manifest in the young or in the strong. Instead, ailments like heart disease, high blood pressure, and cancer, all of which can be related to poor long-term nutritional habits, don't usually affect people until they are much older. Why worry about things today that won't affect you until later in life? A lot of consumers will delay acting upon expert nutritional advice because they can't see any immediate connection to their daily life. It is only when it is too late, like while recovering from a heart attack or stroke, that consumers wish they had been eating better and taking better care of themselves through exercise.

The easy accessibility of convenience foods has made poor nutrition the effortless choice for multitudes of people every day for the past 80 years; that's going to be a hard trend to turn around. In the United States, "life, liberty, and the pursuit of happiness" translates into candies, ice cream, hamburgers, and French fries.

If you're confused about proper nutrition, consider yourself in good company. This text will allow you to make informed choices for yourself and better recommendations to your future customers.

The proper amounts of nutrients needed for good health are still undergoing verification. Theories are proposed, and studies are initiated to prove or disprove those theories; then, more theories, more studies, and more proof. It will take years to add verifiable knowledge to the study of nutrition, and it may take even longer to change consumers' perceptions about health and diet.

One reaction to the ever-changing information regarding nutrition and health may be to accept the three undeniable nutritional guidelines, the rules that everyone can agree on: (1) All dietary fats must be controlled, (2) salt must be used only for specific purposes, and (3) above all, a balanced diet must be consumed.

SUMMARY

The Art of Nutritional Cooking

Convincing modern consumers that the health benefits of nutritionally prepared foods outweigh dining traditions and habits is a difficult task. Nutritional guidelines seem to change from study to study, and many chefs do not seem committed to making nutritionally prepared foods taste better. It is no wonder that people often do not choose heart-healthy or light fare unless it is medically necessary for them to do so—and even then such choices seem like a sacrifice instead of a reward.

It is equally difficult to teach practicing chefs that good cooking does not depend exclusively on fats and salt for flavor. Traditionally, chefs were taught that fat equals flavor and that salt enhances taste. Dietitians may tell chefs to cut back on fat and salt in the meals they prepare, but someone must teach chefs how to return flavor to nutritionally prepared dishes without relying on salt alone.

The art of nutritional cooking can entice dietitians and chefs to work together to create great-tasting foods based on the nutritional guidelines of low-fat, low cholesterol, controlled sodium, high fiber, and high nutrient values while still satisfying the discriminating tastes of customers. Dietitians are the experts in the realm of healthy eating, and chefs are the experts in the realm of taste and dining appeal. Nutritional cooking is a move toward healthy cooking that encompasses great taste, eye appeal, and satisfaction for the hungry diner.

CASE RESOLUTION

John's food choices are probably pretty poor. Perhaps there's leftover pizza from the night before or bits of leftover cold chicken from a platter they ate from three days earlier. There may or may not be fresh vegetables or fruits to snack on. But I'm sure John could find some canned vegetables and fruit, none of which would be too appealing.

A good choice of snacks could include fresh vegetable sticks (carrots, celery, radishes, broccoli stems) or fresh whole fruit. Other choices that would be better than leftover pizza would be peanut butter and jelly (for a small sandwich) or fresh cheese, lettuce, and tomato for a quick salad.

REFERENCE

Brillat-Savarin, Jean Anthelme. 1984. *The Philosopher in the Kitchen*. New York: Penguin.

REVIEW QUESTIONS

1. What do you think about when ordering food in a restaurant? How do you make choices?
2. Why do nutritional principles take a backseat to other factors in the culinary realm?
3. Name three historically significant events connected with nutritional science. How have these discoveries or research findings contributed to the body of evidence informing nutrition?
4. The media provide frequent reports on scientific findings related to nutrition. What is one current topic you have heard or read about in the media, and how have you changed your diet because of the media report?
5. In your opinion, do media reports improve the way people eat? Explain your reasoning.

6. How do cultural eating practices influence health? Keep in mind the nutritional deficiency diseases reviewed in this chapter.

7. What does food mean to you? Besides using food to satisfy your hunger, do you ever use food to comfort or reward yourself?

8. Describe three culturally specific food or mealtime practices that you or your family follows. How do your practices differ from those of your neighbors?

9. A growing number of people must reduce their salt intake. How can you enhance flavor when preparing food with less salt? Share an example of one recipe you would like to modify to contain less salt.

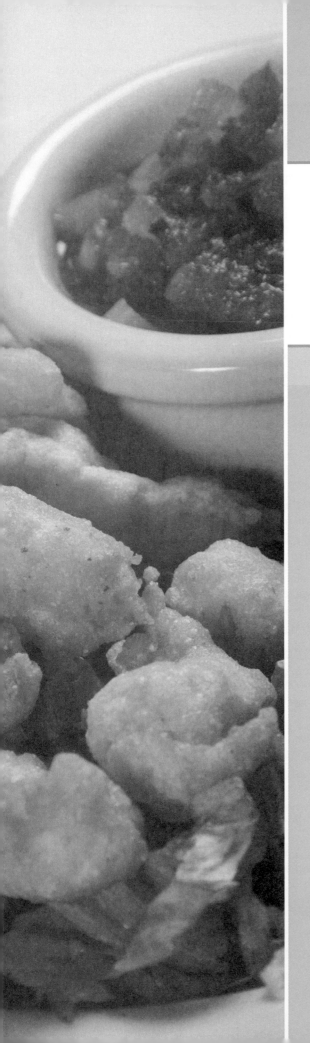

2

Nutritional Guidelines

KEY CONCEPTS

- The Dietary Reference Intakes (DRIs) provide information on specific nutrient needs and are a valuable tool for health professionals.
- The Dietary Guidelines for Americans recommend proper intakes of specific nutrients and foods that are important for reducing the risk of disease.
- My Pyramid, which is the food-guidance graphic, provides food-based guidelines that empower consumers to make wise dietary choices.
- The Nutrition Labeling and Education Act requires manufacturers to present specific information on food labels so consumers can make well-informed purchase decisions.
- International pictorial food guides vary greatly in design but convey similar nutritional advice to consumers: Eat relatively more fruits, vegetables, and whole grains and less foods of animal origin.

The human body requires nutrients for growth, health, and activity. Most of them must come from the diet because our bodies cannot make everything they need to sustain life. Without these nutrients, poor health and disease can result. To combat this, various U.S. government agencies have designed guidelines to educate both consumers and health professionals in meeting nutrient needs. In the United States, these basic nutritional guidelines are presented in the Dietary Reference Intakes (DRIs).

The DRIs list recommended intakes for individual nutrients. Health professionals can use the DRIs to assess the dietary quality of meals in feeding programs like the Special Supplemental Nutrition Program for Women, Infants, and Children (the WIC Program), Head Start, and those used to feed the elderly. In addition, health professionals can use the DRIs to determine the diet quality of individuals who may benefit from adhering to the strict recommendations. Examples include people with diabetes, bodybuilders, and those diagnosed with a diet-related disease.

These nutrient-based guidelines are the foundation for the U.S. Department of Agriculture's (USDA's) food-guidance system, which includes the Dietary Guidelines for Americans and the latest educational graphic, My Pyramid. The USDA designed these food-based guidelines to advise the general public about diet and nutrition. (The DRIs are a tool primarily used by health professionals and scientists.) Another valuable component of nutritional education is the Nutrition Labeling and Education Act of 1990, which requires food manufacturers to display nutritional information on food packages.

This chapter begins with a discussion of the need for dietary guidelines. Then it presents DRI nutrient guidelines, followed by a review of My Pyramid and the Dietary Guidelines for Americans. Because consumers need nutrient labeling to effectively follow nutritional guidelines, this chapter examines U.S. labeling law in depth. The chapter closes by comparing U.S. dietary guidelines to the national dietary guidelines for the seven most commonly served ethnic cuisines.

THINK ABOUT IT

True food allergies are quite uncommon. Most people who claim they are allergic to some type of food actually are not. Milk and dairy, for example, are frequent offenders, especially for minorities. In reality, people are usually intolerant to the carbohydrate—called lactose, or milk sugar—in dairy. An intolerance is different from an allergy. Regardless, if you knew you must avoid an ingredient, like lactose, you would want to know if a food contained any lactose.

Some people do have true allergies to particular foods, such as peanuts. Someone who is allergic to peanuts cannot have even one tiny nut. There are reported cases of consumers eating items they thought were free of peanuts but actually were not, resulting in illness or death. Another example to consider is phenylalanine consumption and phenylketonuria (PKU). An inborn error of metabolism, PKU affects an estimated 1 out of every 10,000 to 14,000 live births. Individuals with PKU must follow highly specialized low-protein diets low in phenylalanine, and infants must consume special formula.

Do you know what would happen to a child with PKU who consumes diet soda? Since some diet sodas contain phenylalanine, the child could be harmed. Thanks to food labels, consumers know when a product contains phenylalanine, as well as peanuts or lactose. How important is it for you to avoid particular food ingredients? You may know someone who carefully reads labels because of an allergy or food intolerance. Imagine how shopping for groceries and dining out must be radically different. For some, it could be life threatening.

CASE STUDY

Smoothies to Die For

Timothy and Julio applied for a new small business loan and were approved. Now they can open the business of their dreams: a smoothie shop—but not just any smoothie shop! They plan to serve fruit drinks made exclusively from organic ingredients and fortified with vitamins and minerals. They want to furnish the healthiest smoothies their city has ever seen.

Both Timothy and Julio are involved in physical fitness and bodybuilding, and they have learned a lot about health and nutrition by reading men's magazines and Web sites. They both take supplements containing megadoses of vitamins and minerals. They plan to add the same supplements to their smoothies.

Organic smoothies sound like a good idea, but what about these megadoses of vitamins and minerals? How much is enough? At what point do nutrients become dangerous? *The resolution for this case study is presented at the end of the chapter.*

NUTRITION IN THE UNITED STATES TODAY

In the United States, dietary inadequacies result from both undernutrition and overnutrition. Even with an ample food supply, there are population groups at risk of vitamin and mineral deficiencies. Vitamins E, A, B_6, zinc, calcium, and folate are commonly underconsumed (Institute of Medicine 1997, 1998, 2000b). For example, the Recommended Dietary Allowance (RDA) for vitamin E is 15 milligrams a day for healthy adults, yet the 1994 Continuing Survey of Food Intakes by Individuals (CSFII) found that the median intake for men and women age 31 to 50 years was 7.5 milligrams a day and 5.4 milligrams a day, respectively (Institute of Medicine 2000b). In other words, men received about one-half and women about one-third the requirement for vitamin E.

Calcium is another nutrient of concern. Adequate consumption is especially important during childhood and adolescence for proper bone growth. The 1994 CSFII reported that the average calcium intake during later childhood and adolescence was approximately two-thirds the requirement for males and one-half for females (Institute of Medicine 1997).

Children and adolescents are particularly at risk of nutrient deficiency due to their elevated rate of growth. Individuals with lower incomes must make wise food purchase decisions in order to prepare healthy meals. In addition, individuals with medical conditions or practices that require restricted diets may be at risk.

Even more important in the United States than the risk of nutrient deficiency is the risk of nutrient excess. Americans are overconsuming **macronutrients**, which are the calorie-containing nutrients—protein, fat, and carbohydrate. Since 1991, obesity has dramatically

MACRONUTRIENT A calorie-containing nutrient, such as carbohydrate, protein, and fat, needed in a relatively large quantity to maintain health.

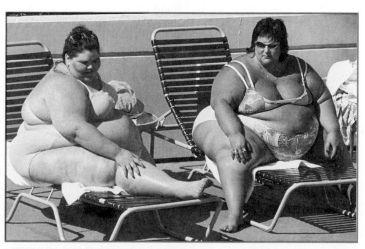

Obesity has become commonplace in the United States.
PhotoEdit Inc.

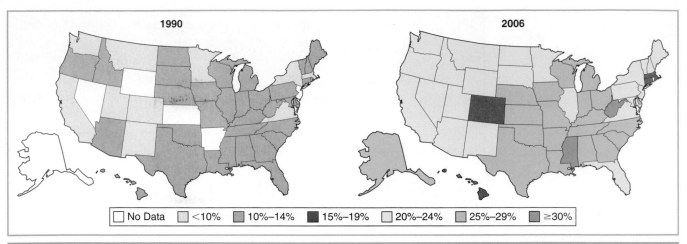

FIGURE 2–1 • OBESITY TRENDS* IN THE UNITED STATES, 1990 AND 2006
*BMI ≥ 30, or about 30 pounds overweight for 5′4″ person
Source: Centers for Disease Control. *Behavioral Risk Factor Surveillance System, 2006.* http://www.cdc.gov/nccdphp/dnpa/obesity/trend/maps/obesity_trends_2006.ppt (accessed June 15, 2008).

increased, in many cases to extreme levels. The Centers for Disease Control and Prevention (CDC) reported that in 1990, obesity rates for adults were below 15% in every state (2006). Sixteen years later, there were no states with obesity rates below 15%, only four states were between 15% and 19%, 24 states had obesity rates between 20% and 24%, 20 states were between 25% and 29%, and two states were reporting adult obesity at or greater than 30% of the population (see Figure 2–1). Overall, adult obesity increased 74% between 1991 and 2001. In the past 20 years, teenage obesity rates have tripled.

Considering that large segments of the population are at risk of obesity, as shown in Figure 2–1, it becomes very important for individuals and food service professionals to buy and prepare food in accordance with the established dietary guidelines.

DIETARY REFERENCE INTAKES

The Dietary Reference Intakes (DRIs) are nutrient-intake guidelines that state the quantity of each essential nutrient that Americans should consume (Tables 2–1 to 2–4). The values are presented for 10 human life stages and are separated by gender.

The original predecessor to the DRIs dates back to 1941, when the Food and Nutrition Board of the Institute of Medicine, National Academy of Sciences published the first RDAs. The information addressed nine essential nutrients: protein, iron, calcium, vitamins A and D, thiamin, riboflavin, niacin, and ascorbic acid (also known as vitamin C) (Davis and Saltos 1999). The RDAs were developed to ensure that American servicepeople involved in the war were adequately nourished. Since then, the RDAs have been reviewed approximately every five years and have been through eleven revisions.

The Institute of Medicine expanded the RDAs into what are now called the Dietary Reference Intakes. The DRIs include four values established for more than 30 nutrients by gender and age categories. The DRIs were gradually released over a period of six years from 1997 to 2002. The four reference values in the DRIs are as follows:

- *Estimated Average Requirement (EAR):* the estimated average requirement for each essential nutrient needed by healthy individuals in the United States.

TABLE 2–1 • DIETARY REFERENCE INTAKES FOR VITAMINS

Recommended Dietary Allowances (RDAs) for Individuals 1 Year Old and Older

Age	Folate (mg/d)	Niacin (mg/d)	B_2 (mg/d)	B_1 (mg/d)	A (mg/d)	B_6 (mg/d)	B_{12} (µg/d)	C (mg/d)	E (mg/d)
Children									
1–3 y	.15	6	.5	0.5	.30	.5	.9	15	6
4–8 y	.20	8	.6	0.6	.40	.6	1.2	25	7
Males									
9–13 y	.30	12	.9	0.9	.60	1.0	1.8	45	11
14–18 y	.40	16	1.3	1.2	.90	1.3	2.4	75	15
19–30 y	.40	16	1.3	1.2	.90	1.3	2.4	90	15
31–50 y	.40	16	1.3	1.2	.90	1.3	2.4	90	15
51–70 y	.40	16	1.3	1.2	.90	1.7	2.4	90	15
>70 y	.40	16	1.3	1.2	.90	1.7	2.4	90	15
Females									
9–13 y	.30	12	.9	0.9	.60	1.0	1.8	45	11
14–18 y	.40	14	1.0	1.0	.70	1.2	2.4	65	15
19–30 y	.40	14	1.1	1.1	.70	1.3	2.4	75	15
31–50 y	.40	14	1.1	1.1	.70	1.3	2.4	75	15
51–70 y	.40	14	1.1	1.1	.70	1.5	2.4	75	15
>70 y	.40	14	1.1	1.1	.70	1.5	2.4	75	15
Pregnant Females									
≤18 y	.60	18	1.4	1.4	.75	1.9	2.6	80	15
19–30 y	.60	18	1.4	1.4	.77	1.9	2.6	85	15
31–50 y	.60	18	1.4	1.4	.77	1.9	2.6	85	15
Lactating Females									
≤18 y	.50	17	1.6	1.4	1.2	2.0	2.8	115	19
19–30 y	.50	17	1.6	1.4	1.3	2.0	2.8	120	19
31–50 y	.50	17	1.6	1.4	1.3	2.0	2.8	120	19

- *Recommended Dietary Allowance (RDA):* the recommended intake for each nutrient that will provide a 97.5% likelihood of meeting the individual's nutrient need. This value is set at 2 standard deviations above the EAR. See Tables 2–1 and 2–2.
- *Adequate Intake (AI):* a recommended intake for nutrients established when insufficient information exists to determine an EAR or an RDA. See Tables 2–3 and 2–4.

TABLE 2–2 • DIETARY REFERENCE INTAKES FOR MINERALS

Recommended Dietary Allowances (RDAs) for Individuals 1 Year Old and Older

Age	Copper (μg/d)	Iodine (μg/d)	Iron (mg/d)	Magnesium (mg/d)	Molybdenum (μg/d)	Phosphorus (mg/d)	Selenium (μg/d)	Zinc (mg/d)
Children								
1–3 y	340	90	7	80	17	460	20	3
4–8 y	440	90	10	130	22	500	30	5
Males								
9–13 y	700	120	8	240	34	1,250	40	8
14–18 y	890	150	11	410	43	1,250	55	11
19–30 y	900	150	8	400	45	700	55	11
31–50 y	900	150	8	420	45	700	55	11
51–70 y	900	150	8	420	45	700	55	11
>70 y	900	150	8	420	45	700	55	11
Females								
9–13 y	700	120	8	240	34	1,250	40	8
14–18 y	890	150	15	360	43	1,250	55	9
19–30 y	900	150	18	310	45	700	55	8
31–50 y	900	150	18	320	45	700	55	8
51–70 y	900	150	8	320	45	700	55	8
>70 y	900	150	8	320	45	700	55	8
Pregnant Females								
≤18 y	1,000	220	27	400	50	1,250	60	12
19–30 y	1,000	220	27	350	50	700	60	11
31–50 y	1,000	220	27	360	50	700	60	11
Lactating Females								
≤18 y	1,300	290	10	360	50	1,250	70	13
19–30 y	1,300	290	9	310	50	700	70	12
31–50 y	1,300	290	9	320	50	700	70	12

TOXICITY The quality or condition of being poisonous.

- *Tolerable Upper Intake Level (UL):* the level up to which 12 nutrients can be consumed without **toxicity** risk.

RDAs are set at a level that is expected to be adequate for 97.5% of the population. Individuals should consume nutrients at a level above the RDA yet below the UL. Keep in mind that as intake levels increase, consumers may eventually reach toxicity. Any food or

TABLE 2–3 • DIETARY REFERENCE INTAKES FOR VITAMINS

Adequate Intakes (AIs) for Individuals 1 Year Old and Older

Age	Biotin (g/d)	Choline (mg/d)	Pantothenic Acid (mg/d)	Vitamin D (μg/d)	Vitamin K (μg/d)
Children					
1–3 y	8	200	2	5	30
4–8 y	12	250	3	5	55
Males					
9–13 y	20	375	4	5	60
14–18 y	25	550	5	5	75
19–30 y	30	550	5	5	120
31–50 y	30	550	5	5	120
51–70 y	30	550	5	10	120
>70 y	30	550	5	15	120
Females					
9–13 y	20	375	4	5	60
14–18 y	25	400	5	5	75
19–30 y	30	425	5	5	90
31–50 y	30	425	5	5	90
51–70 y	30	425	5	10	90
>70 y	30	425	5	15	90
Pregnant Females					
≤18 y	30	450	6	5	75
19–30 y	30	450	6	5	90
31–50 y	30	450	6	5	90
Lactating Females					
≤18 y	35	550	7	5	75
19–30 y	35	550	7	5	90
31–50 y	35	550	7	5	90

nutrient consumed in excess can be toxic, even water (Institute of Medicine 1999). While this information is helpful for health professionals, it presents too much detail for most consumers. For this reason, the Dietary Guidelines for Americans (DGA) were developed. The guidelines provide useful information focusing on specific nutrients linked to specific disease states.

TABLE 2–4 • DIETARY REFERENCE INTAKES FOR MINERALS

Adequate Intakes (AIs) for Individuals 1 Year Old and Older

Age	Calcium (mg/d)	Chromium (mcg/d)	Fluoride (mg/d)	Manganese (mg/d)	Potassium (g/d)	Sodium (g/d)	Chloride (g/d)
Children							
1–3 y	500	11	0.7	1.2	3.0	1.0	1.5
4–8 y	800	15	1	1.5	3.8	1.2	1.9
Males							
9–13 y	1300	25	2	1.9	4.5	1.5	2.3
14–18 y	1300	35	3	2.2	4.7	1.5	2.3
19–30 y	1000	35	4	2.3	4.7	1.5	2.3
31–50 y	1000	35	4	2.3	4.7	1.5	2.3
51–70 y	1200	30	4	2.3	4.7	1.3	2.0
>70 y	1200	30	4	2.3	4.7	1.2	1.8
Females							
9–13 y	1300	21	2	1.6	4.5	1.5	2.3
14–18 y	1300	24	3	1.6	4.7	1.5	2.3
19–30 y	1000	25	3	1.8	4.7	1.5	2.3
31–50 y	1000	25	3	1.8	4.7	1.5	2.3
51–70 y	1200	20	3	1.8	4.7	1.3	2.0
>70 y	1200	20	3	1.8	4.7	1.2	1.8
Pregnancy							
14–18 y	1300	29	3	2.0	4.7	1.5	2.3
19–30 y	1000	30	3	2.0	4.7	1.5	2.3
31–50 y	1000	30	3	2.0	4.7	1.5	2.3
Lactation							
14–18 y	1300	44	3	2.6	5.1	1.5	2.3
19–30 y	1000	45	3	2.6	5.1	1.5	2.3
31–50 y	1000	45	3	2.6	5.1	1.5	2.3

DIETARY GUIDELINES FOR AMERICANS

The Dietary Guidelines for Americans were first published in 1980 by the USDA and the U.S. Department of Health and Human Services. The guidelines provide a framework for nutrient intake as well as the intake of whole foods. They offer advice regarding how consumers should eat to meet the nutrient needs described by the DRIs. Like the DRIs, the guidelines are routinely updated. Since their inception in 1980, they have been updated every five years; they are now in their sixth edition, published in 2005, which emphasizes reducing calorie consumption and increasing physical activity.

The latest report identifies 41 key recommendations, 23 of which are for the general public and 18 for special populations. The recommendations are grouped into nine general topics: Adequate Nutrients within Calorie Needs, Weight Management, Physical Activity, Food Groups, Fats, Carbohydrates, Sodium and Potassium, Alcoholic Beverages, and Food Safety. In addition to energy balance, the new guidelines emphasize the use of food groups to encourage the consumption of fruits, vegetables, whole grains, and milk or milk-equivalent products. The guidelines also suggest limiting fats, sugars, sodium, and alcohol.

The latest revision of the guidelines began in August 2003, when a panel of 13 nutritional and medical professionals was appointed to the Dietary Guidelines Advisory Committee. Committee members were charged with examining the guidelines in relation to current scientific and medical knowledge on the relationship between diet and health. Their first meeting, on September 23, 2003, began the process of evaluating the dietary guidelines. Members directed their energies toward discussing carbohydrates, fatty acids, energy balance and weight maintenance, nutritional adequacy and life cycle needs, food safety, fluid and electrolytes, and **ethanol**. Their final revisions were published January 12, 2005 (Box 2–1).

ETHANOL Alcohol.

MY PYRAMID: THE NEW FOOD GUIDE PYRAMID

As we have seen, the DRIs are nutrient-based guidelines, and the Dietary Guidelines for Americans cover nutrients and foods. On the other hand, My Pyramid, a pictorial model describing the ideal selection of foods to promote good health, provides food-based recommendations and focuses on variety. Even though these recommendations are based on the DRIs, My Pyramid contains information that is more easily applicable to consumers' daily lives. Foods are placed into groups with similar nutrient composition. Eating from each of the groups will ensure that most people's nutrient needs are met.

In 2005, the USDA released My Pyramid. It contains six food groups from which to build a healthy, balanced diet. Before 2005, there were other food guides (Figure 2–2). From 1956 to 1992, the Basic Four was the most widely used pictorial food guide. As its name suggests, it contained only four food groups: meats, dairy, fruits and vegetables, and breads and grains. The Basic Four was followed by the Food Guide Pyramid, which split the fruit and vegetable group into two separate categories, a division that helped emphasize the importance of fruits and vegetables (Figure 2–3). The Food Guide Pyramid's six groups were fats, oils, and sweets; grain products (breads, cereals, rice, and pasta); vegetables; fruits; milk, yogurt, and cheese; and meat (meat, poultry, fish, dry beans, eggs, and nuts).

The Food Guide Pyramid used to educate consumers from 1992 to 2005 was criticized by some nutritional experts. One of the most notable critics was Walter Willett, a doctor from the Harvard School of Public Health, who argued that the pyramid contained major flaws. Willett and his colleagues from Harvard published a book in 2001, *Eat, Drink, and Be Healthy: The Harvard Medical School Guide to Healthy Eating*, describing their objections to the Food Guide Pyramid. Willett suggested that

BOX 2–1 • DIETARY GUIDELINES FOR AMERICANS, 2005

KEY RECOMMENDATIONS FOR THE GENERAL POPULATION

Adequate Nutrients within Calorie Needs

- Consume a variety of nutrient-dense foods and beverages within and among the basic food groups. Choose foods that limit the intake of saturated and trans fats, cholesterol, added sugars, salt, and alcohol.

- Meet recommended intakes within energy needs by adopting a balanced eating pattern, such as the U.S. Department of Agriculture (USDA) Food Guide or the Dietary Approaches to Stop Hypertension (DASH) Eating Plan.

Weight Management

- To maintain body weight in a healthy range, balance calories from foods and beverages with calories expended.

- To prevent gradual weight gain over time, make small decreases in food and beverage calories and increase physical activity.

Physical Activity

- Engage in regular physical activity and reduce sedentary activities to promote health, psychological well-being, and a healthy body weight.

- Achieve physical fitness by including cardiovascular conditioning, stretching exercises for flexibility, and resistance exercises or calisthenics for muscle strength and endurance.

Food Groups to Encourage

- Consume a sufficient amount of fruits and vegetables while staying within energy needs. Two cups of fruit and 2 1/2 cups of vegetables per day are recommended for a reference 2,000-calorie intake, with higher or lower amounts depending on the calorie level.

- Choose a variety of fruits and vegetables each day. In particular, select from all five vegetable subgroups (dark green, orange, legumes, starchy vegetables, and other vegetables) several times a week.

- Consume 3 or more ounce-equivalents of whole-grain products per day, with the rest of the recommended grains coming from enriched or whole-grain products. In general, at least half the grains should come from whole grains.

- Consume 3 cups per day of fat-free or low-fat milk or equivalent milk products.

Fats

- Consume less than 10% of calories from saturated fatty acids and less than 300 milligrams per day of cholesterol. Keep trans-fatty acid consumption as low as possible.

- Keep total fat intake between 20% and 35% of calories, with most fats coming from sources of polyunsaturated and monounsaturated fatty acids, such as fish, nuts, and vegetable oils.

- When selecting and preparing meat, poultry, dry beans, and milk or milk products, make choices that are lean, low-fat, or fat-free.

- Limit intake of fats and oils high in saturated and/or trans-fatty acids, and choose products low in such fats and oils.

Carbohydrates

- Choose fiber-rich fruits, vegetables, and whole grains often.

- Choose and prepare foods and beverages with little added sugars or caloric sweeteners. Use the amounts suggested by the USDA Food Guide and the DASH Eating Plan.

- Reduce the incidence of dental caries by practicing good oral hygiene and consuming sugar- and starch-containing foods and beverages less frequently.

Sodium and Potassium

- Consume less than 2,300 milligrams (approximately 1 teaspoon of salt) of sodium per day.

- Choose and prepare foods with little salt. At the same time, consume potassium-rich foods, such as fruits and vegetables.

Alcoholic Beverages

- Those who choose to drink alcoholic beverages should do so sensibly and in moderation—defined as the consumption of up to one drink per day for women and up to two drinks per day for men.

- Alcoholic beverages should not be consumed by some individuals, including those who cannot restrict their alcohol intake, women of childbearing age who may become pregnant, pregnant and lactating women, children and adolescents, individuals taking medications that can interact with alcohol, and those with specific medical conditions.

- Alcoholic beverages should be avoided by individuals engaging in activities that require attention, skill, or coordination, such as driving or operating machinery.

- To avoid microbial foodborne illness:
  - Clean hands, food contact surfaces, and fruits and vegetables. Meat and poultry should not be washed or rinsed.
  - Separate raw, cooked, and ready-to-eat foods while shopping, preparing, or storing foods.
  - Cook foods to a safe temperature to kill microorganisms.
  - Chill (refrigerate) perishable food promptly and defrost foods properly.
  - Avoid raw (unpasteurized) milk or any products made from unpasteurized milk, raw or partially cooked eggs or foods containing raw eggs, raw or undercooked meat and poultry, unpasteurized juices, and raw sprouts.

the graphic painted all fats as bad, all complex carbohydrates as good, all proteins as the same, dairy products as essential, and potato as a suitable food to choose often. Furthermore, the tool provided no guidance on weight, exercise, alcohol, or vitamins. He compiled a list of seven changes that people could make to improve their health (Willett 2001):

1. Watch your weight.
2. Eat fewer bad fats and more good fats.
3. Eat fewer refined-grain carbohydrates and more whole-grain carbohydrates.
4. Choose healthier (that is, leaner) sources of protein.
5. Eat plenty of vegetables and fruits, but not a lot of potatoes.
6. Use alcohol in moderation.
7. Take a multivitamin for insurance.

In 2003, the USDA initiated a broad-based review and update of the old pyramid's food patterns. They examined current nutritional standards and incorporated those as a framework to help consumers assess and improve their diets. The USDA suggested completing the revisions in three phases:

1. Gather information through technical research, professional input, and consumer research.
2. Update the food guide recommendations.
3. Develop new revised graphics for educational purposes.

The USDA solicited written comments from the public on proposed changes to the Food Guide Pyramid between September 11 and October 27, 2003. The revised graphic, called My Pyramid, debuted in early 2005 (Figure 2–4). It reflected information gathered by the expert panel responsible for revising the Dietary Guidelines for Americans.

Many of the changes to the Food Guide Pyramid that were suggested by Willett and others were incorporated into My Pyramid. In the old graphic, all fats and oils were considered harmful and thus limited. In contrast, My Pyramid encourages liquid oils (monounsaturated and polyunsaturated oils) and suggests a recommended intake for all age levels. Saturated fats, which are solid at room temperature, are limited in My Pyramid. Vegetable and fruit intake is still encouraged with My Pyramid, and all carbohydrates are not considered equal. The current recommendation is that whole grains make up half of the servings of grains.

My Pyramid also includes an illustration of an individual climbing stairs, encouraging exercise and thus energy balance. Along this same concept of balance, My Pyramid provides individual serving suggestions for each food group according to age, gender, and activity level. To receive your personalized recommendations, access the My Pyramid calculator at http://www.mypyramid.gov/.

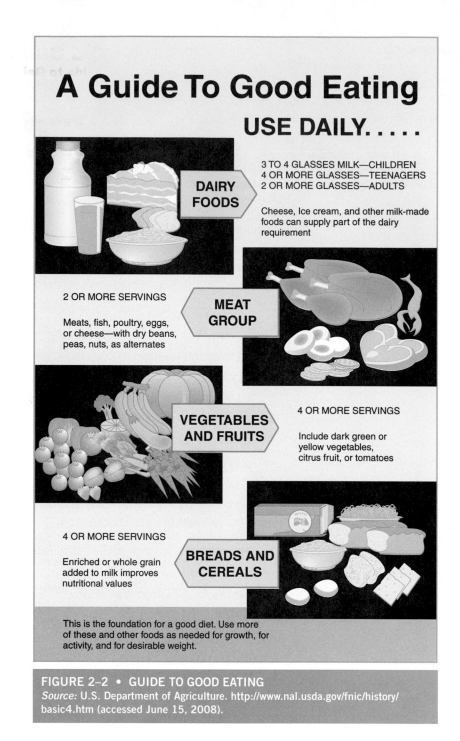

A Guide To Good Eating
USE DAILY.....

DAIRY FOODS

3 TO 4 GLASSES MILK—CHILDREN
4 OR MORE GLASSES—TEENAGERS
2 OR MORE GLASSES—ADULTS

Cheese, Ice cream, and other milk-made foods can supply part of the dairy requirement

2 OR MORE SERVINGS

MEAT GROUP

Meats, fish, poultry, eggs, or cheese—with dry beans, peas, nuts, as alternates

VEGETABLES AND FRUITS

4 OR MORE SERVINGS

Include dark green or yellow vegetables, citrus fruit, or tomatoes

4 OR MORE SERVINGS

Enriched or whole grain added to milk improves nutritional values

BREADS AND CEREALS

This is the foundation for a good diet. Use more of these and other foods as needed for growth, for activity, and for desirable weight.

FIGURE 2–2 • GUIDE TO GOOD EATING
Source: U.S. Department of Agriculture. http://www.nal.usda.gov/fnic/history/basic4.htm (accessed June 15, 2008).

Even with regular revisions of the dietary guidelines based on scientific updates, consumers still sometimes find it difficult to make proper food selections in the grocery store. To aid them in making healthy food choices, U.S. food labeling laws have been enacted.

FOOD LABELING

You have most likely noticed nutrition labels on food packaging. Perhaps this information influenced you to purchase and consume the product or to let it remain on the store shelf. Food labels inform consumers about nutrition and empower them to make better dietary choices.

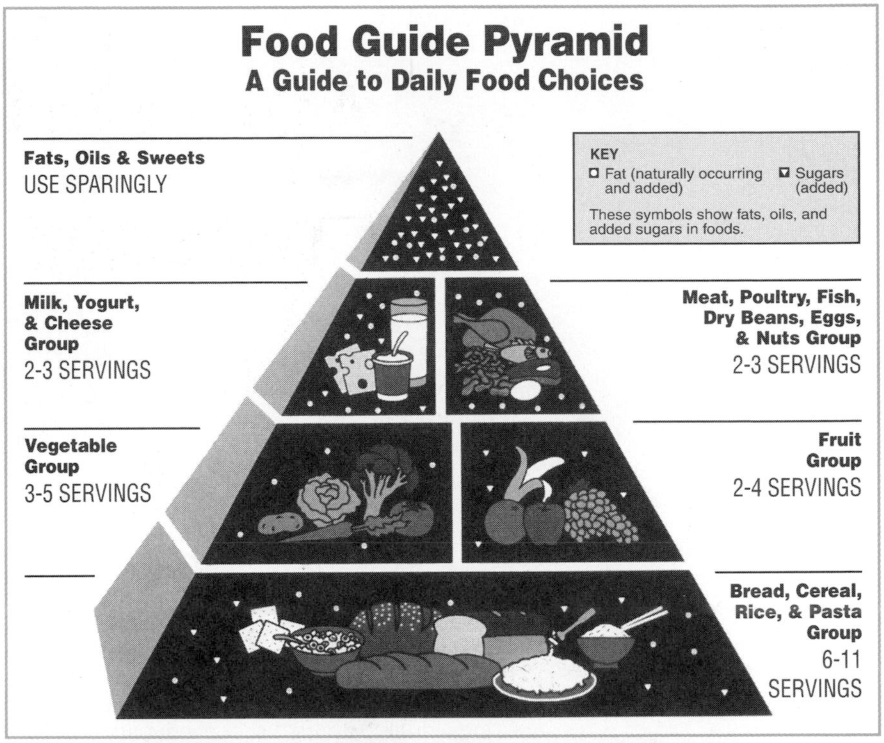

Food Guide Pyramid
A Guide to Daily Food Choices

Fats, Oils & Sweets
USE SPARINGLY

KEY
□ Fat (naturally occurring and added)   ▽ Sugars (added)
These symbols show fats, oils, and added sugars in foods.

Milk, Yogurt, & Cheese Group
2-3 SERVINGS

Meat, Poultry, Fish, Dry Beans, Eggs, & Nuts Group
2-3 SERVINGS

Vegetable Group
3-5 SERVINGS

Fruit Group
2-4 SERVINGS

Bread, Cereal, Rice, & Pasta Group
6-11 SERVINGS

FIGURE 2–3 • FOOD GUIDE PYRAMID
Source: U.S. Department of Agriculture. http://www.cnpp.udsa.gov/FGP.htm (accessed June 18, 2008).

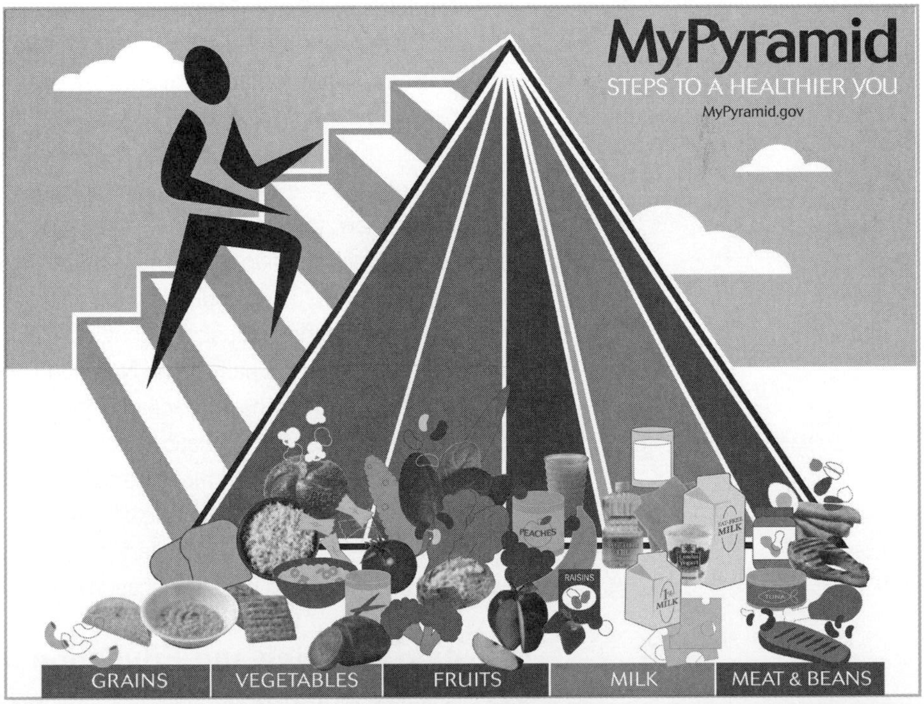

MyPyramid
STEPS TO A HEALTHIER YOU
MyPyramid.gov

GRAINS   VEGETABLES   FRUITS   MILK   MEAT & BEANS

FIGURE 2–4 • MY PYRAMID
Source: U.S Department of Agriculture. http://www.mypyramid.gov/downloads/MiniPoster.pdf (accessed June 15, 2008).

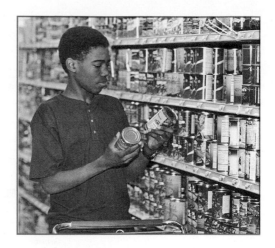

A buyer compares labels on canned groceries.
PhotoEdit Inc.

Americans are utilizing food labels. Surveys taken during the 1980s showed that four out of five Americans paid attention to ingredient and nutritional information on food labels (Bender and Derby 1992). Studies conducted in the 1990s confirm that about 3/4 of the U.S. population read food labels. Label use, however, is not uniform across demographic groups. Adults under 35 years of age have significantly higher label use, as do women and individuals with high school education (Neuhouser et al. 1999).

Since early civilization, people have been concerned about the quality and safety of foods. In 1202, an early English food law called the Assize of Bread outlawed the adulteration of bread with nonstandard ingredients. In the United States, food regulations date back to colonial times. More recently, in 1906, Congress passed the original Food and Drug Act. This law prohibited adulterated foods, drinks, and drugs from interstate commerce. In 1938, Congress passed the Federal Food, Drug, and Cosmetic Act, which defined **standards of identity** for packaged foods. For example, to be labeled ice cream, the product must contain at least 10% milk fat and no less than 20% milk solids and must weigh at least 4.5 pounds per gallon. Any product with less than 10% milk fat must be called by another name, such as ice milk.

Apart from standards of identity, the Federal Food, Drug, and Cosmetic Act authorized factory inspections to ensure proper product manufacturing and handling. Furthermore, as defined in the law, food companies were prevented from making claims on labels relating food to disease. In addition, many states had individual requirements on nutrition labeling and food standards. This resulted in no universal standard for claims like "low-fat" and "reduced-fat," creating confusion among consumers. To clarify and better inform the American consumer, Congress passed the Nutrition Labeling and Education Act (NLEA) in 1990.

The NLEA requires that all packaged foods bear standardized nutrition labeling and that all health claims meet the regulations prescribed by the Department of Health and Human Services. Lawmakers took the measure a step further to address supplements. In 1994, the Dietary Supplement Health and Education Act (DSHEA, pronounced "De-Shay") was established to regulate the labeling of dietary supplements. This law, further described in the following section, mandated the classification of dietary supplements as foods instead of drugs.

STANDARD OF IDENTITY A government standard that defines what ingredients a product must contain in order to be called a particular name.

Nutrition Labeling and Education Act of 1990

With the Nutrition Labeling and Education Act, the Food and Drug Administration (FDA) and the U.S. Department of Agriculture required nutrition labeling for most foods and championed the consumer's cause in the fight against false or misleading food labeling. Before the NLEA, consumers found it difficult to tell the difference between food product marketing and nutrition hype. Catch phrases like *low-fat, no cholesterol, reduced-calorie, and high-fiber* were found on food packages and advertisements but had no standard meaning.

Besides defining key terms, the NLEA required that almost all manufactured food products display accurate information on their exterior packaging following the USDA's accepted nutritional guidelines. Some foods were made exempt from food-labeling laws, including fresh vegetables and fruits, raw meats, foods produced by small businesses, and foods with labels too small to display the information on the package.

Consumers are encouraged to use the information on the food label to make wise dietary choices. Most health professionals consider the FDA food label to be a triumph. Not only is it informative, it is also easy to understand. The label provides dietary information that addresses major diet-related health problems in our society, such as cardiovascular disease, high blood pressure, cancer, osteoporosis, tooth decay, and iron deficiency. Consumers can examine the total fat, saturated fat, cholesterol, sodium, and fiber contents of a product and compare brands to select the one best suited to their particular diet. Portion sizes, while not necessarily consistent with what consumers typically eat, are uniform and allow easy comparison of similar foods.

Required Product Identification, Ingredient, and Nutrient Information

Food labels must provide fundamental product information, such as the name and address of the manufacturer, the product name, the content weight, the sell-by date, and a list of ingredients. Ingredients, listed in descending order by weight, are present if a product contains more than one ingredient. For example, a package of dried cherries containing only cherries does not need an ingredient list. A chocolate candy bar does require an ingredient list because it contains more than one ingredient.

Nutrition Facts Panel

The Nutrition Facts panel lists serving size, servings per container, calories per serving, calories from fat, and micronutrient information (Box 2–2). The law requires the panel to conform to the example shown in the photo below. An exception is made for labels with less than 3 inches of vertical space or when there are fewer than 40 square inches of labeling space available. In these cases, an abbreviated linear table may be used. If fewer than 12 square inches of labeling space is available, nutritional information is not required. The

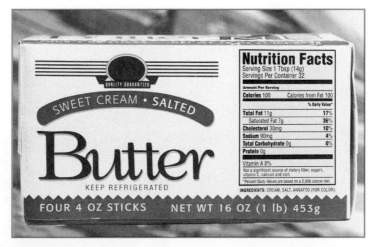

This photograph of packaged butter shows how the nutrition label is displayed.

PhotoEdit Inc.

Nutrition Facts

Serving Size 1 cup (228g)
Servings Per Container 2

Amount Per Serving	
Calories 250	Calories from Fat 110

	% Daily Value*
Total Fat 12g	18%
Saturated Fat 3g	15%
Trans Fat 1.5g	
Cholesterol 30mg	10%
Sodium 470mg	20%
Total Carbohydrate 31g	10%
Dietary Fiber 0g	0%
Sugars 5g	
Protein 5g	
Vitamin A	4%
Vitamin C	2%
Calcium	20%
Iron	4%

* Percent Daily Values are based on a 2,000 calorie diet.
Your Daily Values may be higher or lower depending on
your calorie needs:

	Calories:	2,000	2,500
Total Fat	Less than	65g	80g
Sat Fat	Less than	20g	25g
Cholesterol	Less than	300mg	300mg
Sodium	Less than	2,400mg	2,400mg
Total Carbohydrate		300g	375g
Dietary Fiber		25g	30g

The Nutrition Facts panel
required on most food labels.
U.S. Food and Drug Administration

EXCHANGE LIST A list of foods
with similar nutrient profiles based
on calorie, protein, carbohydrate,
and fat content.

TRANS-FATTY ACID A type of
unsaturated fat made solid via hydrogenation. Shortening, for example, contains trans-fatty acid,
or trans fat. Foods like meat and
butter naturally contain trans fat.

DAILY VALUE The representative
daily requirement for each nutrient. The Daily Value is based on
two sets of standards: the Reference Daily Intakes and the Daily
Reference Values.

serving size is stated in common household measures, such as cup, tablespoon, or teaspoon, along with the metric equivalent, and is based on the amount people normally
choose. If these common measures are not applicable, then alternative units are used, including piece, tray, and jar.

These are not necessarily the same serving sizes seen in diabetic **exchange lists**,
USDA Dietary Guidelines for Americans, or My Pyramid. However, the standard serving size
assists shoppers by allowing them to compare "apples to apples" when deciding between
products and brands.

In July 2003, the FDA published an amendment to its regulation on nutrition labeling,
which required manufacturers to declare **trans-fatty acids** on the nutrition label of conventional food and dietary supplements. All manufacturers had to comply by including trans-
fat content by January 1, 2006.

The history of this regulation is a remarkable one, resulting from the political action of
Michael Jacobson and the Center for Science in the Public Interest (CSPI). CSPI petitioned
the FDA regarding trans fat based on scientific evidence that trans fat increased the risk of
developing coronary heart disease. Studies demonstrated that intake of trans-fatty acids,
similar to saturated fatty acids, increases low-density lipoprotein (LDL) cholesterol—the
"bad" cholesterol—in the blood. Increased levels of LDL cholesterol increase the risk of
developing coronary heart disease. With this additional information, consumers will have
another tool to help maintain a healthy diet.

Daily Values (DVs)

The amounts of most of the nutrients on the food label are shown as a **Daily Value (DV)**. The
DV indicates how much of a nutrient is found in one serving of a particular food product.

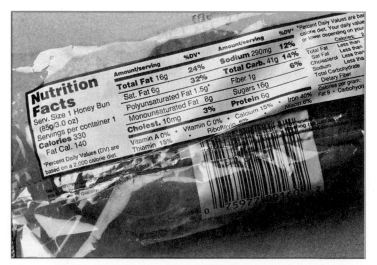

Alternate Nutrition Facts panel for smaller labels.
PhotoEdit Inc.

TABLE 2–5 • REFERENCE DAILY INTAKES (RDIs)

Nutrient	Amount	Nutrient	Amount	Nutrient	Amount
Vitamin A	5,000 IU	Riboflavin	1.7 mg	Iodine	150 µg
Vitamin C	60 mg	Niacin	20 mg	Magnesium	400 mg
Calcium	1 g	Vitamin B_6	2 mg	Zinc	15 mg
Iron	18 mg	Folic acid	.4 mg	Selenium	70 µg
Vitamin D	400 IU	Vitamin B_{12}	6 µg	Copper	2 mg
Vitamin E	30 IU	Biotin	300 µg	Manganese	2 mg
Vitamin K	80 µg	Pantothenic acid	10 mg	Chromium	120 µg
Thiamin	1.5 mg	Phosphorus	1 g	Molybdenum	75 µg
Chloride	3,400 mg				

Note: Based on the National Academy of Sciences' 1968 Recommended Dietary Allowances.

REFERENCE DAILY INTAKES (RDIs) A set of standards for the intake of most vitamins and minerals based on the Recommended Dietary Allowances (RDAs).

DAILY REFERENCE VALUES (DRVs) A set of standards for other nutrients, including fat, cholesterol, and sodium.

DVs are listed as a percentage of the daily requirement based on a 2,000-calorie diet. For example, if one serving of a food provides 100 milligrams of calcium and the daily requirement is 1,000 milligrams, the label would show 10% of the DV. The Daily Values are based on two sets of standards, the **Reference Daily Intakes (RDIs)** (Table 2–5) for nutrients that have an RDA and the **Daily Reference Values (DRVs)** (Table 2–6) for nutrients that do not have an established RDA. Figure 2–5 provides a summary of acronyms.

The RDIs and DRVs are the actual standards for nutrients required each day, yet they do not appear on the food label. The label shows only the DV, which is a percentage of the standard for each nutrient listed. Presenting the DVs as a percentage avoids the complexity of including individual nutrient measures on the label (e.g., retinol equivalents, grams, milligrams, and micrograms).

TABLE 2–6 • DAILY REFERENCE VALUES (DRVs)

Food Component	DRV
Fat	65 g
Saturated fatty acids	20 g
Cholesterol	300 mg
Total carbohydrate	300 g
Fiber	25 g
Sodium	2,400 mg
Potassium	3,500 mg
Protein[a]	50 g

[a]The DRV for protein does not apply to all populations.
Note: Based on 2,000 calories a day for adults and children over 4 only.

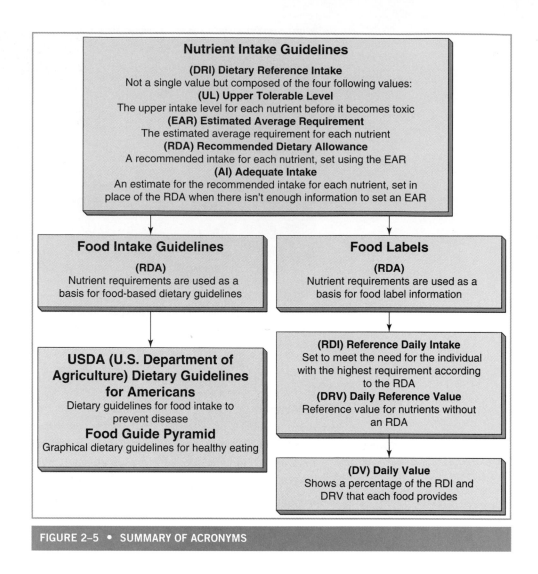

Nutrient Intake Guidelines

(DRI) Dietary Reference Intake
Not a single value but composed of the four following values:
(UL) Upper Tolerable Level
The upper intake level for each nutrient before it becomes toxic
(EAR) Estimated Average Requirement
The estimated average requirement for each nutrient
(RDA) Recommended Dietary Allowance
A recommended intake for each nutrient, set using the EAR
(AI) Adequate Intake
An estimate for the recommended intake for each nutrient, set in place of the RDA when there isn't enough information to set an EAR

Food Intake Guidelines

(RDA)
Nutrient requirements are used as a basis for food-based dietary guidelines

Food Labels

(RDA)
Nutrient requirements are used as a basis for food label information

USDA (U.S. Department of Agriculture) Dietary Guidelines for Americans
Dietary guidelines for food intake to prevent disease
Food Guide Pyramid
Graphical dietary guidelines for healthy eating

(RDI) Reference Daily Intake
Set to meet the need for the individual with the highest requirement according to the RDA
(DRV) Daily Reference Value
Reference value for nutrients without an RDA

(DV) Daily Value
Shows a percentage of the RDI and DRV that each food provides

FIGURE 2–5 • SUMMARY OF ACRONYMS

No Daily Value percentage is listed on the label for trans-fatty acids because present knowledge regarding trans fat does not show that any amount of intake is desirable.

Reference Daily Intakes

Reference Daily Intakes are given for vitamins and minerals that have an established RDA. They are set as the highest requirement for each nutrient for individuals four years of age and older, as recommended by the 1968 RDAs. RDIs provide information that allows consumers to make informed dietary choices. Vegetarians, for example, can use the information if they are concerned about getting enough iron in their diets; people on low-calorie diets can use it to make sure that their calcium intake is sufficient. Although the RDIs and resulting DVs are only required on food labels for vitamins A and C, calcium, and iron, other nutrients may be listed on a voluntary basis. Most of the RDIs are thought of as minimum intake requirements.

Dietary Reference Values

The Dietary Reference Values are given for those nutrients and food components for which an RDA has not been established. Some of the DRVs are maximum intake levels, specified as a percentage of calories based on a 2,000-calorie diet. For example, the USDA Dietary

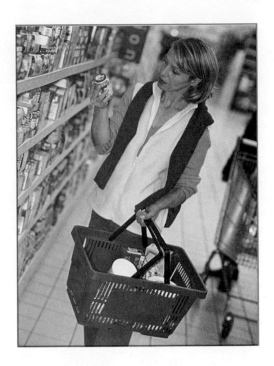

A woman reviews nutritional information on a food label while grocery shopping.
Photo Researchers, Inc.

Guidelines suggest that fat consumption be kept to 30% of daily calories or less. The DRVs are based on a 2,000-calorie diet, so fat intake should be no more than 30% of 2,000 calories, or 600 calories. Since fat provides approximately nine calories per gram, dividing 600 calories by 9 calories per gram produces a DRV of 65 grams.

Other DRVs are also set as a percentage of total calories: 10% for saturated fat, 10% for protein, and 60% for carbohydrates. The DRVs give nutrient content information that health-conscious consumers can use. For example, people on the Atkins diet can use the carbohydrate information to make sure they do not consume too many carbohydrates, and professional athletes can use the same information to ensure they ingest enough carbohydrates when carbohydrate loading.

One Size Does Not Fit All

Food labels give an amount higher than the RDA for some individuals because the DV is set at the required amount for the individual with the highest nutrient need. The DVs may slightly overstate the nutrient needs of some individuals because they are set as the highest requirement for each nutrient for Americans four years of age and over. For example, if an adult male who needs 800 milligrams of calcium according to the DRI consumes a product containing 80% of the Daily Value for calcium, he would actually be getting 100% of his daily calcium requirement because the Daily Value is set at 1,000 milligrams.

Keep in mind that the DVs are set for the person with the greatest need according to the 1968 RDAs. Many consumers may still comfortably use the DVs as a general guideline, but this is not necessarily so for everyone. The age group with the highest requirement for calcium, for instance, should consume 1,300 milligrams per day instead of the 1,000 milligrams that the food label uses as the standard.

Although the Daily Values are based on a 2,000-calorie diet, which is thought to cover most moderately active women and sedentary men, a second reference level of 2,500 calories is given at the bottom of the Nutrition Facts panel for more active people. Many women and the elderly may need fewer than 2,000 calories per day. Those who consume fewer than 2,000 calories per day should note that the DV for certain nutrients, such as fat, may not be applicable to their calorie intake. A summary of nutrient labeling terms is shown in Table 2–7.

CALCULATING ACTUAL VITAMIN CONTENT USING INFORMATION ON THE FOOD LABEL

Although the actual content of certain nutrients, such as fat, is given in grams, vitamins and minerals are shown only as a percentage of the DV. To obtain the actual content of a vitamin or mineral, one must convert the DV percentages found on a food label into actual nutrient content. Without the data in Table 2–5, you would not have the information necessary to perform this calculation. For example, let's assume that a study is publicized suggesting that 120 milligrams of vitamin C is ideal for cigarette smokers. A smoker learns of this study's findings and subsequently aims to consume 120 milligrams of vitamin C per day. She reviews the food label of a fruit juice to find that it contains 125% of the Daily Value (DV) of vitamin C. Does this product provide 120 milligrams of the vitamin? As shown in Table 2–5, the Reference Daily Intake (RDI) for vitamin C is 60 milligrams. The actual vitamin C content of the fruit juice is 125% of 60 milligrams, or 75 milligrams. This amount is not close to the 120 milligrams suggested in the study, but the smoker now knows how much vitamin C to consume from other foods to reach her 120-milligrams goal. She does not need to calculate the actual amount of vitamin C she consumes if she knows the RDI. Given that the RDI for vitamin C is 60 milligrams and she wants 120 milligrams, she should simply aim for a daily vitamin C consumption of 200% of the DV.

TABLE 2–7 • NUTRIENT INTAKE AND FOOD-LABELING STANDARDS

Reference	Abbreviation	Description
Nutrient Intake Standards		
Dietary Reference Intake	DRI	Most updated nutrient-based guideline; has four reference values: RDA, UL, EAR, AI.
Recommended Dietary Allowance	RDA	Recommended intake for individual nutrients to prevent deficiency.
Tolerable Upper Intake Level	UL	Intake level up to which nutrient intake is without risk of toxicity.
Estimated Average Requirement	EAR	Average requirement for each nutrient for the U.S. population.
Adequate Intake	AI	Recommended intakes for nutrients without an RDA.
Food Labeling Standards		
Daily Reference Value	DRV	Recommendations for macronutrients based on 2,000-calorie diet; provides the reference amount used to establish the DV.
Reference Daily Intake	RDI	Recommendations for micronutrients based on 1968 RDA; provides the reference amount to establish the DV.
Daily Value	DV	The reference amount shown on food labels; a percentage of the DRV and RDI in one portion/serving

Nutrient Content Claims

In addition to the required information on food labels, manufacturers may include voluntary information. This information, however, must conform to certain standards. The NLEA permits the use of nutrient content claims that assist consumers in making wise food choices. Nutrient content claims are descriptors used on the label that refer to the level of a certain nutrient the food contains. These particular claims describe the level of a nutrient or dietary substance in the product using terms like *free, high,* and *low,* or they compare the level of a nutrient in a food to that of another food, using terms such as *more, reduced,* and *lite.*

To make these statements, food companies must meet standards set forth by the NLEA. Regulations apply primarily to those nutrients with established Daily Values. Examples of standards are listed in Table 2–8.

Health Claims

In addition to the nutrient content claims, the NLEA required the FDA to review 10 diet-disease relationships that could be used as health claims on food product labels. Of the initial 10 claims reviewed, 8 were approved. Since 1990, an additional 4 have been approved,

TABLE 2–8 • NUTRIENT CONTENT DESCRIPTORS ALLOWED ON FOOD LABELS

Term	Definition
More	Contains 10% or more of the DV compared to the reference food
Good source	Contains 10–19% of the DV for a particular nutrient per serving
High or excellent source of	Contains 20% or more of the DV for a particular nutrient per serving
Healthy	Individual foods must contain • less than 3 g fat • less than 1 g saturated fat • less than 60 mg cholesterol • less than 360 mg sodium and must contain at least 10% DV from one of the following: vitamin A, vitamin C, iron, calcium, protein, or fiber
Fresh	Raw foods that have not been frozen or heated

Nutrient	Free	Low	Reduced/Less
All nutrients	Synonyms for *free*: *zero, no, without, trivial source of, negligible source of, dietarily insignificant source of*. Definitions for *free* for meals and main dishes are the stated values per labeled serving.	Synonyms for *low*: *little* (*few* for calories), *contains a small amount of, low source of*.	Synonym for *reduced/less*: *lower* (*fewer* for calories). *Modified* may be used in statement of identity. Definitions for meals and main dishes are the same as for individual foods on the basis of per 100 g.
Calories (cal)	Less than 5 cal per reference amount and per labeled serving.	40 cal or less per reference amount (and per 50 g if reference amount is small). Meals and main dishes: 120 cal or less per 100 g.	At least 25% fewer calories per reference amount than an appropriate reference food. Reference food may not be "low calorie." Uses term *fewer* rather than *less*.
Total fat	Less than 0.5 g per reference amount and per labeled serving. Meals and main dishes: less than 0.5 g per labeled serving. Not defined for meals or main dishes.	3 g or less per reference amount (and per 50 g if reference amount is small). Meals and main dishes: 3 g or less per 100 g and not more than 30% of calories from fat.	At least 25% less fat per reference amount than an appropriate reference food. Reference food may not be "low-fat."
Saturated fat	Less than 0.5 g saturated fat and less than 0.5 g trans-fatty acids per reference amount and per labeled serving. Meals and main dishes: less than 0.5 g saturated fat and less than 0.5 g trans-fatty acids per labeled serving. No ingredient that is understood to contain saturated fat except as noted below.[a]	1 g or less per reference amount and 15% or less of calories from saturated fat. Meals and main dishes: 1 g or less per 100 g and less than 10% of calories from saturated fat.	At least 25% less saturated fat per reference amount than an appropriate reference food. Reference food may not be "low saturated fat."

[a]Except if the ingredient listed on the food label has an asterisk that refers to footnote (e.g., "*adds a trivial amount of fat").

Note: Reference amount = reference amount customarily consumed.

Small reference amount = reference amount of 30 g or less or 2 tablespoons or less (for dehydrated foods that are typically consumed when rehydrated with water or a diluent containing an insignificant amount, as defined in 21 CFR 101.9(f)(1), of all nutrients per reference amount, the per 50 g criterion refers to the prepared form of the food).

Source: Code of Federal Regulations 21CFR101. 2002. *Food Labeling.* http://www.cfsan.fda.gov/~dms/flg-toc.html.

raising the total claims allowed to 12 (Table 2–9). A health claim has two essential components: (1) a substance (food, food component, or dietary ingredient) and (2) a disease or health-related condition. The NLEA designated a lengthy, complex FDA petition process for claims to receive approval.

In 1997, the Food and Drug Administration Modernization Act was passed to improve the process allowing certain U.S. government bodies to publish authoritative statements on

TABLE 2-9 • HEALTH CLAIMS ALLOWED ON FOOD LABELS

Health Claim	Date Approved
Calcium and osteoporosis	January 1993
Sodium and hypertension	January 1993
Dietary fat and cancer	January 1993
Dietary saturated fat and cholesterol and risk of coronary heart disease	January 1993
Fiber-containing grain products, fruits, and vegetables and cancer	January 1993
Fruits, vegetables, and grain products that contain fiber, particularly soluble fiber, and risk of coronary heart disease	January 1993
Fruits and vegetables and cancer	January 1993
Folate and neural tube defects	March 1996
Dietary sugar alcohol and dental caries	December 1997
Soluble fiber from certain foods and risk of coronary heart disease	February 1998
Soy protein and risk of coronary heart disease	October 1999
Plant sterol/stanol esters and risk of coronary heart disease	September 2000

Source: Code of Federal Regulations 21CFR101. 2002. *Food Labeling.* http://www.cfsan.fda.gov/~dms/flg-toc.html.

food labels (Table 2–10). Then, in 2003, the FDA announced its Consumer Health Information for Better Nutrition Initiative. This measure allows manufacturers to use qualified health claims in cases where emerging evidence supports a relationship between a food or a food component and a disease or a health-related condition. Currently, eight qualified health claims are permitted (Table 2–11). Together, the different types of health claims allowed on food labels total 22.

NLEA Requirements for Restaurants

Proper nutrition is important in the restaurant industry. Over the past 30 years, dining away from home has increased. Restaurants in the United States provide 70 billion meals and make 440.1 billion dollars in sales (National Restaurant Association 2004). Currently, 46% of the food dollar is spent away from home. With the restaurant industry contributing such a large percentage of the American diet, it is important that the industry provide nutritious food options.

Originally, officials exempted restaurants from food-labeling regulation. However, in June 1996, a U.S. district court ordered the FDA to apply the NLEA regulations to

TABLE 2-10 • AUTHORITATIVE STATEMENTS PUBLISHED BY U.S. GOVERNMENT BODIES

Authoritative Statement	Date Approved
Potassium and risk of high blood pressure and stroke	October 2000
Whole-grain foods and risk of heart disease and certain cancers	December 2003

Source: Code of Federal Regulations 21CFR101. 2002. *Food Labeling.* http://www.cfsan.fda.gov/~dms/flg-toc.html.

TABLE 2-11 • APPROVED QUALIFIED HEALTH CLAIMS

Approved Qualified Health Claim	Date Approved
Omega-3 fatty acids and coronary heart disease	October 2000
0.8 mg folic acid and neural tube birth defects	October 2000
B vitamins and vascular disease	November 2000
Phosphatidylserine and cognitive dysfunction and dementia	February 2003
Selenium and cancer	February 2003
Antioxidant vitamins and cancer	April 2003
Nuts and heart disease	July 2003
Walnuts and heart disease	July 2003

Source: Code of Federal Regulations 21CFR101. 2002. *Food Labeling.* http://www.cfsan.fda.gov/~dms/flg-toc.html.

restaurant menu labeling. This was in response to a lawsuit that consumer groups had levied against the FDA claiming gross misrepresentation on restaurant menus regarding "low-fat" and "heart healthy" recipe claims. The court ruled in favor of the consumer group and required restaurants to comply with FDA labeling regulations. For restaurants, this means that health claims for any menu items must be backed up with nutritional information for those items to fully inform consumers. See Figure 2–6. The restaurant

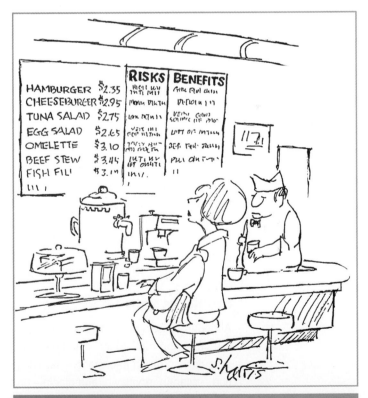

FIGURE 2–6 • THE NLEA REQUIRES RESTAURANTS TO PROVIDE INFORMATION ABOUT FOOD PRODUCTS WHEN MAKING NUTRITIONAL CLAIMS
Source: ScienceCartoonsPlus.com

must be prepared to show that their claims comply with the NLEA definitions. For example, if a restaurant claims that its dressings are reduced fat the restaurant must document that it is.

Unlike food products purchased in the grocery store, restaurants are not required to show complete nutritional information or provide nutritional information on labels. Restaurants must present nutritional information in a "reasonable" manner—such as notebook, poster, or brochure.

However, with concern growing over the obesity epidemic, many Americans did not believe that the NLEA food labeling regulations for restaurants were sufficient. Therefore, in November 2003, the Menu Education and Labeling Act was brought before Congress.

This amendment ensured that consumers would receive information about the nutritional content of restaurant food as well as foods that made health claims. The bill required restaurants with 20 or more outlets to provide nutritional information that is understandable to customers. The bill required the saturated fat, trans-fatty acids, total calories, and sodium content of menu items be made available to customers in a public manner. Additional nutritional information could also be provided. The National Restaurant Association (NRA) released a statement responding to the proposed legislation (2003). A portion of this statement follows:

> If the aim is to effectively address the complex issue of obesity in America, this legislation mandating nutrition labeling for restaurants clearly misses the target. . . . There can be no feasible, one-size-fits-all application of menu labeling legislation. Currently the great majority of quick service chain restaurants have been proactively providing nutritional information to their customers without intrusive government mandates for some time. The restaurant industry remains an industry of choice driven by demand and many restaurants with standardized menus do provide nutritional information for customers through a system that is most workable for their business and their customers through brochures, posted signs, web sites and 1-800 numbers, making this legislation redundant.

In a letter to the FDA, the NRA stated that the inherent variability in nutritional values in restaurant foods forces caution in mandating labeling. Furthermore, the organization contends that the legislation was impractical because of the wide variety of choices at many restaurants. Consider a sandwich shop with 15 possible ingredients for a sandwich. Patrons can order this particular sandwich in 1.3 trillion combinations (National Restaurant Association 2003). Although providing nutritional information in restaurants would be problematic, the NRA supports the FDA proposal for *voluntary* labeling.

Problems with Food Labeling

Although most health professionals consider the FDA food label to be a triumph, it is not without some tribulations. The first is the lack of space on the label. Because of its small size, only so much information fits. The government no longer requires B vitamin information—thiamin, riboflavin, and niacin—on food labels. Certain illnesses associated with B vitamin deficiencies have been eliminated for the most part because several foods were part of an enrichment campaign. Flour, breads, and cereals, for example, were enriched with B vitamins. (See Chapter 3 for more information.)

Consumers must still use caution when nutrient content descriptors are used. Terms like *lite* and *less fat* could actually be high in fat. These terms refer to a standard product.

If the reference foods are very high in fat, then terms like *lite* and *less fat* may still describe foods that do not fit into a low-fat diet plan. For example, a lite frank may supply 66% of its calories from fat because the standard frank provides almost all its calories from fat. A 40% less-fat frank may still provide 69% of its calories from fat. Although it is true that these hot dogs are a better choice than the standard frank, a lite or low-fat frank may still not meet consumer expectations for nutritional quality. Another food product, like sliced turkey, may be a better choice with its lower fat content.

Product manufacturers are permitted to label processed meats as *lean* if they supply less than 10 grams of fat per 100-grams serving. Yet upon closer inspection, you notice the label shows 50% of the total calories from fat. How can a product be labeled *lean* and still contain 50% fat? The fat content for a *lean* frank is set at a maximum of 10 grams, irrespective of calorie content. So as the total number of calories decreases and the calories from fat remain the same, the percentage of calories from fat increases.

Consider the following example:

	Meat A (100 g)	Meat B (100 g)
Total calories	180	270
Calories from 10 g fat	90	90
Calories from fat (%)	50%	33%

Although all foods labeled *lean* contain less than 10 g of fat per 100 g of food, lower-calorie foods contain a greater percentage of calories from fat. If fat is not supplying the calories, another macronutrient—protein or carbohydrate—must.

So even with the food-labeling laws, there are still apparent inconsistencies between label descriptions and some consumer perceptions and expectations. A lean or lite version of a product may still be very high in fat if the standard product is almost entirely fat. Although the food laws provide definitions and standards for what can be stated on a food label, it is still up to the consumer to use the information wisely and to look past the descriptors to the nutrient information that the package provides.

There is another point of concern specific to the labeling of processed meats. When a hot dog package states that the contents are 97% fat-free, most consumers assume that only 3% of the calories are from fat. This is not true. Confusion is caused by stating the percentage of fat by total weight rather than as the percentage of calories from fat. Considering weight alone, the hot dog's major component is water. Actually, this is true for many foods. By using the total weight as the measurement, meats appear to be leaner than they are (Figure 2–7). On the Nutrition Facts label, however, fat is stated in calories instead of weight.

For example, if a hot dog label shows that the product is 97% fat-free, it may actually derive 30% of its calories from fat (Figure 2–8). The front side of the package states fat as a percentage of the entire weight, but this is not the same as percentage of calories. If the hot dog is 90% water and 7% protein and carbohydrate, it contains only 3% fat by total weight. But if the percentage of fat from calories is calculated, this same hot dog contains 70% calories from protein and carbohydrate and 30% from fat.

The key is that most foods are mostly water. So if a shopper wants to choose a hot dog that derives less than 30% of its calories from fat, he or she must choose a product that is at least 97% fat-free by weight. A meat product that is 93% fat-free may derive more than 50% of its calories from fat. Expressing fat percentage by weight may be the greatest deception still allowed on the U.S. food label. Consider this example: If expressing fat content as a percentage of weight were standard practice for dairy products, half-and-half could be labeled 90% fat-free when 75% of its calories come from fat; sour cream 80% fat-free with 75% of its calories from fat; and heavy whipping cream 66% fat-free with 100% of its calories

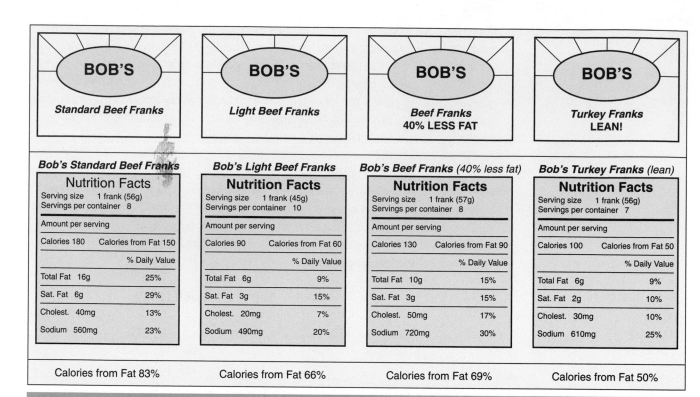

Bob's Standard Beef Franks

Nutrition Facts

Serving size   1 frank (56g)
Servings per container 8

Amount per serving

Calories 180   Calories from Fat 150

% Daily Value

Total Fat 16g	25%
Sat. Fat 6g	29%
Cholest. 40mg	13%
Sodium 560mg	23%

Calories from Fat 83%

Bob's Light Beef Franks

Nutrition Facts

Serving size   1 frank (45g)
Servings per container 10

Amount per serving

Calories 90   Calories from Fat 60

% Daily Value

Total Fat 6g	9%
Sat. Fat 3g	15%
Cholest. 20mg	7%
Sodium 490mg	20%

Calories from Fat 66%

Bob's Beef Franks (40% less fat)

Nutrition Facts

Serving size   1 frank (57g)
Servings per container 8

Amount per serving

Calories 130   Calories from Fat 90

% Daily Value

Total Fat 10g	15%
Sat. Fat 3g	15%
Cholest. 50mg	17%
Sodium 720mg	30%

Calories from Fat 69%

Bob's Turkey Franks (lean)

Nutrition Facts

Serving size   1 frank (56g)
Servings per container 7

Amount per serving

Calories 100   Calories from Fat 50

% Daily Value

Total Fat 6g	9%
Sat. Fat 2g	10%
Cholest. 30mg	10%
Sodium 610mg	25%

Calories from Fat 50%

FIGURE 2–7 • NUTRIENT CONTENT DESCRIPTORS ON HOT DOG LABELS AND THE CORRESPONDING PERCENTAGES OF CALORIES FROM FAT

coming from fat. Even soft-spread margarine could be labeled 50% fat-free, though 100% of its calories come from fat.

Another conundrum in food labeling is the polyunsaturated fat listing. Looking at a label, you see this type of fat listed only as a single value. But it is composed of two families—omega-6 fatty acids and omega-3 fatty acids. Current nutritional science shows us

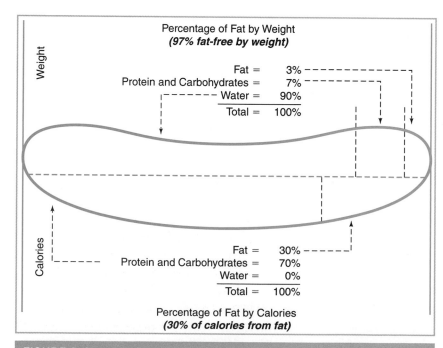

Percentage of Fat by Weight
(97% fat-free by weight)

Fat =	3%
Protein and Carbohydrates =	7%
Water =	90%
Total =	100%

Weight

Calories

Fat =	30%
Protein and Carbohydrates =	70%
Water =	0%
Total =	100%

Percentage of Fat by Calories
(30% of calories from fat)

FIGURE 2–8 • FAT CONTENT OF A HOT DOG

that polyunsaturated fat is preferable to saturated fat. Yet all polyunsaturated fats are not the same. Excessive dietary intake of the omega-6 type of polyunsaturated fat, found in many plant oils, may actually contribute to **atherosclerosis** and other medical conditions (Okuyama, Tetsuyuki, and Watanabe 1997; Hennig, Toborek, and McClain 2001).

Increasing consumption of omega-3 polyunsaturated fat may reduce the risk of coronary heart disease (Sidhu 2003). Consumers wishing to lower their heart disease risk would benefit by having this information on the food label. (See Chapter 4 for more information.)

One final concern with food labeling is how ingredients are listed for oil. If a particular type of oil is not always used consistently in a product, several options may be stated on the ingredient label. In such cases, it is impossible for the label to provide specific information on the type of polyunsaturated fat the food contains. Different oils contain different types of fat. When manufacturers routinely use a specific oil, they can more clearly state ingredients and nutrition facts.

INTERNATIONAL DIETARY GUIDELINES

The United States has long been a multicultural society comprising immigrants from around the globe. Taking one look at the vast range of food Americans eat illustrates this diversity. In light of this, food service establishments commonly offer a variety of ethnic cuisines. *Ethnic Cuisines II*, a report prepared for the National Restaurant Association, surveyed U.S. consumers in relation to "trial of" and "attitudes" about diverse ethnic cuisines. The seven most frequently consumed ethnic cuisines in the United States, ranked from most to least, are Italian, Mexican, Chinese, German, Greek, Japanese, and French (C&R Research 2000). (Chinese cuisine, ranked separately as Cantonese and Mandarin-Hunan-Szechwan, is reported here as Chinese.)

Comparing pictorial food guidelines from these countries, one can see significant variation. Food guide graphics are designed to capture culturally familiar shapes that best communicate nutritional messages to the intended audiences (Gatenby, Hunt, and Rayner 1995; Achterburg et al. 1992). Differences abound. To some cultures, the pyramid's base is most important because it provides support; yet to others, the pinnacle is. Most Americans understood the sweet and fat group at the top of the former Food Guide Pyramid to signify less consumption, members of other cultures might see that group as the most prized and, consequently, the most consumed.

Countries may also have different goals and key concepts to communicate to their populations. Balance, variety, and moderation were desired properties in the U.S. pyramid shape selection (Achterburg et al. 1992), whereas specific quantitative recommendations were more important for other countries. Pyramid and circle/plate images are common worldwide, but some countries developed unique images. France employs a boat graphic, and Italy created an image of undulating arrows.

With variation in image selection and design also comes variation in portion size recommendations. After all, there is no one single way to eat. Some graphics, like China's, are quantitatively based and include specific serving recommendations in units, grams, bowls, or spoons. Others are qualitative guides, like Mexico's. Its provides broad recommendations to eat from each group everyday, moderately or lots.

Besides variation in the main graphic and whether it has a quantitative or qualitative philosophy, the pictures may also group foods differently. For instance, classification systems may either unite or separate fruits and vegetables, while other systems differ in their decision to include fat, sweets, beverages, or dairy groups, or not. Potatoes, for example, are often placed in different food groups. Some guides categorize them with grains. The United States and China consider them to be vegetables; Greece places potatoes in their own group. Japan, on the other hand, leaves off potatoes entirely. Legumes are another food with variation. All of the guides reviewed include legumes, and Mexico even counsels consumers to enjoy them with grains for a complete protein. One may see legumes with vegetables, dairy, protein, or grains or in their own group. Considering their high protein values, legumes are treated like meat-based protein foods, and with their high carbohydrate content they share characteristics of vegetables and grains. It is easy to see why there is no single approach for grouping legumes in various diet schemes.

Neither Mexico nor Japan separated fat or sweets into their own groups, but France and Greece did. The U.S. and remaining guides contain only fat groups. Authorities and scientists have discussed how to handle fat in the development of many food guides. Some chose not to include it as a separate group in an effort to discourage ingestion. Food guide graphics containing fat groups often stress the importance of choosing low-saturated-fat varieties. Greece encourages low-saturated-fat consumption by making olive oil a food group all its own. France is unique in its separation of animal fat from vegetable fat, but its graphic does not use the separate groups to encourage vegetable fat consumption. My Pyramid displays oil as a required category and discusses limiting fat.

Differences are seen in other graphics too. Lettuce varieties are included in every guide. Carrots appear in five guides; tomatoes in three; cabbage in three. Guides pick culturally specific vegetables appropriate for their audiences: China includes bok choy, Mexico depicts cactus and squash blossoms, and Japan illustrates lotus root. Even though every guide contains milk, dairy foods are separated as their own group in some guides, whereas in others it is a protein food, particularly those with lower dairy consumption. Water and tea are pictured in Japan's fan. France shows water. Greece includes wine.

Countries around the world have established guidelines to help people meet their nutritional needs and to improve their health. Recommendations vary. Some address specific nutrient needs, and others provide broader food-based guidelines. It is important for professionals in the hospitality industry to understand the nutritional needs of the consumer and the governmental guidelines that have been created to ensure that the nutritional needs of the population are being met.

SUMMARY

Nutrient Values for Everyone

In the United States, dietary inadequacies result from both undernutrition and overnutrition. Even with an ample food supply, some population groups are at risk of vitamin and mineral deficiencies.

Children and adolescents are particularly at risk of nutrient deficiency due to their elevated rate of growth. Individuals with lower incomes must make wise food purchase decisions in order to prepare healthy meals. In addition, individuals with medical conditions or cultural practices that require restricted diets may be at risk, especially if they are eliminating entire food groups from their daily intake.

The Dietary Reference Intakes (DRIs) are nutrient-intake guidelines that state the quantity of each essential nutrient that Americans should consume. The values are presented for 10 human life stages and are separated by gender.

The Dietary Guidelines for Americans (DGA) were first published in 1980 by the U.S. Department of Agriculture and the U.S. Department of Health and Human Services. The guidelines provide a framework for the intake of nutrients as well as whole foods. They offer advice regarding how consumers should eat to meet the nutrient needs described by the DRIs.

My Pyramid, a pictorial model describing the ideal selection of foods to promote good health, provides food-based recommendations focused on variety. Even though these recommendations are based on the DRIs, My Pyramid contains information that consumers can easily apply to their daily lives. Foods are placed into groups with similar nutrient content. Eating from each of the groups will meet nutrient needs.

The Federal Food, Drug, and Cosmetic Act helped to define food standards and ingredient identity on packaged foods. The act authorized factory inspections to ensure proper product manufacturing and handling and prevented food companies from making claims on labels relating food to disease. Before the law was enacted, many states had individual requirements on nutrition labeling and food standards. The lack of a universal standard for claims like "low-fat" and "reduced-fat" created confusion among consumers. To clarify and better inform the American consumer, Congress passed the Nutrition Labeling and Education Act (NLEA) in 1990.

The NLEA requires that all packaged foods bear standardized nutrition labeling and that all health claims meet the regulations prescribed by the U.S. Department of Health and Human Services.

CASE RESOLUTION

The body needs vitamins and minerals to carry out important health functions, but it needs them in only very small amounts. Eating a varied and balanced diet is the best way to consume all the nutrients the body needs. Healthy people can supplement their good diet with a multivitamin/mineral tablet providing 100% of each nutrient. Beyond 100% could be wasteful if the body does not need extra nutrients. In addition, too much of some vitamins and minerals may even be harmful.

Remember: Enough is good; more is not.

REFERENCES

Achterburg, C., I. R. Contento, M. A. Hess, L. Rendon, and A. L. Baldinger. 1992. An evaluation of dietary guidance graphic alternatives: The evolution of the Eating Right Pyramid. *Nutrition Review* 50: 275–92.

Bender, M. M., and Derby, B. M. 1992. Prevalence of reading nutrition and ingredient information on food labels among adult Americans: 1982–1988. *Journal of Nutrition Education* 24: 292–97.

Centers for Disease Control and Prevention. 2006. 1985–2006 prevalence of obesity among U.S. adults by state. http://www.cdc.gov/nccdphp/dnpa/obesity/trend/maps/obesity_trends_2006.ppt (accessed June 15, 2008).

Chinese Nutrition Society. 1999. Dietary guidelines and the food guide pagoda for Chinese residents: Balanced diet, rational nutrition, and health promotion. *Nutrition Today* 34(3): 106–15.

C&R Research. 2000. Ethnic cuisines II. Prepared for the National Restaurant Association, Washington, DC.

Davis, C., and E. Saltos. 1999. Dietary recommendations and how they have changed over time. *Agriculture Information Bulletin*, no. 750: 33–50.

Food and Drug Administration. 1996. *Food Labeling Questions and Answers. 2: A Guide for Restaurants and Other Retail Establishments*. Washington, DC: U.S. Government Printing Office. http://www.cfsan.fda.gov/~lrd/tpmenus.html.

Department of Health and Human Services. 2003. Food labeling: Trans fatty acids in nutrition labeling, nutrient content claims, and health claims. *Federal Register* 68 (July 11): 414–33.

Gatenby, S., J., P. Hunt, and M. Rayner. 1995. The format for the national food guide: Performance and preference studies. *Journal of Human Nutrition and Dietetics* 8: 335–51.

Hennig, B., M. Toborek, and C. J. McClain. 2001. High-energy diets, fatty acids, and endothelial cell function: Implications for arteriosclerosis. *Journal of the American College of Nutrition* 20: 97–105.

Institute of Medicine. 1997. *Dietary Reference Intakes for Calcium, Phosphorus, Magnesium, Vitamin D and Fluoride*. Washington, DC: National Academies Press.

Institute of Medicine. 1998. *Dietary Reference Intakes for Thiamin, Riboflavin, Niacin, Vitamin B_6, Folate, Vitamin B_{12}, Pantothenic Acid, Biotin and Choline*. Washington, DC: National Academies Press.

Institute of Medicine. 1999. *Dietary Reference Intakes: A Risk Assessment Model for Establishing Upper Intake Levels for Nutrients*. Washington, DC: National Academy Press.

Institute of Medicine. 2000a. *Dietary Reference Intake: Applications in Dietary Assessment*. Washington, DC: National Academies Press.

Institute of Medicine. 2000b. *Dietary Reference Intakes for Vitamin C, Vitamin E, Selenium, and Carotenoids*. Washington, DC: National Academies Press.

Menu Education and Labeling Act. 2003. HR 3444, 108th Cong., November 5.

National Restaurant Association. 2004. Restaurant industry forecast: Executive summary. Washington, DC: National Restaurant Association. http://www.restaurant.org/research/forecast.cfm.

National Restaurant Association. 2003. NRA opposes one-size-fits-all labeling law for restaurant menus: Unnecessary regulations put undue burden on nation's favorite restaurants, news release, November 5. http://www.restaurant.org/pressroom/pressrelease.cfm?ID=758 (accessed July 17, 2008).

Neuhouser, M. L., A. R. Kristal, and R. E. Patterson 1999. Use of food nutrition labels is associated with lower fat intake. *Journal of the American Dietetic Association* 99: 45–53.

Okuyama, H., K. Tetsuyuki, and S. Watanabe. 1997. Dietary fatty-acids: The N-6/N-3 balance and chronic elderly diseases; excess linoleic acid and relative N-3 deficiency syndrome seen in Japan. *Progress in Lipid Research* 35: 409–57.

Sidhu, K. S. 2003. Health benefits and potential risks related to consumption of fish or fish oil. *Regulatory Toxicology and Pharmacology* 38: 336–44.

Supreme Scientific Health Council. 1999. Dietary guidelines for adults in Greece. Ministry of Health and Welfare. http://www.nut.uoa.gr/english/ (accessed July 4, 2002).

U.S. Department of Agriculture, Center for Nutrition Policy and Promotion. 2003. Notice of availability of proposed Food Guide Pyramid daily food intake patterns and technical support data and announcement of public comment period. *Federal Register* 68 (September 11): 535–36.

U.S. Department of Agriculture. MyPyramid.gov. http://www.mypyramid.gov (accessed July 17, 2008).

U.S. Department of Agriculture. 2005. *Dietary Guidelines for Americans*, 6th ed. Washington, DC: U.S. Government Printing Office.

U.S. Department of Agriculture. http://www.nal.usda.gov/fnic/history/basic4.htm (accessed June 15, 2008).

Willett, W. C. 2001. *Eat, Drink, and Be Healthy: The Harvard Medical School Guide to Healthy Eating.* New York: Fireside.

REVIEW QUESTIONS

1. How can a package state that a hot dog contains only 3% fat when the hot dog derives 30% of its calories from fat?
2. Are Americans receiving adequate amounts of nutrients? Consider macronutrients and micronutrients in your answer.
3. Explain the Dietary Reference Intake. Review its four main values.
4. What do the Daily Values indicate? What are they based on? If you followed a 1,600-calorie diet, would the Daily Values apply to you?
5. What laws are in place to ensure that consumers receive appropriate information on food labels and food packaging? Do you feel that the procedures need improvement?
6. Select three guidelines from the Dietary Guidelines for Americans. Describe how you could incorporate the recommendations into your daily routine to improve your health. Make one recommendation to improve the dietary guidelines themselves.
7. Compare and contrast My Pyramid, the newest U.S. food graphic, with food graphics from two other countries. Highlight two key points for each graphic.
8. How are ingredients listed on a food label?
9. Define "low-fat."
10. After reviewing arguments for and against restaurant menu labeling for nutritional content, explain your position on the issue. Do you think consumers would benefit from having nutritional information on restaurant menus?

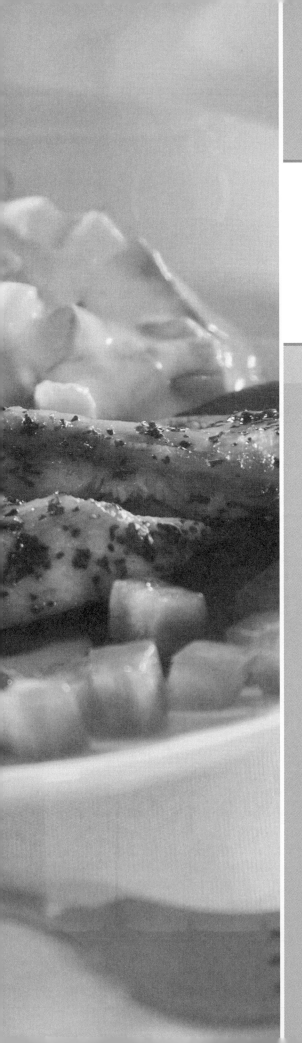

3

Carbohydrates

KEY CONCEPTS

- Carbohydrates are an important energy source.
- Enzymes are needed to digest carbohydrates.
- Lactose intolerance affects the ability of certain individuals to digest lactose, which is the natural sugar in dairy.
- Fiber, although not a nutrient, is essential in maintaining good health.
- There are two categories of fiber: insoluble and soluble.
- Glycogen acts as a stored energy source.
- Insulin and glucagon are hormones that regulate blood sugar.

Carbohydrates, as an energy powerhouse, allow the body to function and perform physical activity. Carbohydrates are organic compounds made of carbon (C), oxygen (O), and hydrogen (H). Each gram of carbohydrate supplies, on average, four calories of energy.

Energy, contained in the chemical bonds of plants, is placed there during photosynthesis. The sun's energy combines carbon dioxide (CO_2) with water (H_2O) to build carbohydrates, which animals and humans consume for food. This is known as the *carbon cycle* (Figure 3–1).

Starches and sugars are the major energy-yielding carbohydrates, and they are found in a range of foods, including cane, beet, and fruit sugars; molasses; honey; flour; cornstarch; rice; and potatoes. These foods contain varying amounts of carbohydrate (Table 3–1).

Even though carbohydrates are a main energy source, not all provide calories. Fiber, for instance, is an indigestible carbohydrate and thus provides little energy for humans. Yet it is essential for the normal functioning of the gastrointestinal tract.

THE ENERGY CYCLE

Energy from the sun gives us food to eat, heat for our homes, shelter from the elements, and clothing to keep us warm. How can this be? Through a process called *photosynthesis*, green plants capture energy from the sun. Plants use this energy to build glucose, a carbohydrate, by taking carbon dioxide from the air and water from the ground. The sun's energy is locked in the chemical bonds of glucose. Glucose is then used by the plant for its own energy needs or is stored as sugar or starch for future use. Some of the glucose is also used to build the structure of the plant by connecting large numbers of glucose molecules together into a fiber called *cellulose*. Cellulose fiber provides the structure for a stalk of celery and the trunk of a tree, for example. So the wooden chair we sit on, the wooden desk we write on, and the wooden pencil we write with are all composed of the sugar glucose. Clothes made from cotton are also glucose. This glucose, however, is in an indigestible form.

We also heat our homes with sugar when we burn wood. Energy from the sun is locked in the chemical bonds in the wood's structure. When wood is burned, the carbohydrate bonds are broken and the energy from the sun is released into our homes as heat. This same sunlight energy is released in our bodies when we digest and then metabolize sugar and starch. The carbohydrates that we digest are combined with oxygen and broken down into water (H_2O) and carbon dioxide (CO_2), which we exhale through respiration. The plants take in CO_2 and H_2O to build carbohydrates, and the cycle continues.

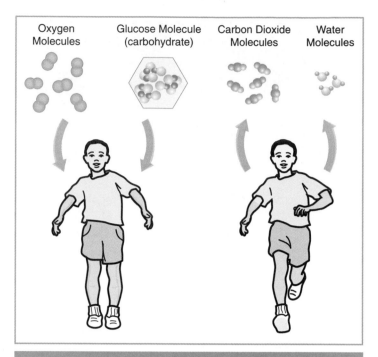

FIGURE 3–1 • THE CARBON CYCLE

Carbohydrates also function in combination with protein to form various compounds in the body that have metabolic activity, such as sugars that form the backbone structure of DNA and RNA. If there is not enough carbohydrate present in the diet, protein is used for energy before building and renewing body cells. Therefore, in this case, carbohydrate

TABLE 3–1 • CARBOHYDRATE CONTENT OF FOODS (GRAMS)

Food	Starch	Sugar	Fiber
Meat, poultry, and fish	—	—	—
Eggs	—	—	—
Fat	—	—	—
Seeds, 1/2 cup	30.0	—	2.0–6.0
Beans, 1/2 cup	20.0	—	5.0–8.0
Nuts, 1/2 cup	20.0	—	2.0–5.0
Bread, 1 slice, or cooked whole grains, 1/2 cup	15.0	—	2.5
Processed grains, 1/2 cup	15.0		1.0
Vegetables, 1/2 cup	5.0	<1.0	1.5
Fruits, 1/2 cup	—	15.0	1.5–3.0
Milk, 1 cup	—	12.0	—
Sugar, 1 teaspoon	—	5.0	—

Note: The amount of starch and sugar is based on the Exchange Lists for Meal Planning, the American Diabetes Association and the American Dietetic Association, 1995; fiber figures are estimates.

"spares" protein. A high-carbohydrate meal, on the other hand, increases the release of serotonin, a neurotransmitter. Serotonin has a calming effect on the body.

THINK ABOUT IT

Have you ever purchased something only to find out later that it was not what you thought you were buying? This happens to everyone at some point. Food labels are designed to prevent this type of deception when buying food. Regardless of what you see on the front of the package—the fancy marketing photos, the scientific-sounding language, and the urgent messages promising to improve your health—you should make it a habit it check out the back. Examine the list of ingredients and the nutrition profile to inform your purchase.

The next time you see "wheat bread," take a peak at the label. What's the first ingredient you see? How much fiber is in each serving? Have any colorings been added to the bread? Wheat bread is not the same as *whole-wheat* bread, but not everyone realizes that. Wheat bread could be plain old refined bread turned brown with caramel or another food coloring. Informed consumers can make better choices.

CASE STUDY

Potent Seeds

Amelia is working on her senior research project in experimental foods. Her task is to modify a recipe, improve its nutritional profile, and maintain taste. She has discovered that milled flaxseeds are useful in baking; they can replace some of the fat and provide fiber and a mild nutty flavor. Amelia prepares flaxseed banana muffins and brings them to school for a taste test, but she fails to mention the muffins' extremely high fiber content. Each muffin has 12 grams of fiber.

What is the main concern? Will these muffins be harmful to anyone's health? *The resolution for this case study is presented at the end of the chapter.*

MONOSACCHARIDE A simple sugar. Glucose, fructose, and galactose are monosaccharides.

DISACCHARIDE A sugar comprising two monosaccharides. Maltose, sucrose, and lactose are disaccharides.

GLUCOSE A simple sugar that is a major energy source for humans.

FRUCTOSE Fruit sugar. Fructose is the sweetest monosaccharide.

GALACTOSE A simple sugar found in milk. Galactose is a constituent of lactose.

DEXTROSE Another name for glucose.

CLASSIFICATION OF CARBOHYDRATES

Carbohydrates are classified by the number of sugar molecules they contain. Those that contain a single sugar molecule, monosaccharides, and 2 molecules, disaccharides, are classified as sugars. Oligosaccharides contain 3–9 molecules, and polysaccharides, starches and fiber, contain 10 or more sugar molecules (Table 3–2).

Monosaccharides and Disaccharides (Sugars)

Sugars are classified as **monosaccharides** and **disaccharides**. The main monosaccharides are **glucose**, **fructose**, and **galactose**. The chemical formula for all three monosaccharides is $C_6H_{12}O_6$, or 6 carbon molecules, 12 hydrogen molecules, and 6 oxygen molecules. Glucose is widely distributed in nature and is found in fruits, vegetables, honey, and tree sap. **Dextrose** is another name for glucose.

Fructose is often called fruit sugar, or levulose. The sweetest tasting of the monosaccharides, it is found in fruits and vegetables, in the nectar of flowers, in honey, and in

TABLE 3–2 • THE MAJOR DIETARY CARBOHYDRATES		
Class (DPª)	**Subgroup**	**Components**
Sugars (1–2)	Monosaccharides	Glucose, galactose, fructose
	Disaccharides	Sucrose, lactose, maltose, trehalose
	Polyols	Sorbitol, mannitol xylatol
Oligosaccharides (3–9)	Malto-oligosaccharides	Maltodextrins
	Other oligosaccharides	Raffinose, stachyose, fructo-oligosaccharides
Polysaccharides (>9)	Starch	Amylose, amylopectin, modified starches
	Nonstarch polysaccharides	Celluloses, hemicelluloses, pectins, guns

ªDP = Degree of polymerization

Source: Adapted from World Health Organization (WHO). 1997. *Carbohydrates in Human Nutrition: Report of a Joint FAO/WHO Expert Consultation.* Rome, Italy: FAO Food and Nutrition Paper 66.

LACTOSE Milk sugar.

MALTOSE Malt sugar produced during fermentation.

SUCROSE Table sugar.

molasses. Galactose is primarily found in **lactose**, or milk sugar. Small amounts of galactose are found in apples, bananas, pears, carrots, peas, sweet potatoes, and some other fruits and vegetables. Legumes and cereals also contain small amounts of galactose.

Disaccharides are two-unit sugars: **maltose**, **sucrose**, and lactose. Maltose comes from the breakdown of starch. It is also found in sprouting grain, malted cereals, malted milk, and corn syrup. Sucrose is table sugar made from sugar cane or sugar beets, and it is found in some fruits, vegetables, cakes, and pies. Lactose, as already mentioned, is milk sugar.

Sugars are important to culinary students for more than the sweetness they add to foods. During the baking process, they are involved in browning reactions, and they can act as shortening agents in baked goods like muffins.

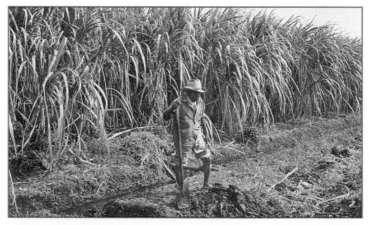

The sugar cane harvest.
Dorling Kindersley Media Library

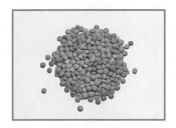 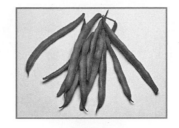 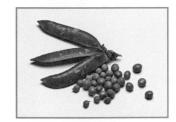

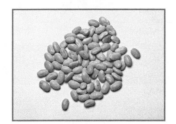 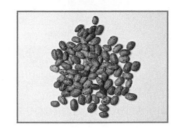 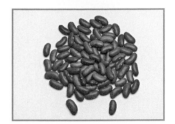

Beans and dried peas are a good source of carbohydrates. From left to right: (top row) Lentils, green beans, and shelling peas; (bottom row) great northern beans, pinto beans, and red kidney beans.
Pearson Education/PH College

Oligosaccharides

OLIGOSACCHARIDE A carbohydrate made up of three to nine linked monosaccharides.

Oligosaccharides are composed of three to nine monosaccharides. The human body does not produce enzymes to dismantle these carbohydrate chains. Common oligosaccharides include maltodextrins, raffinose, stachyose, and fructooligosaccharides (FOSs). Maltodextrins, composed solely of glucose, can be broken down by enzymes in the digestive tract. Raffinose and stachyose are composed of glucose, fructose, and galactose molecules. FOSs are composed of only glucose and fructose. These last three oligosaccharides are not digested by enzymes in the intestinal tract but are acted on by intestinal bacteria, which may cause intestinal gas. Many beans and legumes contain significant amounts of these compounds.

Despite this sometimes unpleasant side effect, oligosaccharides may bestow certain health benefits to the consumer. For example, human breast milk, which contains oligosaccharides, may enhance infant health and provide health benefits later in life.

PROBIOTIC Promoting the growth of healthful microorganisms in the intestine.

Probiotic health benefits are obtained from consuming many of the compounds in this group; FOSs are an example. They are thought to promote the growth of beneficial bifidobacteria in the intestine while inhibiting the growth of pathogenic bacteria (World Health Organization 1997).

Polysaccharides

POLYSACCHARIDE A complex carbohydrate composed of several monosaccharides joined together.

Polysaccharides, or complex carbohydrates, are composed of chains of 10 or more monosaccharides, usually glucose. Polysaccharides are classified in two categories. The first is starch, which is digestible and includes amylose and amylopectin; the second is nonstarch, which is nondigestible and includes fiber and gums. Examples of polysaccharide-containing foods are those made from grains (such as bread, crackers, pasta, and cereal), beans, potatoes, other **tubers**, nuts, and seeds. Well-known grains include wheat, rye, oats, rice, barley, and corn. Less commonly used grains are millet, spelt, quinoa, and amaranth.

TUBER The fleshy part of a root or underground stem. A potato is a tuber.

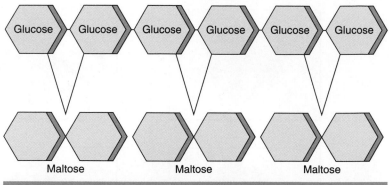

FIGURE 3–2 • GLUCOSE IS BROKEN DOWN INTO MALTOSE MOLECULES THROUGH DIGESTION

Digestion of Starches

The body must convert all carbohydrates to glucose before using them for energy. Starch, the digestible part of polysaccharides, comprises many glucose units that must be broken apart. Digesting starch divides it into the double sugar, maltose (Figure 3–2).

Starch is composed of two kinds of molecules, amylose and amylopectin. Amylose consists of glucose units joined to form linear chains (Figure 3–3a). Amylopectin consists of many short chains of glucose units that form branches containing up to 2,000 units of glucose (Figure 3–3b). Starch is typically 17% to 28% amylose.

Wheat starch and cornstarch are at the higher end of the range, at about 26%; potato starch is at 21%; and tapioca is at the lower end with about 17% amylose. Amylopectin makes up the remainder of the starch (McWilliams 2001). In the dry starch granule, molecules of linear amylose twist and intertwine around the branches of amylopectin. Each type of starch conveys different cooking properties. Starches with lower amounts of amylose, such as potato and tapioca, tend to be better thickening agents. And although cornstarch may not be as strong a thickening agent when cooking, it forms a very firm gel when cooled.

Starch digestion begins in the mouth with an enzyme called **salivary amylase**, or *ptyalin*. This process hydrolyzes, or separates, cooked starch into shorter polysaccharides.

SALIVARY AMYLASE An enzyme secreted in the mouth that converts starch to sugar.

**Starch
Amylose**

Starch Amylopectin

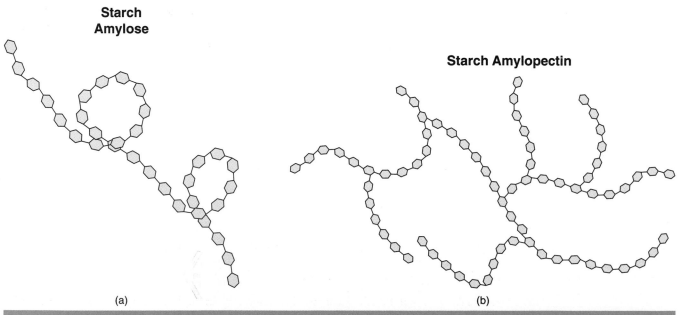

(a)

(b)

FIGURE 3–3 • STARCH AMYLOSE AND AMYLOPECTIN.

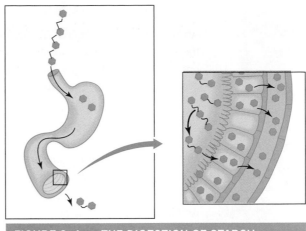

FIGURE 3–4 • THE DIGESTION OF STARCH

CHYME The liquefied mass of partially digested food that moves from the stomach to the duodenum.

PANCREATIC AMYLASE An enzyme from the pancreas that digests carbohydrate.

Food does not remain in the mouth long enough for much digestion to take place there. Salivary amylase that mixes with the food continues to work in the stomach until stomach acids mix with the food to halt starch digestion. The next major activity for starch does not occur again until it enters the first part of the small intestine, called the *duodenum*. By now, starch is a liquefied food, known as **chyme**. **Pancreatic amylase**, a digestive enzyme secreted from the pancreas, breaks down the starch into dextrin, which contains six glucose molecules. Dextrin is then further divided into maltose (Figure 3–4).

Finally, maltose is broken down into two units of glucose that can be used for energy. The breakdown process, mentioned above, is called *hydrolysis* because it is literally splitting the bond by the addition of water (*hydro-* means "water"; *-lysis* means "division" or "separation").

Digestion of Sugars

Specific enzymes, located on the intestinal wall, split disaccharides into monosaccharides. The enzyme maltase, for instance, acts on maltose, and as you might expect, sucrase acts on sucrose, and lactase on lactose. The resulting monosaccharides, also called *simple sugars*, are glucose, fructose, and galactose. Maltose yields two units of glucose when digested; sucrose yields glucose and fructose; and lactose yields glucose and galactose (Figure 3–5). The chemical formula for all three monosaccharides is identical ($C_6H_{12}O_6$), but the chemical bonds are different.

disaccharide + enzyme = monosaccharides

maltose   + maltase = glucose + glucose
sucrose   + sucrase = glucose + fructose
lactose   + lactase = glucose + galactose

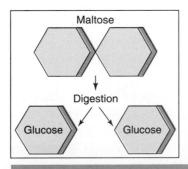
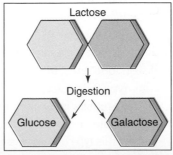
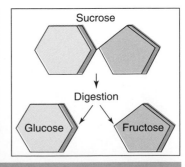

FIGURE 3–5 • THE DIGESTION OF SUGAR

Carbohydrates **49**

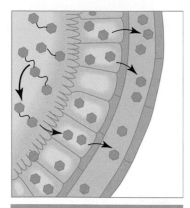

FIGURE 3–6 • THE ABSORPTION OF SUGAR

OXIDIZE To combine with oxygen.

GLYCOGENESIS The metabolic process of converting glucose into glycogen for energy storage.

HORMONE A substance produced in one part of the body that acts elsewhere in the body.

Absorption of Sugars

Absorption of some glucose occurs to a limited extent through the lining of the mouth and the stomach. Primary absorption is in the small intestine where cells take up glucose for energy. Any absorbed glucose that is not immediately required for energy is carried to the liver for glycogen storage (Figure 3–6).

Fructose and galactose go to the liver for conversion into glucose. Only glucose can be used as an energy source; fructose and galactose, in their original forms, cannot.

The bloodstream carries glucose to all parts of the body, where it passes into tissues and cells by way of fluids surrounding the cells. Glucose is **oxidized** in the cell in a long series of chemical processes culminating in the production of energy, carbon dioxide, and water. The waste from this chemical equation—carbon dioxide—is expired by the lungs. And in keeping with the spirit of efficiency, the body converts and stores excess carbohydrate as fat. Some carbohydrate may also assist in the formation of amino acids, the building blocks of protein. Over half of an individual's daily caloric intake should come from carbohydrates. If the proper amount of carbohydrate is lacking in the diet, the liver will convert amino acids and fatty acids to carbohydrate to supply energy. If less than 15% of a person's total daily calories come from carbohydrate foods, the brain may not be supplied with the energy it requires, resulting in dizziness and fatigue. Some individuals on high-protein diets have experienced these symptoms.

Glucose Storage as Glycogen

The liver converts some glucose into a starch, called *glycogen*, for storage. Besides glycogen, glucose can also be converted into amino acids or fatty acids. Glycogen, in turn, can then be converted back to glucose and released when the body needs additional energy. Muscle cells store some glucose as glycogen for use during physical activity. The process of converting glucose to glycogen is referred to as **glycogenesis**.

One-third of the body's glycogen is stored in the liver. The remaining two-thirds is stored in muscles as an emergency energy supply, which can last for two to three hours of intense activity.

Glucose Utilization and Hormonal Regulation

Once glucose is absorbed through the intestinal lining, it enters the bloodstream where it is regulated by **hormones**. After a meal, glucose in the blood stimulates the pancreas to release the hormone insulin, which allows the entry of glucose into the cells. When glucose levels are high, insulin also triggers the liver to remove glucose from the blood and produce glycogen from the excess glucose. If there is not enough insulin, the blood sugar will rise too high, a condition known as *diabetes*.

There are two types of diabetes. Type 1 diabetes, sometimes referred to as *insulin-dependent diabetes*, is when the body does not produce any insulin and individuals must take insulin injections. The classic early symptoms of type 1 diabetes are excessive thirst and frequent urination. There is no cure for this type of diabetes, and patients must take insulin for the rest of their lives.

Type 2 diabetes, sometimes referred to as *non-insulin-dependent diabetes*, does not typically require insulin. In this condition, the body produces insulin, but the insulin does not facilitate the uptake of sugar into the cell as it should, and blood sugar rises. The symptoms of this type of diabetes are not as noticeable as those of type 1, and many individuals go for years without knowing they have the disease. Type 2 diabetics may require oral medications and in special cases insulin injections. Obesity accounts for 95% of the cases of

HYPOGLYCEMIA A condition characterized by a low level of blood sugar.

diabetes in the United States. Although there is no cure for type 1 diabetes, many individuals with type 2 may be cured simply by losing excess weight.

A normal fasting blood sugar level is less than 100 milligrams per 100 milliliters of blood. It takes approximately one to two hours after a meal for the blood sugar to return to fasting (premeal) levels.

Apart from concern over excess glucose levels, some individuals must also prevent low levels of glucose. Inordinate amounts of insulin result in **hypoglycemia,** or too little sugar in the blood. While too much glucose is undesirable, too little is as well.

A number of medical and health factors cause hypoglycemia, such as overconsumption of alcohol, liver failure, and certain medications. Symptoms that health professionals look for are irritability, nervousness, and shakiness. Severe hypoglycemia can lead to unconsciousness. To combat extremely low glucose levels, dietitians recommend a nutritional plan comprising six small meals per day. Each small meal should contain small amounts of refined grains and greater amounts of protein. A sample meal plan is shown in Box 3–1.

GLUCAGON A hormone that raises blood sugar.

ADRENALINE A stress hormone secreted by the adrenal glands.

Glucagon, another hormone produced by the pancreas, acts in opposition to insulin, breaking down the liver's glycogen. This process releases glucose when blood glucose levels are low. **Adrenaline,** also called *epinephrine,* is a hormone produced by the adrenal glands that stimulates the breakdown of liver glycogen into glucose to pass into the tissues for use. Adrenaline also changes muscle glycogen into glucose during exercise to provide energy. If the glucose is metabolized too quickly, as when an athlete is sprinting, lactic acid is formed in the process. Some of the lactic acid can be reconverted to glycogen and stored in the liver for later use.

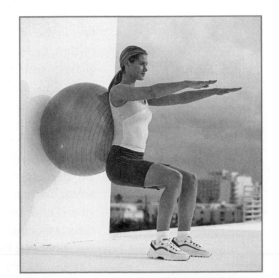

Adrenaline changes muscle glycogen into glucose during exercise.
Russell Sadur © Dorling Kindersley

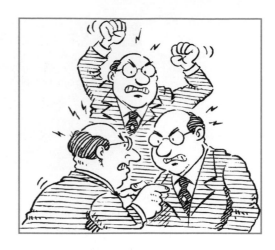

Stress and adrenaline surge.
Images.com

Stress is one of the signals that release adrenaline. This stress trigger ensures that energy is available in the case of emergencies. Excessive stress can cause an adrenaline surge, and the adrenal gland can become exhausted with repeated stress. Hypoglycemia may result. Individuals with this type of hypoglycemia can experience the following symptoms: fatigue, headache, irritability, visual disturbances, shortness of breath, dizziness, rheumatoid-type pains, backache, digestive disturbances, shakiness, and numbness in the arms and legs.

Waiting too many hours between meals can also induce hypoglycemic symptoms. Whether diagnosed with a medical condition, such as diabetes, or not, it is better to eat on a fairly regular schedule to avoid hypoglycemia and its resulting complications. When hypoglycemic, individuals may overeat secondary to the overwhelming feeling of hunger.

Glycemic Index

The glycemic index of a food measures the degree to which the food causes glucose in the blood to rise. For example, if very refined foods, such as white bread or corn syrup, are consumed alone, blood sugar will rise quickly (Box 3–2). These foods contain a large amount of glucose, which is digested and absorbed rapidly. Therefore, white bread and corn syrup are said to have a very high glycemic index. If these foods are modified in ways that slow the digestion and absorption of glucose, the glycemic index of the food is lower. This can happen in a couple of ways.

Removing fiber from a food through processing causes the glycemic index of that food to rise. If the fiber is not removed in processing (as in whole-wheat flour, whole-grain muffins, and so on), the fiber will replace some of the starch, thus reducing the amount of glucose available to the body. Fiber also slows digestion, resulting in a lower glycemic index. Foods that are high in soluble fiber, such as oatmeal, digest even more slowly and have a substantially lower glycemic index. Furthermore, if flour is mixed with fat, the glycemic index is reduced even more. An example is bread dipped in olive oil. Processing flour into pasta also reduces the glycemic index of the food.

As the percentage of carbohydrate in a food or meal decreases, the glycemic index also decreases. Beans and legumes contain a higher percentage of protein compared to bread; therefore, they have a much lower glycemic index. Nuts, because they are higher in fat and have less carbohydrate, have a low glycemic index. Meats that contain little to no carbohydrates have a very low glycemic index.

Changing the type of carbohydrate also changes the glycemic index. Milk products contain galactose, and fruit contains fructose; both of these sugars lower the glycemic

BOX 3–2 • LISTING OF FOOD BY GLYCEMIC INDEX

Kidney/white beans	13
Peanut butter	22
All-Bran	38
Green peas, frozen, boiled	39
Milk, whole	40
Corn chips, plain, salted	42
Apple juice, unsweetened	44
Macaroni, plain, boiled	45
Banana, raw	46
Rice, parboiled	48
Coca-Cola,	53
Pound cake	54
Sucrose (table sugar)	58
50% cracked wheat bread	58
Angel food cake	67
Mars Bar	68
Bagel, white	72
Gatorade	78
Enriched white bread	77
Cornflakes	77
Pretzels, oven-baked, traditional	83

Source: Adapted from K. Foster-Powell, S. Holt, and J. Brand-Miller. 2002. International table of glycemic index and glycemic load values. *American Journal of Clinical Nutrition* 76 (1): 5–56.

index of food. These sugars must first go to the liver after digestion and absorption before being converted to glucose. This requirement greatly lengthens the time from when food is ingested to when the glucose gets to the bloodstream.

Interest in the glycemic index of foods has been increasing. Scientists and healthcare professionals are exploring applications of the glycemic index to diabetes. Promoters of high-protein diets (such as the Zone Diet) use the glycemic index in their work too.

CARBOHYDRATE-RELATED DISORDERS

CELIAC DISEASE A disorder in which the body is unable to metabolize gluten. Celiac disease leads to nutrient deficiencies.

GLUTEN A plant protein found in wheat, rye, and barley.

MICROVILLI Small finger-like projections on the intestinal wall that expand the surface area and thus increase absorption of nutrients.

We have learned that sugars require the proper corresponding disaccharide enzyme for digestion. In certain health conditions, metabolism is distorted in the absence of the required enzymes. Diseases that damage the intestinal lining, such as **celiac disease**, are associated with enzyme deficiency.

Celiac disease is an inherited intolerance to **gluten**, a protein in wheat, rye, and barley. Consumption of gluten causes an autoimmune reaction in the intestinal lining, and the tiny **microvilli** are destroyed, reducing the available surface area for nutrient absorption. This reduced absorptive capacity may lead to nutrient deficiencies, and individuals with celiac disease may experience gas, bloating, and diarrhea. Following a gluten-restricted diet alleviates symptoms; therefore, chefs must develop awareness of food ingredients containing gluten in the event that they serve customers with celiac disease. Even trace amounts of gluten may excite a reaction in sensitive individuals. Besides the grains mentioned earlier, spice preparations, soy sauce, soups, cereals, and vegetarian soy products may contain gluten.

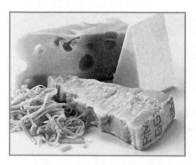

Hard cheese has little lactose if aged for 60 days.
Simon Smith © Dorling Kindersley

The disaccharide lactose, found in milk, may cause digestive problems in some individuals who are deficient in lactase, the essential enzyme needed to digest lactose. Populations around the world experience diminished lactase levels. For instance, in locales where milk is not a safe food or where it is unavailable, inhabitants do not possess the capacity to digest milk. This circumstance, called *lactose intolerance*, is a genetic condition passed on to future generations and is predominantly found in populations with low milk consumption. Much of the world's population is lactose intolerant.

Physicians diagnose lactose intolerance by giving milk to the patient and administering a hydrogen breath test. The presence of hydrogen, usually not found in the breath, indicates lactose intolerance. Lactose, usually not found in the lower intestine, causes overgrowth of intestinal bacteria that form lactic acid, fatty acids, and hydrogen gas. Flatulence (gas), nausea, bloating, diarrhea, and cramps are associated with lactose intolerance and are natural by-products from bacterial growth and osmotic activity drawing water into the intestine. Increased osmotic pressure, caused by the lactose, results in increased motility, pain, and diarrhea.

Many lactose-intolerant people do not develop symptoms until ingesting the amount of lactose in two glasses of milk, about 24 grams. The lactose-intolerance test uses the amount of lactose in about a quart of milk.

Lactose is mostly found in whey (the liquid part of milk). Therefore, hard cheeses made from milk curd have little lactose if aged for 60 days and can be eaten with relative safety. Cream, ice cream, and milk chocolate, on the other hand, contain large amounts of lactose. Although whole milk is better tolerated than skim milk, milk in general causes fewer problems if it is taken with a meal. Yogurt containing active cultures is well tolerated in individuals who have mild lactose intolerance. Frozen yogurt, as well as many commercial yogurts, contain little or no lactobacillus bacteria and are therefore not recommended for those with lactose intolerance. The culture content of yogurt varies. Acidophilus milk is not well tolerated because the bacteria do not occur naturally in the milk; instead, they are grown in a separate medium and added later. Thus they do not ferment the lactose to lactic acid.

Although calcium absorption is not influenced by lactose intolerance, milk products are usually avoided by those who develop symptoms. Fortunately, individuals may obtain calcium from other natural sources. Calcium-rich foods, besides milk, include collard

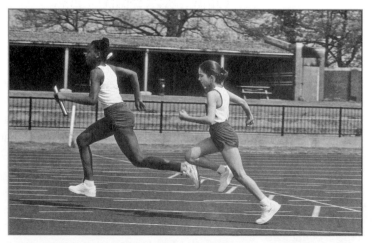

Athletes can store and release energy as needed by manipulating their diets for increased muscle glycogen.
John Garrett © Dorling Kindersley

greens, turnip greens, mustard greens, kale, small fish with edible bones (sardines, for example), salmon, beans (particularly soybeans), and tofu (soybean curd).

For those wishing to consume dairy, lactase is available commercially over-the-counter in pill or liquid form. Consumers can add lactase to milk or ingest it along with the milk products to combat lactose intolerance.

Some individuals, although they produce lactase, are still intolerant of dairy products because they are not able to metabolize galactose, a condition known as **galactosemia**. Dietitians plan a galactose-restricted diet for infants born with this condition. Low-galactose infant formulas are now available (Gropper, Gross, and Olds 1993).

GALACTOSEMIA A genetic disorder in which the body is unable to metabolize galactose. Galactosemia can lead to mental retardation if untreated.

CARBOHYDRATE LOADING FOR SPORTS

Athletes engaging in endurance sports know the importance of carbohydrate foods for energy. They have learned how to manipulate their diets to increase muscle glycogen, which then stores and releases extra energy when needed.

Research shows that depleting the muscle of glycogen by increased exercise and decreased carbohydrate consumption makes the muscles inclined to make an abnormally high amount of glycogen. Subsequently, when a high-carbohydrate diet is consumed and exercise is held to a minimum, the body will store more glycogen than it normally would.

There are various methods to achieve this glycogen loading. One two-phase method is shown in Table 3–3.

Each phase lasts three days and begins one week before the activity or sport. The total number of calories consumed in each phase should be equal.

A sample daily diet containing approximately 4,000 calories might offer as many as 16 servings of starchy foods during the loading phase, whereas the depletion phase would feature as much as 18 ounces of animal protein and 12 tablespoons of fat. Both phases would include moderate servings of fruits and vegetables and adequate liquids. It is easy to see why Phase I of this diet, which may be high in cholesterol and saturated fat, is subject to criticism. Several precautions must be taken if the diet is used at all. The depletion phase should contain at least 100 grams of carbohydrates to prevent hypoglycemic symptoms, and the loading phase should not contain candy and sweet sodas, which may cause stomach bloating.

Controversy exists concerning the merits of glycogen loading. Athletes are better able than most to turn fatty acids into energy and thus may not need the energy from excess glycogen. Glycogen holds water, which adds extra weight and may hinder athletic performance. However, the athlete might need this reserve of water, so this could be considered an advantage as well as a disadvantage.

TABLE 3–3 • TWO-PHASE METHOD FOR GLYCOGEN LOADING	
Phase I: Depletion	**Phase II: Loading**
4–6 Days Before Competition	*1–3 Days Before Competition*
1. Increased exercise	1. Decreased exercise
2. Low-carbohydrate meal plan	2. High-carbohydrate meal plan

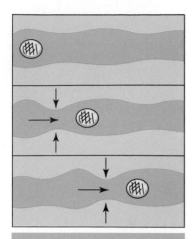

FIGURE 3–7 • THE FUNCTION OF FIBER IN THE INTESTINAL TRACT (PERISTALSIS)

DIGESTING FIBER

Certain ruminant animals, like cattle and sheep, digest cellulose fiber through their intestinal bacteria. This occurs in the human intestine to some extent also, releasing small amounts of energy when the intestine's bacteria produce short-chain fatty acids from fiber.

THE WHOLE-WHEAT BERRY

The wheat grain, which is also known as the *whole-wheat berry*, is composed of a starchy pulp on the interior (endosperm), an external fiber husk (bran), and the high-fat and nutrient-rich germ.

The fibrous outer husk, which protects the berries in nature, supplies needed fiber for human digestion. The germ, if replanted the following season, becomes the new plant and produces its own berries. The endosperm is the berry's energy source, which nourishes the new plant to maturity. Together in nature they each have a specific function, and in human digestion they each add to a healthy diet.

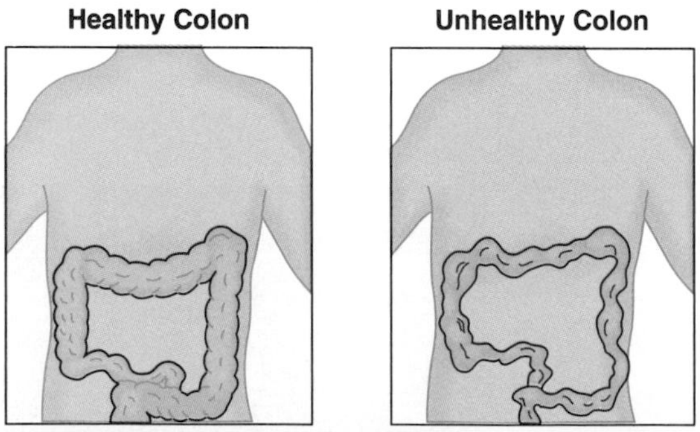

FIBER

Although fiber is carbohydrate, it is not digested by humans. Consequently, fiber is not a source of energy. The human intestine does not have the capacity to digest fiber to any significant degree. The main advantage of fiber is that it is not digested by human intestinal enzymes. The intestine, which is a muscle more than 20 feet long, functions by contracting rhythmically to propel its contents in a process called *peristalsis* (Figure 3–7). Indigestible fiber substances enhance intestinal muscle fitness and carry harmful wastes from the body.

Consider when we swallow. Food moves down the esophagus by this rhythmic contraction. The food is digested in the stomach and intestines, where the nutrients are absorbed. When dietary fiber content is low, there will be little material remaining in the small intestine after absorption. With nothing to move, the intestinal muscle becomes flabby and out of shape. This is no different than putting your arm in a sling and not using it for a length of time. Without use, the arm muscles begin to wither. If the arm is exercised, muscle tone returns. The intestinal muscle functions in the same way. A low-fiber diet gives the intestinal muscle less exercise, and the muscle becomes weak. Conversely, a high-fiber diet gives the intestine more exercise by requiring rhythmic contractions to move fiber along the intestine's length. In this manner, fiber keeps the intestinal muscle fit (Figure 3–8).

The Discovery of Fiber

As vitamins and minerals were being discovered in the early 1900s, authorities thought that fiber was unnecessary for health. At that time, it became common practice to refine flour by removing the bran and the germ from the whole-wheat berry before grinding it, thereby increasing its shelf life. The germ, which contains most of the fat in wheat, can cause flour to go rancid when left at high temperatures for long periods of time. Removing the germ removed the fat and increased the shelf life of the flour, which was the desired outcome. Unfortunately, the wheat's fiber (bran), vitamins, and minerals were discarded in the process (Table 3-4).

There were some health professionals, albeit not in the mainstream, who thought fiber was important for health. One notable person was a preacher-physician who took a religious proverb about marriage and applied it to the removal of bran and germ from the whole-wheat kernel. He said, "What God has joined together let no man put asunder." His name was Sylvester Graham, the developer of the graham cracker.

The original graham cracker was made as a way to reintroduce whole wheat into the American diet (Burrows and Wallace 1999). The cracker Dr. Graham developed bears very little resemblance to today's graham cracker. The whole-grain flour found in the original is almost nonexistent in today's version.

Healthy Colon   **Unhealthy Colon**

FIGURE 3–8 • HEALTHY AND UNHEALTHY COLONS

TABLE 3–4 • AMOUNT OF VITAMINS FOUND IN THE WHOLE-WHEAT KERNEL (%)			
Vitamin	Bran	Germ	Endosperm
B_1	33	64	3
B_2	42	26	32
B_3	86	2	12
B_6	73	21	6
Pantothenic acid	50	7	43

Besides Dr. Graham, there were others in the early 1900s who thought fiber should be returned to the American diet. Following Graham was another advocate of whole grains who developed whole-grain cereals because he, too, thought fiber enhanced health. Instead of a cracker, he developed a revolutionary new product, cornflakes.

As with graham crackers, the cornflakes of today are more refined and don't contain nearly the fiber of the original version. These crisp dry flakes could be hydrated using a grain beverage and then consumed fairly quickly. The inventor of cornflakes ran one of the largest hospitals in the United States at the time and started a cereal company that bears his name, Dr. John Harvey Kellogg.

Yet the medical community as a whole did not acknowledge the importance of fiber in human health for another 50 years. Several years after Dr. Kellogg died, another doctor, Dennis Burkitt, noticed that officers in the Royal British Navy were suffering from many diseases that the inhabitants of developing countries were not.

These degenerative diseases included colon cancer, diverticulitis, and hiatus hernia. He saw an association between the low fiber content in the British diet and an increase in degenerative disease.

Burkitt's theory on the relationship between low fiber intake and disease was published in 1975, and the high-fiber era began (Burkitt 1975). When his observations were published, the medical community began to take notice of the importance of fiber, and new connections began to surface between chronic disease and the lack of fiber in the diet.

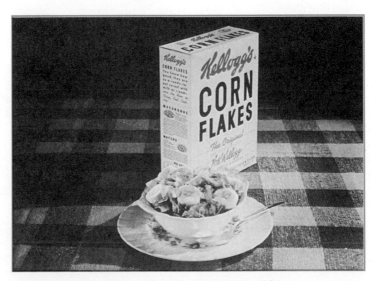

In the early 1900s Corn Flakes were the new health treat.
Getty Images Inc.—Hutton Archive Photos

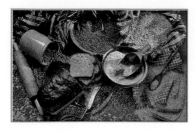

Whole-wheat products are great sources of vitamins, minerals, and fiber.

Photo Researchers, Inc.

The Classification of Fiber

Dietary fiber is categorized by its solubility in water; it is termed *insoluble fiber* or *soluble fiber*. The insoluble fibers are lignin and the celluloses (both cellulose and most of the hemicelluloses) that are found in the cell walls of plants. The soluble fibers are some of the hemicelluloses, pectin, gums, and mucilages. Fiber within plant cells is sometimes referred to as *storage polysaccharides* and includes gums, algal polysaccharides (such as alginate carrageenan), and mucilages (Table 3–5). There is a synthetic fiber, methylcellulose, which is a gummy product resulting from the introduction of the methyl group into cellulose.

All plants have more than one type of fiber. The amounts of soluble and insoluble fiber vary from plant to plant. More insoluble fiber is found in whole wheat, corn, bran, vegetables, and the skins of fruit. More soluble fiber is found in dried beans, oats, barley, sweet potatoes, carrots, citrus fruits, and apples.

For food-labeling purposes, the Institute of Medicine recently provided a specific definition of what should be called fiber in food. It defines *total fiber* as the combination of dietary and functional fiber. **Dietary fiber** is the edible, indigestible component of carbohydrates and lignin naturally found in plant food. **Functional fiber** refers to fiber sources that have health benefits similar to those of dietary fiber but are isolated or extracted from natural sources or are synthetic. Pectin extracted from citrus peel for making jelly is an example of functional fiber (Institute of Medicine 2002).

DIETARY FIBER Edible but indigestible fiber that is found in plants.

FUNCTIONAL FIBER Isolated, extracted, or synthetic fiber.

The Properties of Fiber in Food Products and Human Digestion

The different types of fiber express different characteristics in food products and in human digestion. Pectin is used in pie fillings, jams, and jellies. Commercial pectin is usually extracted from citrus products for use as a thickening agent. Natural sources of pectin include orange pulp, sweet potatoes, apples and other fruits, and vegetables. Purified pectin, used to thicken yogurt, is not palatable and causes nausea if consumed in large amounts.

The food industry uses gums extensively to affect food texture. Examples include oat gum extracted from oat bran, guar gum from the Indian cluster bean, and mucilage from seaweed. Cellulose absorbs water and swells like a sponge. It increases stool's bulk and softness and is important for bowel regularity.

Sources of Fiber

Removing the peels from fruits and vegetables reduces the amount of fiber eaten. Juices, for instance, contain only a small fraction of the fiber found in the whole fruit or vegetable. Dates,

TABLE 3–5 • TYPES OF FIBER AND THEIR FUNCTIONS IN THE PLANT	
Type of Fiber	**Plant Function**
Insoluble	
Cellulose	Cell wall
Lignins	Woody part of plants
Soluble	
Hemicelluloses	Cell wall
Pectin	Intercellular cement
Gums and mucilages	Secretions

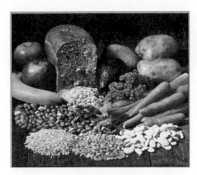

Foods containing whole wheat.
Photo Researchers, Inc.

figs, prunes, and raisins are very high in fiber. Melons and berries also have a high fiber content, but they have less sugar and are lower in calories than dates, figs, prunes, and raisins.

The lowest-calorie high-fiber foods are vegetables, such as celery, cucumbers, mushrooms, zucchinis, and string beans. Iceberg lettuce is mostly water and has very little fiber content.

When food shopping, choosing products with high-fiber grains can be confusing because a brown color does not always reflect the presence of bran. Caramel is added to some products to deepen the color. Consumers must examine the ingredient list to determine if the product is whole grain. Ingredients are listed on packaging by weight in descending order, so the first ingredient listed on the label is present in the largest amount. When selecting bread, make sure the first ingredient is whole-wheat flour (or another whole grain) instead of wheat flour or bleached flour. Healthy-sounding names, like *cracked wheat*, *oat*, or *seven-grain bread*, may not be whole grain. If the first ingredient is bleached wheat flour and the seven grains are farther down the list near salt, the product probably has too little of the seven grains to make any difference.

With careful inspection, you can find excellent high-fiber whole-grain breads, cereals, and crackers. But an overwhelming number of breads on the market are simply made from refined wheat flour. Even rye bread and rye crackers usually contain very little whole-rye flour. A wise consumer reads ingredient lists on food labels, checking the percentage of the recommended daily values for fiber. The fiber content of a serving of bread can range from almost nothing to 10% of the daily requirement.

When developing a taste for healthier grain products, you may enjoy whole-grain breads by toasting them or by adding jam to soften the taste of the whole grain. Choosing partial whole-grain products is an amenable way to start including whole grains in the diet. Whole-grain flour can replace some of the refined flour in baking, thus adding nutrients without completely changing the taste of the food. Whole-grain pastry flour makes a softer crumb for cakes and pies than regular whole-wheat flour.

Selecting a high-fiber diet may be easier and tastier than you think. It is much more than eating a bowl of bran cereal. Fiber-containing foods are quite palatable and tasty. Refer to the sample meal plan in Box 3–3.

Healthy but Problematic Beans

Beans of many varieties provide water-soluble fiber, protein, minerals, and the important vitamin folic acid. Many people, however, are concerned about the flatulence, or intestinal

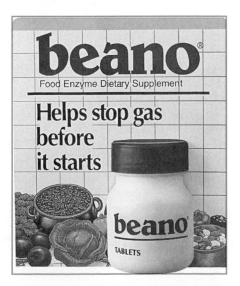

Gas-relieving pills are now available.
GlaxoSmithKline plc

TABLE 3–6 • A SAMPLE OF THE ESSENTIAL NUTRIENTS LOST IN THE REFINING OF WHEAT

Element	Loss (%)
Wheat	28.0
Ash	75.5
Calcium	60.0
Phosphorus	70.9
Magnesium	84.7
Potassium	77.0
Sodium	78.3
Chromium	40.0
Thiamine	77.1
Riboflavin	80.0
Niacin	80.8
Vitamin B_6	71.8
Pantothenic acid	50.0
Folate	66.7
Tocopherol	86.3
Manganese	85.8
Iron	75.6
Cobalt	88.5
Copper	67.9
Zinc	77.7
Selenium	15.9
Molybdenum	48.0
Betaine	22.8
Choline	29.5
Average Nutrient Loss	*65.2*

Source: Adapted from Schroeder, H. A. 1991. Losses of vitamins and trace minerals resulting from processing and preservation of foods. *The American Journal of Clinical Nutrition* 24: 562–573.

gases, that beans produce. Consumers can prevent gas discomfort by taking a commercial enzyme available in pill or liquid form.

Soaking beans, changing the water before cooking, and rinsing off canned beans also help to prevent gas. Moreover, one type of bean may cause gas, whereas another may not. Because beans are also low in fat, come in many varieties, and are generally inexpensive

BOX 3–3 • SAMPLE HIGH-FIBER DIET

BREAKFAST

1 cup orange juice (with pulp)

1 cup oatmeal

Milk

2 slices whole-wheat toast

Butter

Preserves (jam)

LUNCH

Lean meat on 2 slices whole-wheat bread

Three-bean salad on lettuce

Apple

DINNER

Baked fish

Coleslaw

Carrots

Baked potato

Melon

food choices; they are very versatile and nutritious. For consumers who do not eat beans regularly, introduce them into the diet gradually via soups and salads rather than having whole portions at once.

Psyllium

Psyllium is an herb that is high in soluble fiber and used for its laxative properties. Psyllium grows in India and in the Mediterranean.

Psyllium seed husk is usually made into a powder and used as a medicine to regulate bowels. Individuals taking psyllium must consume plenty of water to ensure proper hydration; otherwise, it could pull water from the body. Health professionals recommend that healthy people eat a balanced diet with high-fiber foods rather than take psyllium seed products.

A balanced diet provides necessary nutrients along with adequate fiber. Many other components in fruits, vegetables, and grains, in addition to fiber, protect against disease. This is another reason to eat a variety of plant-based foods rather than taking fiber supplements.

There are reports of some allergies to psyllium. One psyllium-containing cereal was removed from the market for this reason.

Locust Bean

Locust bean is processed into locust bean gum and carob. Locust bean gum is a thickener that comes from the bean; carob is a chocolate substitute that comes from the husk. Carob, with its high pectin and lignin content, grows on trees in the Middle East, Spain, Morocco, Greece, and Cyprus. It is also found in southern regions of the United States. It takes 15 years before the trees bear carob fruit, which is a glossy, brown pod 4 to 12 inches in length and 1 to 2 inches wide. Each pod contains numerous hard seeds in a sticky, sweet membrane. When this sticky part dries, it resembles peanut brittle and is enjoyed by some ethnic groups.

In research studies, locust bean gum has been reported to decrease low-density lipoprotein (LDL) and very-low-density lipoprotein (VLDL) cholesterol by binding bile acids,

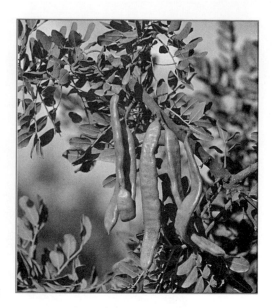

Locust beans.
Nature Picture Library

but it has no effect on glucose. In large amounts, it causes temporary flatulence and increased stool bulk. Carob was actually used in ancient times as a laxative. Locust bean gum is used as a food additive and helps the texture of commercial products by making them thicker. An example is ice cream, which may have gum agents added as well.

Flaxseed

Flaxseed is a source of soluble (mucilage) and insoluble (lignins) dietary fiber. The omega-3 fatty acid in flaxseed provides another benefit. (See the discussion of the health benefits in Chapter 5.) Whole flaxseed keeps well in a cool, dry place. Ground flaxseed should be kept refrigerated or frozen to prevent rancidity.

Cooks use flaxseed as an egg replacer in baking because it acts as a binder. Flaxseed is boiled in water and then simmered until the water becomes viscous, resembling raw egg whites. This procedure takes about five minutes. Individuals with an egg allergy may use this flaxseed preparation to enjoy some of their favorite recipes sans egg. To replace one egg, use 1 tablespoon of flaxseed to 1/3 cup water.

Replacing the flour in muffins and oatmeal cookies with 30% to 50% ground flaxseed produces an acceptable product. The fat in the recipe should be reduced by 35% to compensate for the flaxseed's own natural oil (Alpers and Sawyer-Morse 1996).

Other Fiber-Containing Foods

Rice bran has half the soluble fiber of oat bran and can be found in some cakes and cereals. Corn and barley also contain soluble dietary fiber. Nuts, packed with heart-healthy oil, provide fiber too; however, they are high in calories and should be consumed in moderation. A nut butter spread, such as almond butter or peanut butter, on whole-wheat bread packs a lot of fiber (Table 3–7).

For all practical purposes, animal products do not contain fiber. Meat, poultry, fish, eggs, and milk products are considered fiber-free foods. Of some interest, however, are indigestible polysaccharides of animal origin, called *chitin* and *chitosan*. These are found in the skeletons of insects and in the shells of shellfish. Chitosan can also be produced synthetically. These viscous polysaccharide substances could, in the future, be used as thickeners and stabilizers in processed food. Some diet pills contain chitosan.

TABLE 3–7 • HIGH-FIBER FOODS

Food	Dietary Fiber (g)	Calories
Navy beans, cooked, 1/2 cup	9.5	128
Bran ready-to-eat cereal (100%), 1/2 cup	8.8	78
Black beans, cooked, 1/2 cup	7.5	114
Pinto beans, cooked, 1/2 cup	7.7	122
Artichoke, globe, cooked, 1 whole	6.5	60
Great northern beans, cooked, 1/2 cup	6.2	105
Soybeans, mature, cooked, 1/2 cup	5.2	149
Bran, ready-to-eat cereal, 1 oz.	2.6–5.0	90–108
Sweet potato, baked, with skin, 1 medium	4.8	131
Green peas, cooked, 1/2 cup	4.4	67
Pear, raw, 1 small	4.3	81
Blackberries, raw, 1/2 cup	3.8	31
Potato, baked, with skin, 1 medium	3.8	161
Dates, 1/4 cup	3.6	126
Spinach, frozen, cooked, 1/2 cup	3.5	30
Shredded wheat cereal, 1 oz.	2.8–3.4	96
Almonds, 1 oz.	3.3	164
Apple, with skin, raw, 1 medium	3.3	72
Brussels sprouts, frozen, cooked, 1/2 cup	3.2	33
Whole-wheat spaghetti, cooked, 1/2 cup	3.1	87

Source: U.S. Department of Agriculture. 2005. *Dietary Guidelines for Americans*, 6th ed. Washington, DC: U.S. Government Printing Office.

Recommended Daily Intake for Fiber

The Institute of Medicine Food and Nutrition Board has set the Adequate Intake (AI) for total fiber for adults up to 50 years old at 38 grams for men and 25 grams for women (Institute of Medicine 2002). Most Americans, however, eat only half of that amount because of their dependence on processed foods. The American Cancer Institute recommends 25 to 40 grams of fiber per day. More than 50 grams of fiber daily may decrease zinc, iron, magnesium, and calcium absorption and should be avoided.

The new food labels define a *high-fiber* food as one containing 5 grams or more per serving and a *good* source of fiber as one containing 2.5 to 4.9 grams per serving. Products claiming *more fiber* must have an extra 2.5 grams per serving.

The Health Aspects of Fiber

Cellulose, found in plant cell walls, and hemicellulose, from the cell wall and cell contents, bind water and thereby increase stool bulk and decrease intestinal **transit time**. This gives them a laxative effect.

Wheat bran is the best food source for cellulose, and bran flakes breakfast cereal is therefore a good laxative. Avoiding constipation also helps prevent hemorrhoids, a painful swelling of the veins near the anus.

Cholesterol-Lowering Properties of Fiber

Pectins, gums, and mucilages tend to bind bile salts, cholesterol, and some fatty acids, removing them from the body. Bile salts are made from cholesterol and are usually recycled back to the liver. Their removal, plus the removal of dietary cholesterol, aids in controlling blood cholesterol levels.

The water-soluble fiber in oats and beans lowers LDL. Pectin, guar gum, and oat gum have these unique cholesterol-lowering properties (Brown et al. 1999). Neither cellulose nor hemicellulose has significant cholesterol-lowering effects, though. Gums, on the other hand, provide a high viscosity responsible for the hypocholesterolemic action (lowering cholesterol in the blood).

Some individuals respond favorably to dietary fiber treatment, while others do not. Pectin and guar gum are five times less effective than the medicine cholestryamine in binding bile salts. Therefore medication in addition to diet may be necessary to reduce blood cholesterol levels in some people. The key is to start with diet under a physician's and a dietitian's supervision and progress to prescription medication as directed.

A Harvard study of 43,000 male health professionals found that 29 grams of fiber daily led to a 41% lower risk of heart attack compared to men who ingested only 12 grams of fiber daily (Liebman 1997). Another study demonstrated a decrease in death from heart disease associated with a 6-grams increase in daily fiber from cereal. The effect was independent of any other dietary variables (Committee on Diet and Health 1989).

Blood Sugar Control

Fiber plays a role in controlling blood sugar in diabetes. A highly processed, low-fiber diet is rapidly absorbed in the upper part of the small intestine, creating a rapid rise in blood sugar. The presence of fiber in the diet delays stomach emptying and thus slows sugar absorption. All types of fiber impede the outward passage of sugar from the intestine, but the most effective are the viscous fibers—guar gum and tragacanth.

Pectin and methylcellulose, a gummy product resulting from the introduction of the methyl group into cellulose, are also viscous, but in research studies the use of a special crisp bread made with guar provided the best results. In tests done with natural foods, beans were found to lower blood sugar better than breads and grain products. Individuals with diabetes who followed a diet of high-fiber foods, such as whole-grain cereals, vegetables, and legumes, were able to reduce their intake of insulin.

The Nurses Health Study has followed 80,000 female nurses since 1986. Participants in the study completed dietary questionnaires, and the results showed that the women who ate the most sugar, white bread, and pasta were at higher risk for diabetes than those who reported a high-fiber diet. By 1992, 915 nurses had developed non-insulin-dependent diabetes (Liebman 1997).

Diverticulosis

There is evidence that dietary fiber helps prevent diverticulosis (Figure 3–9), a condition in which tiny pockets form in the colon wall. These pockets, called *diverticula* or *little herniations*, may become inflamed and rupture.

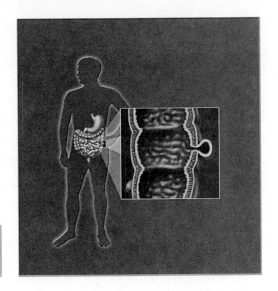

Diverticulitis is the condition in which the diverticula are inflamed. Rupture of diverticula can lead to possible death from sepsis, a severe infection. As explained earlier, fiber increases stool volume, which expands the colon. The filled, expanded colon provides intestinal muscle exercise that may prevent formation of diverticula. Close to half of the U.S. population over age 50 have diverticula, and most are asymptomatic. Not all cases improve with increased fiber intake.

Weight Control and Fiber

Fiber is often used to amplify weight-reducing diets since it is filling and contributes few calories overall. Intestinal bacteria ferment some of the fiber into gas and short-chain fatty acids, which do provide calories in varying amounts, but the calories are insignificant in comparison to other foods. When a person counts calories to manage weight, adding large quantities of fiber-rich foods may be advantageous in expanding dietary volume without adding calories.

There are pros and cons to fiber-rich, low-calorie diets. More study is needed to examine the relationship of fiber to satiety and, ultimately, satiety to weight loss.

Protection against Cancer

Fiber may decrease the risk of colon cancer in many ways. First, by decreasing the transit time of stool that may contain carcinogens, fiber helps lessen the presence of potential cancerous growth. Second, as the bulk in the intestine increases, it will dilute the carcinogens that are present. And finally, fiber helps bind carcinogens for elimination from the body.

The National Research Council reported inconsistent findings with regard to colon and rectal cancer and fiber. In some studies, colon cancer rates did not correlate with fiber intake after controlling for fat intake (Duyff 1996). Nonetheless, fiber can produce intestinal cell changes that may modify risk, and wheat bran may increase the excretion of bile acids and fecal mutagens, substances believed to promote colon cancer.

Some of the soluble fibers found in oat bran, pectin, and guar gum also stimulate the excretion of bile acids. Although findings are inconsistent, fiber-rich foods seem to provide a protective effect. Phytochemicals in vegetables, fruits, and grains may help provide protection against cancer as well. Phytochemicals are natural plant chemicals that include carotenoids, flavonoids, indoles, isoflavones, capsaicin, and protease inhibitors. Researchers are investigating the potential disease protection afforded by these plant constituents.

Carbohydrate Consumption

The consumption of carbohydrate foods in the United States has fluctuated greatly over the past 100 years. The U.S. Department of Agriculture collects consumption data by food category per person per year. Their findings reveal that grain products in the diet have decreased since 1909 from a high of 300 pounds per person to 204 pounds in 1945 and 139 pounds in 1975. But grains are on the upswing. Since 1975, there has been an increase to 200 pounds per person. Sugar usage has shown a steady increase from 84 pounds per person in 1909, 92 pounds in 1945, and 118 pounds in 1975 to 158 pounds per person in 1999. One of the greatest contributors to this increase has been the corn sweetener found in carbonated beverages and sweetened fruit drinks. The use of corn syrup and high-fructose corn syrup has increased from 5 pounds per person in 1909 to 85 pounds per person in 1999 (Bente and Gerrior 2002).

One way the food service industry can help curb this explosion in sugar consumption is to incorporate noncaloric sweeteners in food products. Chefs may also be able to substitute a sweeter sugar in place of one that is less sweet, to reduce total calories (Table 3–8)

TABLE 3–8 • SWEETENERS AND THEIR RELATIVE POTENCY (SUCROSE = 1)	
Sweetener	**Potency**
Sugars	
Fructose	1.2
Sucrose	1.0
Glucose	0.7
Maltose	0.4
Lactose	0.2
Sugar Alcohols	
Xylitol	1.0
Sorbitol	0.8
Noncaloric Sweeteners[a]	
Sucralose (Splenda)	600
Acesulfame-K (Sunette)	150
Aspartame (Equal)	200
Saccharin (Sweet'n Low)	300
Herbal Sweeteners[b]	
Stevioside (from stevia)	300
Glycyrrhizin (from licorice)	50

[a]Approved as sweeteners in the United States.
[b]Not approved as sweeteners in the United States.
Source: Adapted from Heijden, A. V. 1995. *Sweetness: The Biological, Behavioral and Social Aspects.* Brussels: International Life Sciences Institute.

SUMMARY

The Energy Powerhouse

Carbohydrate, as an energy powerhouse, allows the body to function and perform physical activity. Carbohydrates are organic compounds made of carbon (C), oxygen (O), and hydrogen (H). Each gram of carbohydrate supplies an average of four calories of energy.

Starches and sugars are the major energy-yielding carbohydrates, and they are found in a range of foods, including cane, beet, and fruit sugar; molasses; honey; wheat flour; cornstarch; rice; and potatoes. The different food groups contain varying amounts of carbohydrate.

Even though carbohydrates are a main energy source, not all provide calories. Fiber, for instance, is an indigestible carbohydrate and does not provide energy for humans. However, these indigestible fibers are essential for the normal functioning of the gastrointestinal tract.

Starch is comprised of many glucose units, which must be broken apart during the process of digestion in order for the energy they contain to be accessible. Starch digestion begins in the mouth with an enzyme called *salivary amylase*, or *ptyalin*. This process hydrolyzes, or separates, cooked starch into shorter polysaccharides. Food does not remain in the mouth long enough for much digestion to take place there. The salivary amylase that mixes with the food continues to work in the stomach until stomach acids exchange with the food to halt starch digestion. The next major activity for starch does not occur until it enters the first section of the small intestine, called the *duodenum*. By now, starch is a liquefied food, known as *chyme*.

While fiber is also a carbohydrate, it is not digested by humans. Consequently, fiber is not a source of energy. The human intestine does not have the capacity to digest fiber to any significant degree, unlike cows and deer and some other animals. The main advantage of fiber for humans is that it is not digested by human intestinal enzymes but is carried through the digestive system, exercising the intestinal muscle and aiding in the excretion of waste.

All plants have more than one type of fiber. The amounts of soluble and insoluble fiber vary from plant to plant. More insoluble fiber is found in whole wheat, corn, bran, vegetables, and the skins of fruit. More soluble fiber is found in dried beans, oats, barley, sweet potatoes, carrots, citrus fruits, and apples.

CASE RESOLUTION

Although fiber is a healthy addition to most people's diets, too much at once can cause problems. Besides experiencing unpleasant gas from too much fiber, some individuals may suffer cramping, diarrhea, or constipation. Many Americans fall short of getting their recommended fiber intake, and the students in Amelia's class are probably no exception. Going full throttle with fiber is undesirable, however. For that matter, too much of anything at once is unhealthy. Amelia should have mentioned the fiber content of her muffins so her classmates could exercise appropriate caution.

Let us assume that Amelia has not presented her project yet. To notify her classmates, Amelia could easily craft a miniature version of a Nutrition Facts panel with an analysis of her product. This label could emphasize the high fiber content, and Amelia could verbally review the label with her classmates.

REFERENCES

Alpers, L., and M. Sawyer-Morse. 1996. Eating quality of banana nut muffins and oatmeal cookies made with ground flaxseed. *Journal of the American Dietetic Association* 96 (8): 794–96.

Bente, L., and S. A. Gerrior. 2002. Selected food and nutrient highlights of the 20th century: U.S. food supply series. *Family Economics and Nutrition Review* 14 (1): 43.

Brown, L., B. Rosner, W. W. Willett, and F. M. Sacks. 1999. Cholesterol-lowering effects of dietary fiber: A meta-analysis. *American Journal of Clinical Nutrition* 69 (1): 30–42.

Burrows, E. G., and M. Wallace. 1999. *Gotham: A History of New York City to 1898*. New York: Oxford University Press.

Committee on Diet and Health, Food and Nutrition Board, Commission on Life Sciences, and National Research Council. 1989. *Diet and Health: Implications for Reducing Chronic Disease Risks*. Washington, DC: National Academies Press.

Duyff, R. 1996. *The American Dietetic Association's Complete Food and Nutrition Guide*. Minneapolis: Cronimed.

Gropper S., K. Gross, and J. Olds. 1993. Galactose content of selected fruit and vegetable baby foods: Implications for infants on galactose restricted diets. *Journal of the American Dietetic Association* 93 (3): 328–29.

Institute of Medicine and Food and Nutrition Board. 2002. *Dietary Reference Intakes for Energy, Carbohydrate, Fiber, Fat, Fatty Acids, Cholesterol, Protein and Amino Acids.* Washington, DC: National Academies Press.

Liebman, B. 1997. The whole grain guide. *Nutrition Action Health Letter* 24 (2): 8–10.

McWilliams, M. 2001. *Foods: Experimental Perspectives*, 4th ed. Upper Saddle River, NJ: Prentice Hall.

Sandberg A. S., and T. Andlid. 2002. Phytogenic and microbial phytases in human nutrition. *International Journal of Food Science and Technology* 37: 823–33.

World Health Organization. 1997. Carbohydrates in human nutrition: Report of a joint FAO/WHO expert consultation. Rome, Italy: FAO Food and Nutrition Paper 66.

REVIEW QUESTIONS

1. Name the naturally occurring sugar found in milk and the main sugar found in fruit. Why are these sugars, eaten in their natural form, more desirable than processed sugars?
2. Which monosaccharides and disaccharides are listed among the ingredients in many commercially processed foods?
3. How can lactose-intolerant individuals consume a good source of dietary calcium without drinking milk?
4. What is carbohydrate loading?
5. Name five foods that are high in water-soluble fiber.
6. Explain how water-soluble fiber helps lower blood cholesterol levels.
7. What are two other health benefits of water-soluble fiber, and what are the probable mechanisms involved?
8. How does cellulose fiber prevent constipation?
9. How many grams of fiber are recommended in the daily diet?
10. Which three food groups contribute to the daily fiber intake?
11. How is carbohydrate stored in the body?

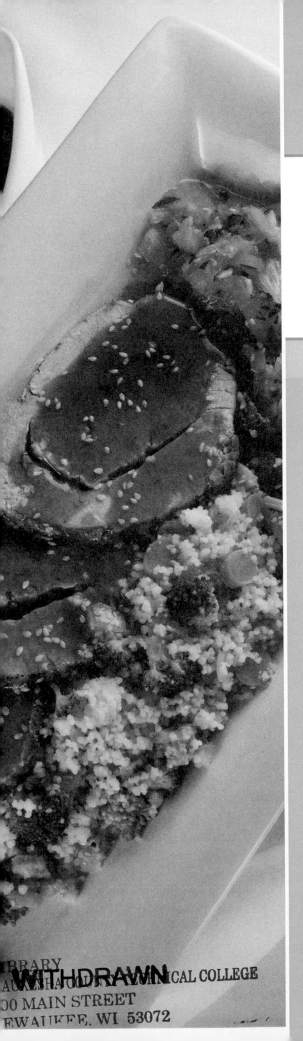

4

Proteins

KEY CONCEPTS

- Protein is required for cell growth and renewal.
- A person's protein requirement varies with age and is based on standard formulas.
- The quality of protein varies between foods.
- Vegetarians can obtain an adequate protein intake by selecting foods wisely.
- Protein quality is determined by the balance of the essential amino acids.

Protein has long been the center of attention in meals. Think about all those juicy steaks, fish, tacos, and holiday birds you have consumed over the years. And now protein's popularity is surging even more with the high-protein, low-carbohydrate diet craze.

Try to picture some traditional foods or meals without protein. It seems bizarre. A jelly sandwich sans the peanut butter? A reuben with only sauerkraut and Swiss cheese? Or what about a summer barbecue with ears of corn and potato salad, but no burgers or hot dogs? Protein, in fact, comes from many sources other than meat and the time-honored featured entrees, but dietary customs and cultural practices have encouraged us over the years to focus on meat.

Let's examine protein further by reviewing some of its functions in human health and cooking. Then we will discuss how the body processes it.

THINK ABOUT IT

Fads come and go all the time. Just look at the fashion industry, home furnishings, and automobiles. There are fads in dieting too: the grapefruit diet; the Miami heart diet; the no-fat diet; the cabbage soup diet; the high-protein, low-carbohydrate diet; the lemon water with paprika diet . . . The list goes on.

Have you tried any of these fad diets to manage your weight or to improve your health? If so, why? Often when a friend or neighbor has success with a "new" diet, we try it too. What works for one person may not work for you, but more importantly, fad diets are not meant to serve as permanent lifestyle enhancements. That is why they usually include some quirky or gimmicky regimen. After two days you simply cannot tolerate it anymore, and then you revert to eating as you did before. Regardless of how others eat or which celebrity is supposedly on a certain fad diet, make your decisions based on science. If something sounds too good to be true, then it probably is. Nutritional science has shown us that moderation, balance, and plenty of variety are the keys to a successful diet. Steer clear of dieting fads.

CASE STUDY

Milk Allergy versus Lactose Intolerance

Chef Phillip Esposito was planning his work for the evening when he received a call from the front-of-the-house manager, Justine Ramos. She relayed a message from a restaurant customer who said he could not consume milk because it upset his stomach. Justine wanted to know if the customer would be okay eating the fresh fruit appetizer, which comes with yogurt dressing.

How should Chef Phillip proceed? What questions should he ask Justine or the customer before determining whether the appetizer would be acceptable? *The resolution for this case study is presented at the end of the chapter.*

PROTEIN A chemical compound composed of amino acids, which in turn are composed of carbon, hydrogen, oxygen, and nitrogen. The term *amino acid* is a derivative of amine, which indicates nitrogen.

CATALYZE To facilitate or speed up a chemical reaction. Enzymes act as catalysts.

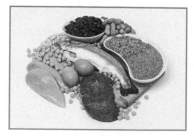

Protein-rich foods include steak, beans, seafood, eggs, nuts, and poultry.
© Dorling Kindersley

WHY DO WE NEED PROTEINS?

Proteins are nutrients that are needed for building body tissue like skin and bones, and they **catalyze** chemical reactions in body cells. Proteins are composed of the elements carbon, hydrogen, oxygen, and nitrogen. Protein is essential for everyone, but it is particularly important for growing infants, children, adolescents, and pregnant and lactating women. It is also needed for new tissue growth after fracture healing, surgery, and burns; and for the renewal of blood cells, intestinal cells, and cells in the rest of the body.

Proteins are composed of basic building blocks called *amino acids*. The human body requires 20 amino acids to produce protein, 9 of which cannot be made by the body and must be obtained in the diet. These are known as "essential amino acids" because it is essential that they be obtained in the diet. The quality of protein is determined by the presence and balance of these 9 amino acids in each food. Animal foods contain a better balance of these amino acids compared to plant foods, but this does not mean that one source is necessarily healthier than the other.

As you already may have suspected, the foods that contain the largest amounts of protein are poultry, fish, shellfish, eggs, milk products, nuts, beans, legumes, and meat. Second to these are grains and vegetables. Fruits also contain protein but in small

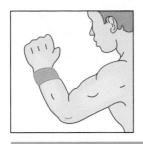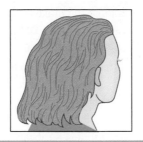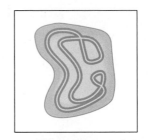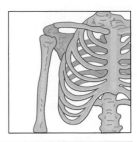

FIGURE 4–1 • PROTEIN FUNCTIONS: MUSCLE, HAIR, ENZYMES, AND BONES

amounts. With the exception of pure sugar, fat, and alcohol, most foods contain some protein, which makes it easy for people to ingest adequate levels. In fact, U.S. diets tend to be too high in protein, but more about that later.

PROTEIN DISCOVERY AND FUNCTION

Protein was discovered in 1838 by Gerardus Mulder, who derived the term from the Greek word *prota,* which means primary. He considered protein a primary constituent of the body (Institute of Medicine 1999). Indeed, the diet must contain protein because the human body cannot produce some of the components needed to make body tissues. Protein functions as one of the main structural components in muscle, bone, hair, nails, and skin (Figure 4–1). Proteins also form the structure in a variety of foods, for example, eggs in custards, gluten in breads, and casein in yogurt.

Protein also functions in the body as enzymes that facilitate hundreds of chemical reactions. Our food is digested, for example, because certain proteins in the digestive secretions act as enzymes. These enzymes break down carbohydrates, fats, and protein into simple compounds that the body can absorb. Moreover, proteins can help make new proteins. Proteins coil into complex structures that bind to specific food components to break them down. These complex coiling structures are shown in the protein that is responsible for mad cow disease, as seen in Figure 4–2.

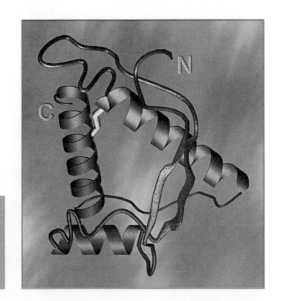

FIGURE 4–2 • THE THREE-DIMENSIONAL STRUCTURE OF THE PROTEIN THAT CAUSES MAD COW DISEASE
Source: Photo Researches, Inc.

DNA Deoxyribonucleic acid. DNA is a major component of chromosomes and carries genetic information.

RNA Ribonucleic acid. RNA is necessary for protein synthesis and the transmission of genetic information.

ANTIBODY A protein produced to fight off intruders called *antigens*.

INSULIN A hormone made of protein in the pancreas that facilitates the uptake of glucose from the blood into cells.

WATER BALANCE The balance between water inside and outside the blood vessels.

ACID/BASE BALANCE The balance in the blood between compounds that give off hydrogen and compounds that receive hydrogen.

AMINO ACID An organic acid that is a building block of protein.

ESSENTIAL A nutrient that is not synthesized in the body and that must be consumed in the diet for good health.

NONESSENTIAL A nutrient that can be made in the body from other nutrients and need not be consumed in the diet.

Some proteins contain minerals like iron, sulfur, iodine, and cobalt. The human body uses mineral-rich proteins to make **DNA**, **RNA**, **antibodies**, enzymes, hemoglobin, and certain hormones (**insulin**, thyroxine, and adrenaline). Protein is also necessary for regulating **water balance** and for **acid/base balance**.

Proteins can be used to supply energy as well as for building muscle. However, our body prefers to use other energy sources, like fats and carbohydrates, first. To be used as energy, protein must be converted to glucose or fatty acids that contain carbon, hydrogen, and oxygen. The nitrogen that is removed from the protein can be excreted in the urine, or the body can use it for the production of other **amino acids**.

AMINO ACIDS: THE STRUCTURE OF PROTEIN

Proteins are created from amino acids. There may be only a few up to many hundreds of amino acids locked together in a single protein. To better visualize amino acids, think of them as white crystalline substances that can be sweet, bitter, or even tasteless.

The human body requires 20 amino acids for proper nutrition. Some of these the body can generate by digesting dietary nitrogen from various protein sources. Others cannot be made in the body and must be ingested directly from food. These are called **essential** amino acids. The ones that the body can make are known as **nonessential** amino acids (Table 4–1).

TABLE 4–1 • ESSENTIAL AND NONESSENTIAL AMINO ACIDS

Nonessential	Essential
Alanine	Isoleucine
Arginine	Leucine
Asparagine	Lysine
Aspartic acid	Methionine
Cysteine	Phenylalanine
Glutamic acid	Threonine
Glutamine	Tryptophan
Glycine	Valine
Histidine	
Proline	
Serine	
Tyrosine	

PROTEIN QUALITY

Scientists and health professionals once believed that people should consume different foods that together contained the essential amino acids in the same meal to enable the body to build tissue. That meant that combinations of grains, nuts, beans, and seeds were recommended for all vegetarian meals, and often in the same dish. Today we know that this is not necessary as long as adequate amounts of the essential amino acids are eaten in the course of a day.

Foods vary in their essential amino acid content. Animal foods usually have a better balance of these amino acids than do plant foods (Box 4–1). There are, however, some exceptions: Gelatin, an animal food product, has a poor balance of the essential amino acids; conversely, soybeans, tofu, and soy milk contain a good balance of the essential amino acids. Almonds, Brazil nuts, buckwheat, and wheat germ contain a better balance of these acids than do most other plant foods, but their protein content is still not of as high a quality as the meat proteins.

COMPLETE PROTEIN A protein containing all essential amino acids in the proper amounts.

A protein that contains all the essential amino acids is a **complete protein** and thus is of higher quality. A protein that does not provide all the essential amino acids is said to be an **incomplete protein** or one of poorer quality.

INCOMPLETE PROTEIN A protein lacking or very low in one or more of the essential amino acids.

Furthermore, a limiting amino acid is one that is provided in an insufficient amount by a protein, which causes the protein to be categorized as less than complete. Currently the FAO and FDA use a protein digestibility corrected amino acid score (PDCAAS) (Institute of Medicine 1999) to assess the quality of protein. This method compares the food's amino acid content to a reference amino acid content that the human body requires. It also takes into account the age of the person consuming the protein and the digestibility of the protein. The dietary value for protein on the Nutrition Facts panel on food labels is based on the PDCAAS.

COMPLEMENTARY PROTEIN A protein that must be combined with another to achieve a better amino acid balance.

Adding the limiting amino acid to a deficient food puts the essential amino acids in a proportion that will foster optimal growth. If two foods having different limiting amino acids are eaten together, their resulting protein value is greater than if the foods had been eaten separately. The proteins in these foods complement each other, thus forming complete proteins called **complementary proteins** (Table 4–2). For example, wheat contains very little of the amino acid lysine, but legumes contain a lot of it; thus legumes and wheat complement each other. Legumes, on the other hand, do not have much of the amino acid methionine, which wheat has in generous quantities; thus peanut butter on toast provides a higher-quality protein than either the peanut butter or toast alone.

BOX 4–1 • PROTEIN EFFICIENCY RATING OF SELECTED FOODS, IN DESCENDING ORDER

Egg (whole)	Soybean meal (low-fat)	Yeast (dried brewer's)
Milk (whole, human)	Rice (whole)	Cottonseed meal
Milk (whole, cow)	Casein	Corn (whole)
Egg albumin	Wheat (whole)	Rye (whole)
Liver (animal)	Potatoes (white, raw)	Buckwheat flour
Meat (beef)	Wheat (gluten)	Peanut flour
Fish (muscle)	Oats (whole)	Peas and beans (dried)
Wheat germ	Barley	

TABLE 4–2 • COMPLEMENTARY PROTEIN CHART: SOME EXAMPLES

Healthy Combinations	Good Food Choices
Grains + milk	Bread and cheese
	Rice and milk (pudding)
	Cereal and milk
	Cheese and rice casserole
	Macaroni and cheese
	Manicotti (pasta + mozzarella)
	Blintz (crepe + cottage cheese)
	Bread pudding
	Tacos with cheese
	Pizza with cheese
Grains + legumes	Falafel and pita bread
	Rice and bean casserole
	Wheat and soy bread
	Lentils and rice
	Corn and soy bread
	Wheat bread and baked beans
	Peas and rice
	Corn tortillas and beans
	Pea soup and toast
	Legume soup and bread
	Peanut butter and bread
	Chickpeas and rice
	Bean burritos
	Peanut butter cookies
	Rice and tofu
	Rice and black-eyed peas
Legumes + milk	Bean soup and milk
	Garbanzo beans with cheese sauce
	Peanut butter soup

TABLE 4–2 • *(continued)*	
Healthy Combinations	**Good Food Choices**
Seeds + grains	Rye bread with caraway seeds
	Rice with sesame seeds
	Sesame bread sticks
	Poppy seed cookies
	Danish with poppy seed filling
Seeds + legumes (hummus)	Chickpeas with sesame seed paste
Nuts + grains	Baklava (Greek pastry with nuts and honey)
	Banana nut bread
	Almond cookies
	Walnut cake
Grains + nuts + seeds	Granola (oats, sunflower seeds, almonds)

Buckwheat has an amino acid composition that is nutritionally superior to that of other cereals. It is high in lysine, the limiting amino acid in wheat and rice. Buckwheat flour is commonly used as a pancake ingredient, which not only increases the protein quality but also makes the final product even more delicious.

Nonessential amino acids are as important as the essential amino acids. They make up 40% of tissue-building proteins and provide nitrogen needed for the synthesis of body compounds such as enzymes, hormones, antibodies, and other nonessential amino acids.

PROTEIN REQUIREMENT

One method of determining the minimum daily protein requirement for the average healthy adult is to use the formula 0.8 × adult body weight in kilograms. The following example calculates this protein requirement for a person who weighs 150 pounds, or 68 kilograms. Divide the weight, in pounds, by 2.2 to determine the number of kilograms.

For Example, calculate the minimum daily protein intake for a 150-pound individual.

Step 1. 150 lb / 2.2 = 68.2 kg

Step 2. 68.2 kg × 0.8 = 54.6 g protein

The method in the preceding example is based on the **Recommended Dietary Allowances (RDAs)** of the Food and Nutrition Board, National Academy of Sciences, and National Research Council.

Athletes have a higher need for protein than do nonathletes. As mentioned earlier, the protein recommendation for healthy adults is 0.8 grams per kilogram of body weight, but for athletes it increases to 1.1 to 1.6 grams per kilogram of body weight. Most Americans consume much more protein than they need (Table 4–3).

So do athletes need to eat extra protein? Many bodybuilders consume large amounts of protein in the belief that it will build more muscle. But consuming protein in amounts far above the 1.6 grams per kilogram of body weight needed may only provide expensive calories that will be used for energy. Certain endurance athletes, however, may benefit from eating a higher-protein diet that may give them a competitive edge.

TABLE 4–3 • GRAMS OF PROTEIN PER PORTION FOR VARIOUS FOOD ITEMS		
Food Type	**Portion Size**	**Grams of Protein per Portion**
Meat, poultry, fish, eggs	1 oz.	7.0
Legumes	1/2 cup	7.0
Milk (whole, skim)	8 oz.	8.0
Bread	1 slice	3.0
Starchy food, such as rice, pasta	1/2 cup	3.0
Vegetable, cooked	1/2 cup	2.0
Vegetable, raw	1 cup	2.0
Fruit	1/2 cup	0.5
Nuts	1 oz.	2.0–6.0

Processed protein foods contain more salt than do fresh protein foods. Canned meats, fish, and beans and processed cheese, for example, are much saltier than fresh meat, fish, beans, and natural cheese. Some protein foods even have sugar added. These include custards, flavored yogurts, some sausages, cold cuts, and cured ham. To achieve optimal health and nutrition, consumers need to choose lean cuts of meat, like the shank, first cut brisket, flank steak, and top round. Because they are lean, these cuts are tougher than fatty ones. Culinary professionals and home cooks can tenderize lean cuts before or during cooking by grinding, pounding, slow cooking, braising, and marinating. It is also a

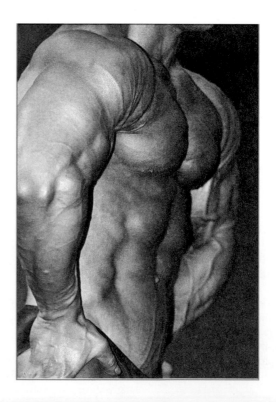

Bodybuilders consume a lot of protein, but is it necessary?
© Kolvenbach/Alamy

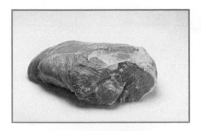

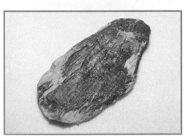

For optimal health, choose lean cuts of beef like flank steak and top rounds for cooking.
Pearson Education/PH College

good idea to experiment with marinades. Marinades contain an acidic ingredient, such as wine, vinegar, molasses, tomato, or some type of fruit, which helps to break down protein strands and partially tenderize the food.

CHOOSING IDEAL PROTEIN FOODS

The best foods to use as protein sources are those low in fat, salt, and sugar. Fish, beans, lentils, skinless chicken, lean meat, skim and low-fat milk, and tofu are good choices. These foods help the consumer avoid cardiovascular disease, cancer, and obesity. Individuals who avoid obesity can lower their chances of developing diabetes, gout, and arthritis.

Calculating Protein in the Diet

A gram of protein has 4 calories. With this fact in mind, calculate the recommended daily protein intake, given an intake of 2,500 calories per day.

Step 1. 2,500 calories/day × 15% (0.15) (recommended percentage of protein) = 375 calories of protein recommended

Step 2. 375/4 calories per gram of protein = 93.75 grams of protein, or approximately 3.3 ounces

Amounts in excess of the recommendation would not be immediately harmful to healthy individuals. Most peoples' bodies can process the protein eaten and any waste products that result from metabolism. But overeating protein on a regular basis may cause health problems in the future. Eating too much protein could reduce fiber intake and produce a diet high in saturated fat, especially if the dietary choices are meats or whole-milk dairy products. Excess protein may also damage the kidneys and bones.

Table 4–4 shows a sample menu that provides a healthy level of protein intake.

Individual calculations are not important if you eat a variety of food and select items from each food group. If, however, you eat a particular food often, it would be prudent to look up its nutrition profile using the food composition tables in the USDA Nutrient Data Laboratory.

So far in this text, we have emphasized keeping protein intake at a healthy level. Sometimes, though, more protein is necessary. Pregnancy and lactation require a daily addition of 25 grams of protein. Furthermore, infants, children, and teenagers need proportionately more protein than do adults to allow for growing bones and muscles. For example, a baby needs 2.2 grams of protein per kilogram of body weight in the first six months of life and 2 grams of protein per kilogram of body weight for the second half of the first year. During this time of rapid growth, a baby will have tripled its body weight by the first birthday. Imagine if adults did this each year!

FOOD IS MORE THAN PROTEIN

Protein does not account for all of a food's calories. Many of the things we eat will contain carbohydrate or fat too. Consider the following. Flesh foods, even lean meats, contain fat. Fat can also be found in whole and skim milk. Carbohydrates are found in

TABLE 4–4 • SAMPLE DAILY PROTEIN TOTAL

Food	Amount	Grams of Protein
Breakfast		
Egg	1	7.0
Toast	2 slices	6.0
Margarine	2 teaspoons	0
Skim milk	8 oz.	8.0
Cooked cereal	1/2 cup	3.0
Orange juice	8 oz.	1.0
Total for breakfast		25.0
Lunch		
Bread	2 slices	6.0
Tuna	2 oz.	14.0
Mayonnaise	1 tablespoon	0
Medium peach	1	0.5
Tossed salad	1 cup	2.0
Cola beverage	8 oz.	0
Total for lunch		22.5
Dinner		
Sautéed chicken	4 oz.	28.0
Potato	1 medium	3.0
Broccoli	1/2 cup	2.0
Rice	1 cup	9.0
Watermelon	1 cup	1.0
Tea	1 cup	0
Sugar	1 teaspoon	0
Total for dinner		43.0
Snack		
Skim milk	1 cup	8
Total for Day		*98.5*

bread, vegetables, and fruits, but not in meats. Nuts are plentiful sources of protein, but they also contain large amounts of fat. Beans are also good sources of protein, yet have virtually no fat; they do, however, contain large amounts of carbohydrates.

Sugars, jellies, syrups, honey, and sweet drinks contain no protein; neither do pure fats and oils. Alcoholic beverages—wine, beer, and distilled spirits—do not contribute to protein intake either.

DIGESTION AND ABSORPTION OF PROTEIN

DIGESTION The process in which food is converted into substances small enough for absorption.

GASTRIN A hormone that stimulates the production of gastric hydrochloric acid.

HYDROCHLORIC ACID An acid that activates pepsinogen.

PEPSINOGEN A precursor to pepsin.

PEPSIN An enzyme found in the digestive process that breaks down protein into polypeptides.

POLYPEPTIDE A compound consisting of linked amino acids.

DUODENUM The first part of the small intestine just beyond the stomach.

DUODENAL Referring to the duodenum, or the beginning of the small intestine.

PANCREATIC Referring to the pancreas, a gland involved in digestion.

TRYPSIN A digestive enzyme from the pancreas.

CHYMOTRYPSIN A digestive enzyme from the pancreas.

DIPEPTIDE A chemical compound consisting of two linked amino acids.

TRIPEPTIDE A chemical compound consisting of three linked amino acids.

ABSORPTION The process of moving smaller nutrients from the intestines into blood for transport throughout the body.

Digestion begins in the mouth, where food is chewed and moistened with saliva. Then the food passes into the stomach. Most digestion of proteins occurs in the stomach and in the small intestine. When food reaches the stomach, a hormone called **gastrin** stimulates the production of **hydrochloric acid**, which activates an enzyme called **pepsinogen**. Pepsinogen converts into **pepsin**, which, in turn, breaks down proteins into smaller parts called **polypeptides** (Figure 4–3).

Some of the still-intact proteins, some polypeptides, and a small amount of amino acids leave the stomach and enter the upper portion of the small intestine, or the **duodenum**. **Duodenal** hormones stimulate the release of **pancreatic** enzymes, which break down the proteins that are still intact. The enzymes **trypsin** and **chymotrypsin**, which come from the pancreas, further break down proteins to form polypeptides. Other intestinal enzymes break down the polypeptides into **dipeptides**, **tripeptides**, and individual amino acids, which is the final step of protein digestion.

Protein digestion, as you can see, is a complicated process that includes many steps and many key players. Magnesium, zinc, copper, and manganese are all essential for the enzyme activity just described. These minerals can be found in foods such as meats, grains, and vegetables.

Once protein is broken down during digestion into small polypeptides and ultimately into amino acids, these amino acids undergo **absorption** into the bloodstream through the lining of the small intestine. Then they enter the portal vein and go to the liver, and from the liver they are dispersed to body tissues.

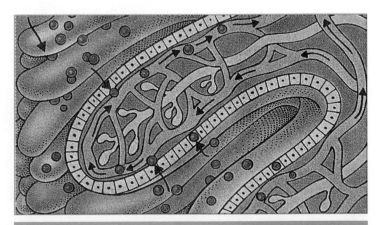

FIGURE 4–3 • THE DIGESTION OF PROTEIN
Source: © Dorling Kindersley

RENNIN An enzyme that coagulates, or curdles, milk.

GELATINASE An enzyme that breaks down gelatin.

KWASHIORKOR Severe protein malnutrition often seen in children from developing countries. Potbelly is one characteristic.

EDEMA Excessive fluid buildup.

MARASMUS Severe protein and calorie malnutrition.

CONSEQUENCES OF INSUFFICIENT DIETARY PROTEIN

Protein-deficiency disease is rarely seen in the Western world because of the availability and variety of protein foods. In the United States, for example, protein is affordable and is enjoyed at almost every meal. High-protein diet weight-loss plans help trigger even more protein consumption than before.

Developing nations often face protein shortages in their diets because high-protein foods are either not available or not affordable. Children are among the people most affected by insufficient protein intake. The symptoms of a mild protein deficiency include lackluster hair and nails. More severe protein deficiency leads to hair that is thin, easily plucked out, and dyspigmented. The parotid glands, located below and in front of each ear, become enlarged. Moderate protein deficiency may also cause the liver to become enlarged.

Kwashiorkor

Kwashiorkor is the protein-deficiency disease usually encountered in developing parts of the world where the diet consists primarily of a limited variety of plant proteins. This disease is characterized by retarded growth, **edema**, peeling skin, anemia, and susceptibility to infection. A child with kwashiorkor may have a large protruding abdomen.

The mortality rate is very high, but the cure is quite simple. Delivering skim-milk powder to developing countries provides protein that can alleviate kwashiorkor. In addition to food assistance, help should include lessons in soybean farming and education about combining plant proteins for better nutrition.

Marasmus

Another major form of nutritional deficiency is **marasmus**. It is characterized by not only a lack of protein, as seen in kwashiorkor, but insufficient calories as well. Children with this form of nutritional deficiency do not display the large abdomen seen in kwashiorkor; rather, they look completely emaciated, displaying very little muscle mass. Children in this condition require adequate protein and calories to regain health.

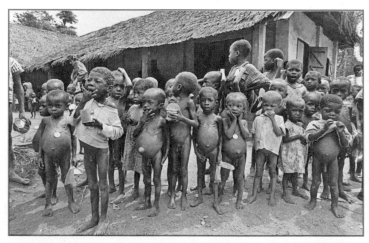

Children in developing third-world countries are prone to develop the protein-deficiency disease known as kwashiorkor.
Getty Images Inc.—Hulton Archive Photos

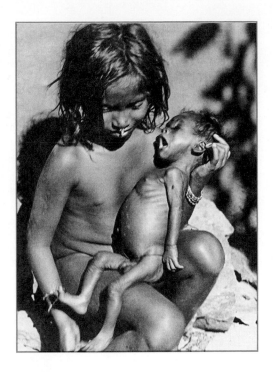

A child suffering from a lack of protein and calories displays signs of marasmus.
Food and Agriculture Organization of the United Nations

PROTEIN COOKERY

Eggs, milk, and meat foods, the major sources of protein, need proper cooking for maximum nutritional value, taste, and dining satisfaction. A general rule for cooking protein foods is to use low to moderate heat whenever possible. Excessive heat will make eggs rubbery, milk curdle, and meat tough.

Cooking processes that use high heat draw water out of protein, which leaves a dry, tough food product. The exceptions are broiling and grilling, in which naturally tender cuts of meat, poultry, and fish are subjected to very high heat but for short periods of time. Other meats cooked at high heat not only will be tough but will also lose a great deal of volume. Their excreted juices collect in the bottom of the pan and evaporate. Custard cooked at a high temperature will "weep," a classic example of overheated protein.

Tender meat cuts, such as tenderloin, rib roast, and sirloin, contain a high amount of **collagen**. Collagen and **elastin** are the two types of connective tissues in muscles. Collagen decomposes and takes on water when cooked, changing to gelatin, which has a tenderizing effect on meat. This reaction is known as **hydrolysis**. Elastin does not react with water and must be ground or chopped to soften it. Meat in which collagen dominates can be cooked at higher temperatures, but only for a brief time (such as in grilling and broiling).

COLLAGEN A protein substance found in connective tissue, bone, cartilage, and tendons.

ELASTIN A protein substance that works with collagen to provide elasticity.

HYDROLYSIS A chemical reaction involving water.

VEGAN A strict vegetarian who eats only plant products.

VEGETARIANISM

Think of the term vegetarianism as an umbrella that covers many different styles of eating (Figure 4–4). All vegetarians avoid animal products to some degree. The typical vegetarian does not eat meat, poultry, or fish. The strict vegetarian, or **vegan,** is an individual who practices a form of vegetarianism that extends to avoiding all animal products, including eggs, milk, and milk products. They may also avoid food ingredients and additives that contain these products. Some subcategories of vegans restrict themselves to uncooked raw food. Fruitarians, for example, eat primarily fruits, but their diet may also contain nuts and some vegetables.

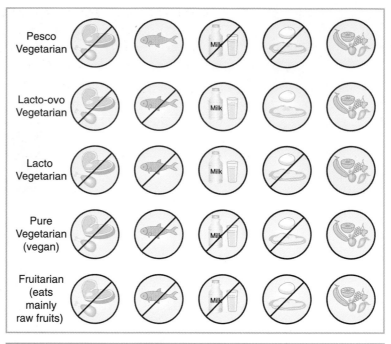

FIGURE 4–4 • TYPES OF VEGETARIANS

LACTO VEGETARIAN A vegetarian who consumes milk and dairy products.

LACTO-OVO VEGETARIAN A vegetarian who consumes milk, dairy products, and eggs.

PESCO VEGETARIAN A vegetarian who consumes fish.

Slightly more liberal than vegans are the **lacto vegetarians**, who eat a diet that includes dairy products (lacto for lactose), such as yogurt and butter, along with plant foods, but no meats or eggs. Some adherents of the Hindu faith practice lacto vegetarianism.

Someone who eats eggs as well as milk and dairy is called a **lacto-ovo vegetarian** (ovo for ovum or egg). A well-planned lacto-ovo diet poses no threat of nutritional deficiencies. As long as a variety of plants, protein-rich foods, and a sensible level of fat are included, followers can easily sustain healthy and active lifestyles.

The term **pesco vegetarian** means that one practices a vegetarian diet allowing fish (pesco for fish). Meat and poultry are excluded. Semivegetarians eat poultry and/or fish in addition to vegetables, but not red meat, veal, or pork; they also sometimes consume dairy and eggs.

BOX 4–2 • MAKING THE VEGETARIAN DIET WORK

Nutritional balance is necessary for both vegetarians and nonvegetarians. Although a vegetarian diet can be a very healthy choice, food selection requires thought to provide adequate nutrition. Consuming a vegetarian diet does not guarantee proper nutrition. A nonvegetarian eating freshly sliced skinned turkey breast with lettuce and tomato on whole-wheat bread and an apple is getting less fat, less sodium, and more fiber than a vegetarian eating a taco salad in a fried taco bowl. Likewise, a meal of French fries, a chocolate shake, and a fried apple pie is vegetarian, but it would not be a healthy choice. Vegetarians can make wholesome, delicious meals that are nutritious in every way. Such meals must be planned, however. The menu for all, vegetarians and nonvegetarians alike, should minimize saturated fat, fried food, high-fat desserts, and whole-milk products.

The U.S. Department of Agriculture's food guide graphic, called My Pyramid, provides recommendations for both vegetarians and nonvegetarians. Vegans, however, would replace cow's milk and more traditional dairy products with those made from soy, almonds, and rice. (Consumers should select vegan milks fortified with vitamin B$_{12}$ and calcium.) Legumes, nuts, and meat substitutes would replace flesh foods in the meat group. They can be used in a variety of recipes, such as soups, casseroles, and salads. Tofu (a soy product) and other soy foods, such as texturized vegetable protein, soy grits, and fermented soy (miso), can also be used. Meat substitutes are usually made with soy protein and sometimes with grains. They are made to resemble meat products, such as hamburgers, sausages, and cold cuts. Many are very salty, so take care to select brands that are not high in salt. More information on vegetarian cooking is found in Chapter 14.

Macrobiotic vegetarians follow a diet based on an ancient Eastern religious culture, which emphasizes whole grains and legumes. Certain foods are thought to be bad combinations (yin and yang). The Zen macrobiotic diet features stages of stringent deprivations because of the lack of balance of some foods with others.

For some people the vegetarian choice is based on religion, ethics, economics, or ecology, while others think it is simply a healthy lifestyle. Whatever the basis of the decision, deciding not to consume animal products usually produces a lower-cost, healthful diet. As with a meat-centered menu, consumers must take care to plan a well-rounded vegetarian menu to ensure proper nutrient levels in the foods consumed.

Health Implications of Vegetarianism

Meat is one of the best sources of complete protein, but it is also one of the greatest sources of saturated fat. Saturated fat is a major food component that increases LDL cholesterol (bad cholesterol) in the body.

Poultry and fish, however, do not contain as much saturated fat and are thus a better source of protein. Eating fresh fish at least twice a week helps increase the omega-3 fatty acid content of the diet to beneficial levels. Omega-3 fatty acids help prevent cardiovascular disease and some types of inflammation (Holub 2002). Although these fatty acids are present in certain plants, fatty fish, such as salmon, tuna, and mackerel, contain them in the largest amounts (more on this in Chapter 5).

If milk is avoided, food must be chosen wisely to get enough calcium and vitamin D in the diet. These nutrients are of particular importance for growing children, adolescents,

---

BOX 4–3 • COMMERCIAL FOOD INGREDIENTS THAT CONTAIN DAIRY

It is difficult to tell which food additives are derived from animals or insects and which are totally vegetarian. The following is a partial list of additives and their sources.

CONTAINS DAIRY

Calcium/sodium caseinate. Commercial source: mineral-animal. An additive that is used as a source of protein and as a replacement for sodium caseinate in low-sodium foods. Used in imitation cheese, creamed cottage cheese, diet foods and beverages, frozen desserts, and vegetable-based whipped toppings.

Simplesse. Commercial source: animal (milk and egg). A fat substitute. Used in margarine, ice cream, salad dressings, and yogurt.

Casein. Commercial source: animal (milk). The principal protein in milk. Used in cereals, breads, imitation cheeses, ice cream, fruit sherbets, and special diet preparations.

Whey. Commercial source: animal (milk). The watery material that remains after most of the protein and fat have been removed from milk. Used in baked goods, ice cream, dry mixes, and processed foods.

CONTAINS ANIMAL OR INSECT

Carmine. Commercial source: animal (insect). A food coloring derived from the dried bodies of female beetles. Used in confections, juices, "New Age" beverages, pharmaceuticals, dairy products, baked goods, yogurt, ice cream, fruit fillings, and puddings.

Cochineal. Commercial source: animal (insect). A food coloring derived from the dried bodies of female beetles. Used in confections, juices, yogurt, ice cream, fruit fillings, and puddings.

Gelatin. Commercial source: animal (cow or hog derived). An animal protein used especially for its thickening and gelling properties. Vegetable or synthetic "gelatins" are found in some foods on the market. Used in puddings, yogurt, ham coatings, marshmallows, sour cream, frozen desserts, cheese spreads, soft drinks, pill capsules, wine, and juice.

Source: Adapted from Bartas, J. M. 1997. *Vegetarian Journal's Guide to Food Ingredients.* Full journal available from the Vegetarian Resource Group, P.O. Box 1463, Baltimore, Maryland 21203 (http://www.vrg.org).

and pregnant women. Infants and toddlers who are allergic to milk protein should stay on fortified infant soy formulas to ensure adequate intake of these nutrients.

In terms of calcium and bone health, some studies have shown that vegetarians absorb and retain more calcium from foods than do carnivores. Calcium intake recommendations for Americans are set high to compensate for the urinary calcium losses that accompany a high intake of animal protein.

The strict vegetarian who eats no flesh, eggs, or dairy products should consume grains and other foods fortified with vitamin B_{12} and vitamin D. Other nutrients can be obtained through a wise selection of beans, nuts, dried peas, and soy products eaten with generous amounts of dark green leafy vegetables, fruits, and whole grains.

Is Vegetarianism the Way to Go?

Vegetarians suffer from less cardiovascular disease and cancer of the colon than people who eat meat regularly. This fact could be attributed to other lifestyle habits, such as regular exercise, not smoking cigarettes, and maintaining a lean body weight, but eating a plant-based diet is no doubt favorable to good health.

Some of the health benefits associated with being a vegetarian are due to the large amounts of fruits and vegetables that they consume. Fruits and vegetables contain **antioxidants**, **phytochemicals**, and fiber that are beneficial in the prevention of cardiovascular disease, cancer, and many digestive disorders.

People who are not vegetarians should try to include lots of fruits, vegetables, and whole grains in their diets. This will ensure intake of the protective elements plants offer. Apart from health benefits, many vegetarians choose their diet because they are concerned about food additives, pesticides, hormones, antibiotics, and the humane treatment of livestock. Articles have been written about the treatment of milking cows and egg-producing chickens, which is less than pleasant (Raymond 1990). These concerns should be important to all people, and animal abuse should be corrected through increased monitoring and legislation. Consumer groups and government agencies can take a leading role in dealing with such issues without espousing vegetarianism. Culinary professionals can also support farmers and producers who abide by healthy, humane farming and slaughtering practices.

ANTIOXIDANT A chemical substance that protects body cells from damage.

PHYTOCHEMICAL A substance in plants that is involved in protecting human health.

SUMMARY

Essential Proteins: One Way or the Other

Proteins are nutrients that are needed for building body tissue like skin and bones, and they catalyze chemical reactions in the body's cells. Proteins are composed of the elements carbon, hydrogen, oxygen, and nitrogen. Protein is essential for everyone, but it is particularly important for growing infants, children, adolescents, and pregnant and lactating women. It is also needed for new tissue growth during fracture healing, surgery, and burns and for renewal of blood cells, intestinal cells, and the rest of the body.

Proteins are composed of basic building blocks called *amino acids*. The human body requires 20 amino acids, 9 of which cannot be made by the body and must be obtained in the diet. These are known as "essential amino acids." The quality of protein is determined by the presence and balance of these 9 amino acids in each food. Animal foods contain a better balance of these amino acids compared to plant foods.

Proteins can be used to supply energy as well as for muscle building; however, our body prefers to use other energy sources, like fats and carbohydrates, first. To be used as energy, protein must be converted to glucose or fatty acids that contain carbon, hydrogen, and oxygen.

A protein that contains all the essential amino acids we need is a complete protein and is thus considered to be of higher quality. On the other hand, one that does not provide all the essential amino acids is said to be an incomplete protein or one of poorer quality. Some of the best protein foods are fish, beans, lentils, skinless chicken, lean meat, skim and low-fat milk, and tofu.

Many people believe that avoiding meat, poultry, and fish is a healthful choice to make. The strict vegetarian who eats no flesh, eggs, or dairy products should consume grains and other foods fortified with vitamin B_{12} and vitamin D. Other nutrients can be obtained through a wise selection of beans, nuts, dried peas, and soy products eaten with generous amounts of dark green leafy vegetables, fruits, and whole grains.

CASE RESOLUTION

There is a difference between protein allergy and lactose intolerance. Chef Phillip must find out if the customer is allergic to the protein in dairy or is intolerant to lactose, which is the natural sugar in milk. If it is a true allergy, the customer should have the fruit with a dairy-free topping; if he's lactose intolerant, the yogurt would probably be safe for him. It's always best to notify customers of the ingredients and let them decide what to eat. Visit the National Dairy Council's Web site (http://www.dairycouncil.org) for more on this topic. Refer specifically to the section on lactose intolerance and misconceptions about dairy.

REFERENCES

Holub, B. J. 2002. Clinical nutrition: 4. Omega-3 fatty acids in cardiovascular care. *Canadian Medical Association Journal* 166 (5): 608–15.

Institute of Medicine. 1999. *The Role of Protein and Amino Acids in Sustaining and Enhancing Performance.* Washington, DC: National Academies Press.

Raymond, J. 1990. Free range eggs. *Vegetarian Journal Reports:* 64, 65, 78–80.

1. What are the best protein foods to choose for a low-fat omnivorous diet?
2. Explain how a person could possibly gain weight on a high-protein diet.
3. What is the significance of nitrogen balance?
4. Calculate the ideal protein requirement for yourself, given your own weight and level of activity. Plan a day's worth of food that meets this requirement.
5. Create new recipes or menu ideas utilizing the concept of complementary protein.
6. Why is it wasteful to eat a high-protein diet?
7. What are the advantages and disadvantages of a vegetarian diet?
8. Create a well-balanced vegan menu that contains adequate protein and nutrients.

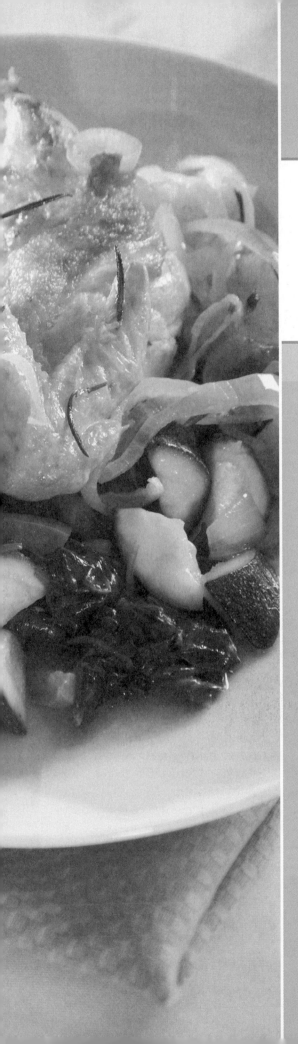

5

Lipids: Fats and Oils

KEY CONCEPTS

- Fats vary in function and structure.
- Saturated fat comes largely from animal sources; unsaturated fat comes from plants.
- Saturated fat increases low-density lipoprotein (LDL) cholesterol; polyunsaturated and monounsaturated fats decrease LDL cholesterol.
- Omega-3 and omega-6 fatty acids must be consumed in balance.
- Fat is a necessary component of the diet.
- Consuming excess saturated fat is a risk factor for certain diseases.
- Trans fats are harmful by-products formed during the hydrogenation of partially hydrogenated unsaturated fat.
- A desirable diet is low in saturated fat, free from trans fat, and moderate in total fat intake.
- Cholesterol serves a vital function in body processes and in health.

There is a great deal of emphasis on monitoring the amount and type of fat and oil in the diet. Some types of dietary fat like the saturated fat found in red meat, butter, and dairy products are less healthy, while the omega-3 oils found in fish and monounsaturated oil in olive oil are health promoting. More recently, health authorities have determined that trans fat in processed food is harmful.

Are some fats or oils bad and others good, or is this just a question of balance? Some of the most popular diets allow large amounts of fat yet control carbohydrates, while others focus on restricting fat and do not restrict carbohydrates.

There is no question that fat plays a very important role in regular bodily functions. Some body fat is essential for cushioning the body's organs, insulating against cold temperatures, transporting fat-soluble vitamins, storing energy, and providing precursors for hormones regulating body functions.

Polyunsaturated fat is the only classification of dietary fat essential for humans. It is needed for healthy skin, normal liver function, cell wall structure, and the synthesis of **eicosanoids**, which are hormone-like substances.

Besides its role in human health, fat also adds taste and texture to food. Because fat is digested slowly, it provides a feeling of satiety. Feeling full longer after eating fat could help consumers reduce their overall daily caloric intake and remain satisfied longer.

In this chapter we look at the different classifications of fats and oils and how fat undergoes metabolism. Then we discuss the possible benefits and risks of consuming fat.

EICOSANOID Hormone-like substances that regulate body functions, including inflammation, vasodilation, platelet aggregation, and immune response.

THINK ABOUT IT

Cardiovascular disease is the number one cause of death in the United States, claiming almost 700,000 lives each year. You may know someone who has cardiovascular disease. Did you ever consider the close connection between the food we eat and heart health? Three variables—salt (sodium) content, amount of fiber, and the amount and type of fat in the diet—can make a profound difference in the health of many individuals. If you were told to reduce or avoid either sodium or fat, how successful would you be? Is it possible to avoid either of these nutrients? What impact do these nutrients have on the enjoyment and pleasure food brings? Fat and salt impart flavor, and without them food tastes different.

CASE STUDY

Cholesterol-Free Margarine?

Gwendolyn is the manager of a large café that specializes in southern cuisine. Her customers enjoy cornbread made in an iron skillet as well as many other traditional recipes. The café offers a selection of pan-fried food and highly seasoned vegetables. Recently, a regular customer informed Gwendolyn that his doctor instructed him to eat margarine instead of butter to reduce his cholesterol intake. But she has been reading that the trans fat in many hydrogenated margarines is not healthy. She has heard about the Mediterranean diet and she knows that the olive oil in this diet is helpful in reducing cholesterol levels, but she wonders if the flavor of the olive oil will change the taste of her southern dishes. She calls her vendor to find out what other oils are available. Gwendolyn discovers that there are many oils available, including soy and canola oils.

Considering that she has other customers with **hypercholesterolemia**, which should Gwendolyn order? *The resolution for this case study is presented at the end of the chapter.*

HYPERCHOLESTEROLEMIA Elevated blood cholesterol, which is a risk factor for heart disease.

CLASSIFICATION OF DIETARY LIPIDS, FATS, AND OILS

LIPID Any of a variety of substances that are soluble in fat but not in water.

TRIGLYCERIDE The most abundant form of fat found in foods and in the body. Triglycerides are composed of glycerol and three fatty acids.

FATTY ACID An organic acid found in animal and plant materials. Three fatty acids combine with glycerol to create a triglyceride.

SATURATED Containing the maximum amount of hydrogen.

MONOUNSATURATED Having a single double bond in its carbon chain.

POLYUNSATURATED Having more than one double bond in its carbon chain.

OMEGA-3 FAT An essential fatty acid that most Americans do not consume enough of. The first double bond is located on the third carbon from the omega end.

OMEGA-6 FAT An essential fatty acid that Americans consume in large quantities. The first double bond is on the sixth carbon from the omega end.

LINOLEIC ACID An omega-6 fatty acid. Examples include corn and sunflower oils.

ARACHIDONIC ACID (AA) An omega-6 fatty acid. Arachidonic acid is the precursor to prostaglandins, substances that activate platelet aggregation, vasoconstriction, and clotting.

ALPHA-LINOLENIC ACID (ALA) An omega-3 fatty acid. Examples include canola oil and flaxseed oil.

Fat is a broad term that has many meanings. Butter and lard are fat, nuts are high in fat, some meats are fatty, and even avocados and olives are high in fat. Most importantly, not all dietary fats are of equal nutritional value.

Lipid is an umbrella term for the group of substances in foods that are insoluble in water. Dietary lipids consist of cholesterol, fats, oils, and phospholipids. A lipid that is solid at room temperature is normally called a *fat*; one that is liquid, an *oil*. Most dietary fats and oils are consumed in the form of **triglyceride**, a glycerol with three **fatty acid** chains of various lengths (Figure 5–1). The type of fatty acid in these chains determines the function and corresponding health benefit or risk. Fatty acid chains can be **saturated**, **monounsaturated**, or **polyunsaturated**. The degree of saturation of the fat is determined by the number of hydrogen atoms on the carbon chain.

Saturated fat has all of the hydrogen it can possibly hold. It is saturated, or full, with hydrogen. This increases the melting point of saturated fats, which makes the fat solid at room temperature. In baked products, saturated fat, such as lard, produces flakey biscuits and pie crusts. Saturated fat holds up during frying and stays fresh longer than unsaturated fat. Consuming too much of certain kinds of saturated fat tends to increase the amount of low-density lipoprotein (LDL) cholesterol—or "bad" cholesterol—in the blood and correspondingly increase the risk of coronary heart disease. This will be discussed later in the chapter.

Monounsaturated fat is missing one hydrogen pair, so its carbon chain is not saturated. This is indicated by a double bond in its chemical structure. Monounsaturated fat is liquid at room temperature. Consuming this type of fat in the diet tends to decrease unhealthy LDL cholesterol and the risk of coronary heart disease.

Polyunsaturated fatty acids likewise are not saturated and have multiple double bonds. A higher number of double bonds indicates a greater degree of polyunsaturation. Polyunsaturated fatty acids are further classified by the location of the first double bond. A fat with the first double bond on the third carbon from the omega end is called an **omega-3 fat**; if the first bond is on the sixth carbon, the fat is an **omega-6 fat**. The location of this first double bond is extremely important in determining the ultimate benefit of the fat.

The main omega-6 fatty acids are **linoleic acid** and **arachidonic acid**. These are found in plant oils, such as corn, safflower, and sunflower. Omega-3 fatty acids are typically found in fish as eicosapentaenoic acid (EPA) and docosahexaenoic acid (DHA). Omega-3 fatty acids are also found in plants in the form of **alpha-linolenic acid (ALA)**. This fatty acid is found in abundance in flaxseed oil and, in lesser amounts, in walnuts, soy products, and

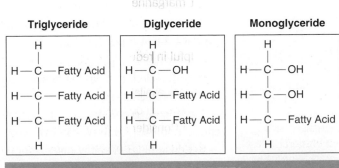

FIGURE 5–1 • THE STRUCTURE OF FATS

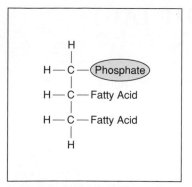

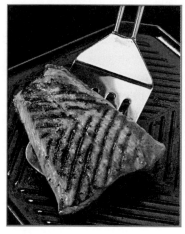

FIGURE 5–2 •
PHOSPHOLIPID STRUCTURE

Grilling is a healthy cooking style.
Dave King © Dorling Kindersley

canola oil. The particular fatty acids that predominate in a food lend it characteristic properties and determine its health effect.

In addition to the triglycerides, there are other dietary lipids. The lipid in the diet that has received the most negative press is cholesterol. It provides a small percent of the total dietary lipid intake, but it is important to consider because of its impact on health. The last category of dietary lipids for discussion is phospholipids (Figure 5–2). These are similar to triglycerides but have one fatty acid replaced by phosphate. The most notable phospholipid in food is lecithin, which we will explore later in this chapter.

Saturated Fat

Most saturated fat in the diet comes from animal products and processed foods. Saturated fats vary in structure and function. Although all fats in this group are completely saturated, and are solid at room temperature, their fatty acid chains differ in length and exhibit different properties.

Lauric and myristic acids are short-chain saturated fats that produce the greatest rise in LDL cholesterol in the blood. Thus they are thought to increase the risk of heart disease (Hajri et al. 1998). But not all saturated fats elevate blood cholesterol to the same extent. Palmitic and stearic acids have longer chains, and their effects on raising blood cholesterol are moderate and neutral, respectively (Grundy, 1994).

Thus it is prudent for culinary professionals to reduce the saturated fat in food preparation. Consumers should consider reduced-fat or low-fat dairy products to reduce saturated fat. Moreover, selecting lean cuts of meat (prepared healthfully) contributes to lowering saturated fat. Healthful meal preparation, such as broiling and grilling, helps remove fat.

Avoiding fried foods is wise because frying oil is either of animal origin or composed of hydrogenated vegetable oils and thus elevates blood cholesterol. Whatever the oil's composition, fried foods in and of themselves are not a healthy choice. Reducing consumption of pastries and fried snack foods is an effective measure to reduce saturated fat intake.

Tropical oils like coconut, palm, and palm kernel oils are highly saturated even though they are plant based. The food industry is responding to concerns about tropical oils by replacing coconut and palm oils with more desirable fats. Palm kernel oil is much more saturated than palm oil. Palm oil is similar in composition to human breast milk fat and in some studies did not raise cholesterol levels. In some parts of the world, coconut oil and palm oil are the main oils consumed, but there is less cardiovascular disease in those areas than in the United States. Other factors besides fat intake, however, affect cardiovascular health.

Polyunsaturated Fatty Acids

Unlike some of the saturated fats, polyunsaturated fatty acids like linoleic acid lower LDL cholesterol levels and are essential in the diet. So for the past few decades, U.S. national nutrition policy has focused on replacing some of the saturated fat in the diet with polyunsaturated fat. As discussed earlier, polyunsaturated fats fall into two main groups: omega-3 and omega-6. Ingesting large amounts of omega-6 oils containing linoleic fatty acid without sufficient omega-3 fatty acids could decrease LDL cholesterol but could also lead to other problems, such as blood vessel constriction and increased blood clotting. The omega-6 polyunsaturated oils, if consumed excessively, also may have a strong promoting effect on tumor growth (Weisburger 1997).

Consuming a healthy balance of the omega-6 and omega-3 fatty acids is important because both compete for the same enzyme to convert them to eicosanoids (Figure 5–3). Both of these produce eicosanoid hormone-like substances that control inflammation

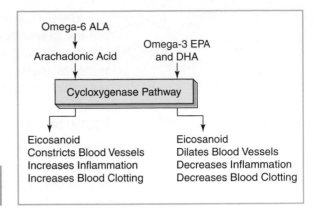

FIGURE 5-3 • EICOSANOID PRODUCTION

response, blood vessel constriction, and blood clotting. But the type of the eicosanoid produced depends on which fatty acid is consumed. If relatively more omega-3 is consumed, the eicosanoids produced will dilate blood vessels, decrease inflammation, and decrease blood clotting. These eicosanoids are additional factors in the diet–heart disease connection because of their effect on blood vessel dilation and blood clotting.

Researchers first found that omega-3 fatty acids might decrease the risk of cardiovascular disease (CVD) in 1971 when the rate of CVD in a Danish population was compared to that of a group of Eskimos (Bang, Dyerberg, and Nielsen 1971). The Eskimos had a very low incidence of cardiovascular disease, yet their diet was very high in animal fat. But the fat in the diet came mainly from fish, whales, and seals, all high in omega-3 fatty acids. The high-omega-3 diet was thought responsible for these findings. Another study showed that the Greenland Eskimos had decreased blood clotting compared to the Danish controls (Dyerberg and Bang 1979). A more recent study of Alaskan Eskimos, consuming a similar diet, showed significantly lower rates of death from cardiovascular disease compared to non-Eskimo controls (Parkinson et al. 1994).

In heart and blood vessel tissue, eicosanoids work in harmony—one dilating and the other constricting blood vessels, and one increasing and the other reducing blood clotting. Inflammation is also partly governed by these eicosanoids (Calder 2002). Inflammation is the body's natural response to infection or injury, usually characterized by pain, redness, and swelling. Blood flow into the affected area increases, allowing antibodies to destroy invading bacteria and promote healing. Inflammation is usually a healthy response to infection but can be damaging if excessive. Scientists now believe that chronic low-grade inflammation plays a role in promoting cardiovascular disease (Ross 1999).

The omega-6 linoleic acids (LA) form the eicosanoids that increase the inflammation seen in sepsis (Blok et al. 1996). The omega-3 fatty acids, eicosapentaenoic acid (EPA), docosahexaenoic acid (DHA), and their precursor, alpha-linolenic (ALA) acid, produce eicosanoids that decrease inflammation. The balance of omega-6 to omega-3 fatty acids determines the degree of inflammation.

Both fatty acids compete for the same enzyme and produce their particular degree of inflammation (Calder 2002). Precise dietary recommendations for those with inflammatory diseases like arthritis, asthma, and psoriasis are not yet available. Yet omega-6 fatty acids are known to produce a strong inflammatory response, while the omega-3 fatty acids produce milder responses. Individuals with inflammatory conditions might want to avoid excessive intake of safflower, sunflower, and corn oils and to use canola or flaxseed oil instead. In the United States, Americans consume large amounts of plant oils that contain omega-6 but relatively little omega-3.

Therefore, in addition to substituting polyunsaturated fat for saturated fat, it is important also to substitute some omega-3 for omega-6 fatty acids. Besides eating the recommended omega-3 oils, consumers should also consider consuming fatty fish. Sardines anchovies, mackerel, herring, salmon, albacore tuna, lake trout, bluefish, and Atlantic halibut contain omega-3 fatty acids, which help balance the omega-6 fatty acids.

Plant Sources of Omega-3

Omega-3 fatty acid (alpha-linolenic acid) from plant sources is converted in the body to EPA and DHA. Flaxseed oil is the most abundant plant source, with omega-3 providing about two-thirds of its total fat content. Canola oil, which is made from rapeseed (a member of the mustard family that has oil-rich seeds, which grows in Canada and the northwestern United States), contains 10% alpha-linolenic omega-3 fatty acids. The predominance of monounsaturated fat and the benefit of alpha-linolenic acid in canola oil make it a good dietary choice. In the past, rapeseed oil, the source of canola oil, was banned by the Food and Drug Administration because it contained erucic acid. Rapeseed oil once contained 30% to 60% of its fatty acids as erucic acid, which is highly toxic. Today, erucic acid makes up only a very small percentage of rapeseed oil.

Walnuts are a good source of alpha-linolenic fatty acid. Four teaspoons of chopped walnuts or 1 1/4 teaspoons of walnut oil gives the equivalent of 300 milligrams of omega-3 fatty acid. Walnuts, however, also contain omega-6 fatty acids. Soybean oil also contains alpha-linolenic fatty acid (omega-3), in addition to generous amounts of linoleic acid (omega-6).

Monounsaturated Fats

The main monounsaturated fatty acid is oleic acid, which is found in many fats. The body produces oleic acid from acetic acid. Animal fats vary in oleic acid content from 20% to 40%. Vegetable oils range from 12% to 75% oleic. The richest source of oleic acid is olive oil, followed by canola oil and then peanut oil. In one study, monounsaturated fat in the diet reduced LDL levels as effectively as polyunsaturated fat (Hodson, Skeaff, and Chisholm 2001). No health problems have yet been associated with oleic acid. Olive and canola oils are recommended as substitutes for corn oil, which was traditionally one of the most popular oils in the kitchen.

A light, tasteless, and odorless form of olive oil is now available for baking and other uses where pronounced flavor is unwanted. Canola oil is also a good choice, particularly because it has a mild odor and flavor. Regarding peanut oil, another monounsaturated oil, not much has been publicized to confirm or refute any possible benefits from its consumption.

Cholesterol

Cholesterol is a substance found in the plaque that produces atherosclerosis. Cholesterol is a fatlike, waxy substance that yields few calories compared to fats. It is classified as a sterol and is made by the liver. Because the human body manufactures cholesterol, obtaining it from the diet is unnecessary.

The liver makes much more cholesterol (approximately 1,000 milligrams per day) than the body gets from food. Foods high in dietary cholesterol are fish eggs (such as caviar and shad roe), brains, liver, egg yolks, shrimp, and sardines.

Milk contains a small amount of cholesterol, most of it in butterfat. Foods made with large amounts of dairy fat, such as cheeses and ice cream, are high in cholesterol. All meats, poultry, and fish contain cholesterol regardless of how lean they may be. Cholesterol is part of the cell membrane of all animal tissue. Plants do not produce cholesterol. Fatty foods of plant origin, such as avocados, olives, nuts, and all plant oils, do not contain cholesterol.

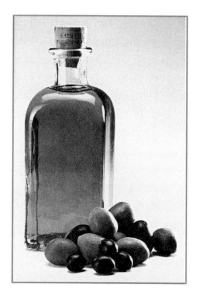

Canola and olive oils are recommended substitutes for less-healthy oils.
David Murray © Dorling Kindersley

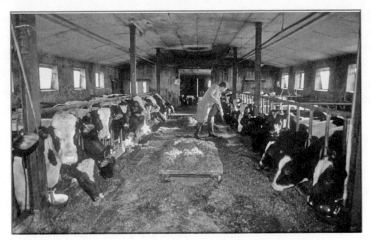

Dairy products can contain a high amount of cholesterol.
Peter Arnold, Inc.

EMULSIFIER An agent that forms a stable mixture of two immiscible liquids.

Although consumers are admonished to lower their cholesterol levels because of associated health risks, cholesterol has many positive functions. It is necessary for hormone production, for vitamin D synthesis, and for making bile. The liver produces about 700 milligrams of cholesterol daily for this purpose alone. Bile functions as an **emulsifier** in fat digestion. Cholesterol is also found in human breast milk, which demonstrates cholesterol's importance in infant development.

One must differentiate between dietary cholesterol and blood cholesterol. High dietary cholesterol does not necessarily convert into high blood cholesterol. America's preoccupation with reducing dietary cholesterol may not be as important in reducing heart disease risk as a number of other factors. Most individuals can eat large amounts of foods that contain a lot of cholesterol and not develop health problems associated with high blood cholesterol levels. (More information on this topic will be presented later in the chapter.) Consumers should speak with a physician to discuss blood cholesterol testing, particularly if a family history of cardiovascular disease or stroke exists.

Lecithin

The last group of lipids to be considered is the phospholipid. These are similar in their chemical structure to triglycerides, but with one of the fatty acids replaced by a phosphate group (see Figure 5–2).

The most important phospholipid is lecithin. Lecithin is used in food products as an emulsifier. An emulsifier allows two ingredients that normally do not mix together to form a stable mixture. The most common example of two ingredients that do not mix is oil and water. Italian dressing with vinegar and oil, as a result, will not remain mixed even after shaking. Adding lecithin produces a stable mixture. Mayonnaise is an example of a stable mixture created by lecithin. The lecithin naturally found in egg yolks allows the oil in the yolk to stay suspended in the watery component and provides nonstick sprays their functionality.

LINGUAL LIPASE An enzyme formed in the salivary glands that digests minimal amounts of fat in the mouth.

GASTRIC LIPASE An enzyme in the stomach that digests fat.

BILE A fat emulsifier made in the liver and stored in the gallbladder.

DIGESTION OF FAT

Fat digestion begins in the mouth with the chewing and mechanical breaking down of food. Some enzymatic digestion of fat occurs in the mouth by the action of **lingual lipase** and in the stomach via **gastric lipase**. But most fat is digested in the small intestine. When fat leaves the stomach, **bile** is released from the gallbladder. The liver produces

PANCREATIC LIPASE An enzyme made in the pancreas and released in the intestine that digests fat into free fatty acids.

INTESTINAL LIPASE An enzyme that hydrolyzes fat into fatty acids and glycerol.

MONOGLYCERIDE An organic compound derived from glycerol with only one fatty acid.

LIPOPROTEIN A fat unit containing protein on the outermost layer to transport it through water.

CHYLOMICRON A lipoprotein unit, containing triglycerides and cholesterol, that is transported from the intestines ultimately to the blood.

bile and stores it in the gallbladder until needed (that is, when food enters the intestine). Bile emulsifies fat by dividing large conglomerations of it into smaller pieces, allowing **pancreatic lipase** and **intestinal lipase** to break it down. These enzymes remove fatty acid chains from the triglyceride, forming a **monoglyceride** (see Figure 5–1). The monoglycerides and individual fatty acids are then absorbed into the intestinal cells. Inside the cells, the triglycerides are reassembled. Triglycerides would have a difficult time traveling through the water-based human body, so they are packaged into vessels called **lipoproteins**. Just as oil- and water-based foods do not mix, as we have seen, fat does not mix with water, but proteins do; therefore, fat is wrapped in protein and carried throughout the body.

Chylomicrons are the lipoproteins made in the intestinal lining that carry fat from the intestine via the lymph system to the bloodstream and eventually to the liver. The liver processes the fat for distribution throughout the body.

METABOLISM OF LIPIDS

As discussed earlier, triglycerides and cholesterol are packaged by the liver into lipoproteins that carry them throughout the body. After the individual dietary fats are processed by the liver, they enter the bloodstream and are distributed throughout the body.

As these lipids are transferred to the body cells, the lipoprotein that carries them shrinks and becomes low-density lipoprotein (LDL). LDL distributes cholesterol and usually is collected and reprocessed by the liver after it has done its job. Excess LDL circulating in the bloodstream begins to distribute cholesterol in the blood vessels where it should not be.

At the same time there are other lipoproteins collecting fatty acids and cholesterol. High-density lipoprotein (HDL) contains little cholesterol; it continually collects cholesterol from the body and takes it back to the liver for processing. HDL is the vehicle that clears cholesterol from the blood. Simply put, LDL distributes cholesterol, whereas HDL collects cholesterol (Figure 5–4).

Balance between the two lipoproteins, LDL and HDL, is necessary to maintain health, and HDL is important in the prevention of cardiovascular disease. People who have inadequate amounts of HDL (less than 40 milligrams per deciliter for men and less than 50 milligrams per deciliter for women) may be at risk for coronary heart disease.

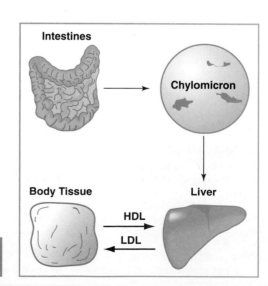

FIGURE 5–4 • CHOLESTEROL AND FAT DISTRIBUTION

GRAIN-FED VERSUS GRAZED LIVESTOCK

Animal feed that is high in grain is also high in omega-6 fatty acids. Grain-fattened animals have much higher levels of saturated fat than do animals fed mostly by grazing. Alternatively, if animal feed contains flaxseed, a food high in omega-3 fatty acids, the resulting beef, pork, chicken, or eggs will also contain high levels of omega-3 fatty acids.

You may have heard about "good" and "bad" cholesterol. Consumers often inquire when food shopping whether the cholesterol in food is the good or bad type. In fact, there is only one type of cholesterol. The cholesterol in certain foods and in the body is neither good nor bad in and of itself. It is the location of cholesterol in the human body that determines whether it is good or bad. Cholesterol that is located in LDL for distribution is referred to as bad cholesterol; if it is located in HDL, it is called good cholesterol. This is because HDL takes cholesterol back to the liver and LDL distributes cholesterol throughout the body. The key is to keep a healthy balance between distribution and collection, which usually means increasing HDL and decreasing LDL.

So how do we increase HDL and decrease LDL? Very few foods greatly increase HDL. Aerobic exercise, such as running, biking, dancing, swimming, and walking, will increase HDL levels. Avoiding tobacco and maintaining a healthy body weight will help raise HDL too. Low HDL levels are the most serious lipoprotein risk factor for women to develop cardiovascular disease.

As mentioned previously, the body's level of HDL does not respond readily to the food we eat; therefore, dietary attention should focus on LDL. The level of LDL cholesterol is affected greatly by food consumption. But surprisingly, dietary cholesterol has very little effect on the balance between HDL and LDL. Put another way, the cholesterol we eat is not the most important determinant of blood cholesterol. Instead, one of the most powerful ways to decease LDL is to decrease saturated fat and trans-fat intake.

Remember, saturated fat is typically found in animal products. Therefore choosing low-fat dairy products and lean meats is beneficial for reducing consumption of animal fat. Increasing intake of polyunsaturated or monounsaturated fats or substituting them for saturated fat will also decrease LDL. Thus soybeans, nuts, legumes, seeds, and beans are good alternatives to animal foods. Other foods like olive oil, avocado, oat bran, and garlic are also effective in lowering LDL.

FUNCTIONS OF DIETARY FAT IN MAINTAINING HEALTH

Most dietary fat provides energy, while excess dietary fat is stored as body fat. Dietary fat is also necessary for transporting fat-soluble vitamins, storing them in the body, and insulating the body against the cold. Fat adds taste to food and produces a feeling of fullness as well. Dietary fat is not the villain it is portrayed to be in the media. Polyunsaturated fat, for example, is essential. For a few decades public policy has been to reduce total fat consumption. Today, however, some health organizations do not recommend reducing total fat; instead, they favor balancing the type of fat consumed.

DIETARY RECOMMENDATIONS

The Dietary Reference Intakes (DRIs) recommend that 20% to 35% of calories come from fat (Institute of Medicine 2002), with the ratio of omega-6 to omega-3 being about 10 to 1. The Adequate Intake (AI) for healthy men is 17 grams omega-6 [linoleic acid (LA)] and 1.6 grams omega-3 [alpha-linolenic acid (ALA)] per day; and for women it is 12 grams LA and 1.1 grams ALA per day (Institute of Medicine 2002). At present, the Western diet contains a ratio of omega-6 to omega-3 closer to 20 or 30 to 1 (Simopoulos 1999). Because the ratio of omega-6 to omega-3 in the traditional

Western diet prior to the fast food era was closer to 4 to 1, some nutrition professionals suggest that this ratio is closer to optimal (Simopoulos 1999). Most Americans would probably benefit from increasing their omega-3 fatty acid intake to maintain a healthier balance.

HYDROGENATION

Hydrogenation is the process of using heat and metal catalysts to add hydrogen to the double bonds of unsaturated fats. This process changes the fat's cooking and baking qualities. For example, margarine is vegetable oil that has been partially hydrogenated to give it the spreading consistency of butter. Another example is shortening, which is liquid oil that has been hydrogenated into a semisolid, giving the product a higher melting point. The hydrogenation process also enhances products' storage qualities, making them last longer on the shelf.

Hydrogenation poses some health concerns. The process forms trans fats, a by-product that does not have the same effect on the body as do normal fatty acids, which occur in the cis form. In cis fats, the hydrogen atoms are on the same side of the carbon chain at the double bond, which makes the fat molecule bent in shape. In trans fats, the hydrogen molecules are on the opposite side of the double bond, which means the molecule is straight and looks like saturated fat (Figure 5–5).

The body perceives the trans fats produced by hydrogenation as being more like saturated fats than unsaturated fats. Thus these fats also raise LDL cholesterol levels in the blood. Some stick margarines can contain as much as 35% trans-fatty acids. Tub margarines and hydrogenated oil may contain up to 20% trans-fatty acids. Most margarines on the market contain trans fat. Those without trans fat advertise this fact, making them recognizable. Trans fat must now be listed on food labels, as required by the Nutrition Labeling and Education Act of 1990, and all foods must show the trans-fat content in the Nutrition Facts panel as of January 2006.

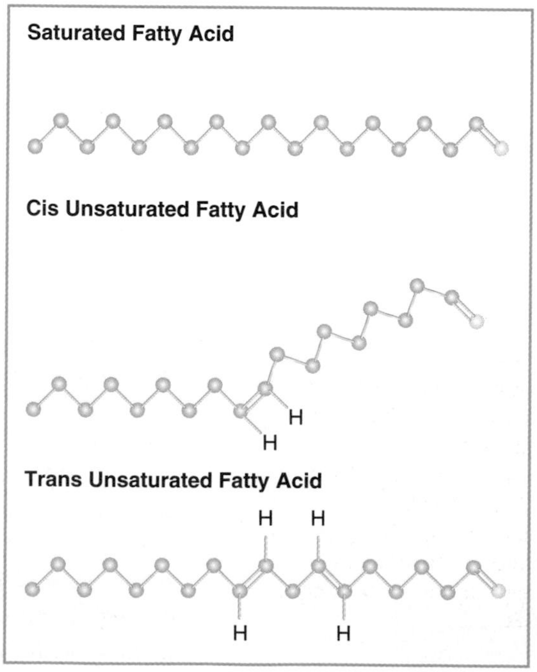

Saturated Fatty Acid

Cis Unsaturated Fatty Acid

Trans Unsaturated Fatty Acid

FIGURE 5–5 • THE SHAPE OF TRANS-FATTY ACIDS

A major meta-analysis reports that trans monounsaturated fat and saturated fat have a similar effect in elevating blood cholesterol levels (Kwiterovich 1997). In the Nurses Health Study, women who consumed the largest quantity of trans-fatty acids had the greatest risk of heart attack.

Although trans fats are generally regarded as unnatural, they do appear in nature in very small amounts. For example, microbes inside cows hydrogenate unsaturated fatty acids, thereby contributing a slight amount of trans fat to butter. Other foods contain small amounts of naturally occurring trans fat. Even so, the Dietary Reference Intake (DRI) report from the Institute of Medicine states there is no safe level of consumption for trans fats and recommends that their consumption be as low as possible (Institute of Medicine 2002).

OXIDATION

Fats may spoil, or turn rancid, in the presence of oxygen. Rancidity is the technical term for the oxidation of fat. For example, fat in whole flaxseed is very stable. But once the seed is ground, however, its oil comes in contact with oxygen in the air and oxidizes. In addition, heat or air used to process items like powdered eggs, powdered milk, whey, and smoked fish and meats may increase oxidation. Many commercially prepared products contain one or more of these processed ingredients. Oxidation also occurs in oils used for deep frying.

Manufacturers reduce oxidation by adding artificial or natural antioxidants that react with oxygen, preventing it from oxidizing fat and making it rancid. EDTA, BHA, and BHT are some of the artificial antioxidants; vitamin E, beta-carotene, vitamin C (ascorbic acid), and selenium are natural antioxidants.

Oxidation of fat is also a process that occurs normally in all body tissues. Many experiments suggest that cholesterol in the body becomes more of a health concern when it is oxidized. Thus cholesterol is susceptible to oxidation in our bodies as well as in food.

TIPS ABOUT FATTY ACIDS

Most current research focuses on the role of fatty acids in heart disease and their effect on the immune system. Some health authorities call for more research before publicly defining the correct amounts of certain fats in the diet.

It may be prudent, however, to replace some of the omega-6 fatty acids with monounsaturated fatty acids and omega-3 fatty acids. For the consumer that means using more olive oil, canola oil, walnuts, and fish in place of corn, safflower, and sunflower oils.

Another important consideration is that food contains a mixture of several fatty acids, and all fatty acids are high in calories. Excess calories contribute to weight gain, and obesity is an independent risk factor for some of the same conditions fatty acids are used to alleviate.

At this point, nutritional science suggests that fat should comprise 20% to 35% of the total daily caloric intake and that saturated and trans fat within that figure should be minimized.

Food labels list the grams of fat and total calories, making it possible to determine the percentage of calories from fat. To make the calculation, you must know that a gram of fat is about 9 calories. So if a bag of chips provides 180 calories with 10 grams of fat, then fat

TABLE 5–1 • AVERAGE FAT CONTENT

Food	Fat
Milk (whole)	8 g per 8 oz
Milk (2% fat)	4 g per 8 oz
Milk (skim)	0 g per 8 oz
High-fat meat	8 g per oz
Meat (medium fat)	5 g per oz
Lean meats, poultry, fish	3 g per oz
Vegetables	0 g per serving
Fruits	0 g per serving
Butter, margarine, oil, or nuts	5 g per teaspoon
Breads and starches without added fat	1 g per slice or 1/2 cup serving

provides 50% of the calories. (For example, 10 grams of fat multiplied by 9 calories per gram equals 90 calories from fat; 90 calories from fat divided by 180 calories equals 50%.) To determine the grams of fat in fresh foods, follow the information in Table 5–1.

FAT REPLACERS

The FDA has approved several fat replacers in processed foods. Simplesse contains 1 to 2 calories per gram compared to 9 calories per gram for regular fat. Simplesse is made from microparticulated protein derived from egg whites or skim milk. It is useful in salad dressings and ice cream but inappropriate for cooking.

Olestra, sold under the brand name Olean, is a fat replacer that has no calories. It is made from sugar and a chemically altered fat that passes unabsorbed through the digestive system. However, Olestra also carries out the fat-soluble vitamins A, E, D, and K and enhances their likelihood of excretion. Furthermore, ingesting too much Olestra can cause diarrhea. Unlike Simplesse, Olestra lends itself to frying and is used in potato chip production.

A third substitute for fat is Salatrim, which contains 5 calories per gram and is only partially absorbed. It is used in commercial baked goods.

Z-Trim is one of the most recent fat substitutes to hit the market. It is made with cellulose from corn bran fiber and is quite versatile. Manufacturers use Z-Trim to replace fat in quick breads, sauces, cookies, and ice cream.

In addition to these fat replacers, several foods contain other ingredients to offset fat. These ingredients include modified food starches, dextrins, cellulose, and gums, which behave as thickeners in fat-free salad dressings. These are also used as texturizers, providing a mouth feel comparable to fat but with fewer calories.

The food manufacturing industry has responded to health authorities' call for lower-fat foods. This trend gives rise to several issues. The first is nutritional merit. Generally, foods that are reduced fat are high in salt, sugar, or corn syrup and low in fruits, vegetables,

DOUBLE THE CALORIES

Although some types of fats are healthy, you should not consume unlimited amounts of them. Remember that fat contains twice the calories of protein or carbohydrates, and excess calories lead to weight gain.

EXPERIMENTAL EXERCISES

1. Look at different types of fat in bottles. Observe the fats at room temperature, heated, and under refrigeration. Discuss the properties of the fats.
2. Find three recipes to create a meal that is high in omega-3 fatty acids.
3. Find a recipe that uses butter and determine which oil to substitute to create the best product.

ASSESSMENT EXERCISE

Calculate the grams of total fat and saturated fat for a day's intake.

and whole grains. Second, consumers may rationalize indulging in larger portions of the reduced-fat items, leaving little room for basic whole foods. Third, the art of cooking delicious, tasty, wholesome food is diminishing in the craze for low-fat and fat-free foods. As a result, children are growing up without ever experiencing the taste of home-cooked food.

Even though convenience foods are handy, consumers can create their own low-fat meals without using fat substitutes. For example, they can make fat-free salad dressings at home with low-fat yogurts, cottage cheese, tofu with herbs, or tomato juice with lemon and spices. Simple substitutions can reduce the fat content of meals. (See Table 5–2.)

TABLE 5–2 • COMPARISON OF HIGH-FAT AND LOW-FAT MEALS

High-Fat	Low-Fat
Breakfast	
Juice	Juice
Cereal	Cereal
Whole milk[a]	Skim milk
Biscuit[a]	Toasted bread
Margarine[a]	Jelly
Coffee	Coffee
Cream[a]	Skim milk
Sugar	Sugar
Lunch	
Salami[a] and bologna[a]	Lean roast beef
Croissant[a]	Rye bread
Mayonnaise[a]	Mustard
Salad with dressing[a]	Sliced tomato on lettuce
Ice cream[a]	Frozen fruit ice dessert
Soda	Soda
Dinner	
Fried chicken[a]	Baked chicken
French fries[a]	Baked potato + 1 teaspoon butter
Spinach in cream sauce[a]	Spinach
Apple pie[a]	Apple sauce
Snack	
Cookies[a]	Low-fat yogurt with fruit
Fruit	

[a]Items contain fat.

SUMMARY

The Health Concerns Surrounding Fats

Lipid is an umbrella term for a group of substances in foods that are insoluble in water. Dietary lipids consist of cholesterol, fats, oils, and phospholipids. A lipid that is solid at room temperature is called a *fat*; one that is a liquid, an *oil*. Most dietary fats and oils are consumed in the form of triglyceride, a glycerol with three fatty acid chains of various lengths. The type of fatty acid in these chains determines the fat's function and corresponding health benefit or risk. Fatty acid chains can be saturated, monounsaturated, or polyunsaturated (see Figure 5–1). The degree of saturation of the fat is determined by the number of hydrogen atoms on the carbon chain.

Some types of dietary fat like the saturated fat found in red meat, butter, and dairy products are less healthy, while the omega-3 oils found in fish and the monounsaturated oil in olive oil are health promoting. More recently, health authorities have determined that trans fat in processed food is harmful.

There is no question that fat plays a very important role in regular bodily functions. Some body fat is essential for cushioning the body's organs, insulating against cold temperatures, transporting fat-soluble vitamins, storing energy, and providing precursors for hormones regulating body functions.

Polyunsaturated fat is the only classification of dietary fat essential for humans. It is needed for healthy skin, normal liver function, cell wall structure, and the synthesis of eicosanoids, which are hormone-like substances. Besides its role in human health, fat also adds taste and texture to food, and because fat is digested slowly, it provides a feeling of satiety. Feeling full longer after eating fat could help consumers reduce overall daily caloric intake and remain satisfied longer.

The main omega-6 fatty acids are linoleic acid and arachidonic acid found in plant oils, such as corn, safflower, and sunflower. Omega-3 fatty acids are typically found in fish as eicosapentaenoic acid (EPA) and docosahexaenoic acid (DHA). Omega-3 fatty acids are also found in plants in the form of alpha-linolenic acid (ALA). They are also found in abundance in flaxseed oil and, in lesser amounts, in walnuts, soy products, and canola oil.

CASE RESOLUTION

It has been known for years that butter, made from animal products, is high in saturated fat and contains cholesterol, which contributes to heart disease. We have been taught for years that margarine does not contain cholesterol and thus is preferred over butter. But now with the new information about the trans fat in many margarines, they may not be the best choice.

Now that Gwendolyn is aware of these facts, she wants to select a healthy oil rather than butter or margarine to season her vegetables and pan-fry her foods. Her first choice is olive oil, but she is concerned about the flavor that olive oil might add to her recipes. She should test the recipes substituting olive oil for the butter, and if the flavor is not compatible, she should try a different oil without the characteristic flavor, such as canola oil. Gwendolyn must strike a balance between serving healthier foods and retaining the flavor of her original recipes.

REFERENCES

Bang, H. O., J. Dyerberg, and A. B. Nielsen. 1971. Plasma lipid and lipoprotein pattern in Greenlandic west-coast Eskimos. *Lancet* 71: 1143–45.

Blok W. L., M. B. Katan, J. W. van der Meer. 1996. Modulation of inflammation and cytokine production by dietary (n-3) fatty acids. *Journal of Nutrition* 126: 1515–33.

Calder, P. C. 2002. Fatty acids and gene expression related to inflammation. In *Clinical Nutrition: Early Intervention,* eds. D. Labadarios and C. Pichard. 19–25. Switzerland: Nestec.

Dyerberg, J., and H. O. Bang. 1979. Hemostatic function and platelet polyunsaturated fatty acids in Eskimos. *Lancet* 2: 433–35.

Grundy, S. M. 1994. Influence of stearic acid on cholesterol metabolism relative to other long-chain fatty acids. *American Journal of Clinical Nutrition* 60: S986–90.

Hajri, T., P. Khosla, A. Pronczuk, and K. C. Hayes. 1998. Myristic acid-rich fat raises plasma LDL by stimulating LDL production without affecting fractional clearance in gerbils fed a cholesterol-free diet. *Journal of Nutrition* 128 (3): 477–84.

Hodson, L., C. M. Skeaff, and W. A. Chisholm. 2001. The effect of replacing dietary AU saturated fat with polyunsaturated or monounsaturated fat on plasma lipids in free-living young adults. *European Journal of Clinical Nutrition* 55 (10): 908–15.

Institute of Medicine. 2002. *Dietary Reference Intakes for Energy, Carbohydrate, Fiber, Fat, Fatty Acids, Cholesterol, Protein, and Amino Acids (Macronutrients).* Washington, DC: Government Printing Office.

Kwiterovich, P. 1997. The effect of dietary fat, antioxidants, and pro-oxidants on blood lipids, lipoproteins, and atherosclerosis. *Journal of the American Dietetic Association* 97: S31–41.

Parkinson, A. J., A. L. Cruz, W. L. Heyward, and L. R. Bulkow. 1994. Elevated concentrations of plasma omega-3 polyunsaturated fatty acids among Alaskan Eskimos. *American Journal of Clinical Nutrition* 59: 384–88.

Ross, R. 1999. Atherosclerosis: An inflammatory disease. *New England Journal of Medicine* 340 (2): 115–26.

Simopoulos, A. P. 1999. Essential fatty acids in health and chronic disease. *American Journal of Clinical Nutrition* 70: S506–9.

Weisburger, J. H. 1997. Dietary fat and risk of chronic disease: Mechanistic insights from experiment studies. *Journal of the American Dietetic Association* S16.

REVIEW QUESTIONS

1. Most dietary fat is consumed in which form?
2. What type of fat is found in plant products?
3. Which class of fatty acid tends to increase blood cholesterol levels?
4. Which foods provide the most dietary cholesterol?
5. Which foods in the milk group are a high-cholesterol source?
6. Explain how coconut oil, which has no dietary cholesterol, can raise blood cholesterol levels.
7. Name the two categories of polyunsaturated fats.
8. What happens when a fat is hydrogenated, and how is trans fat involved?
9. Why might a no-fat or extremely low-fat diet be undesirable?
10. Which lifestyle changes affect HDL cholesterol levels?

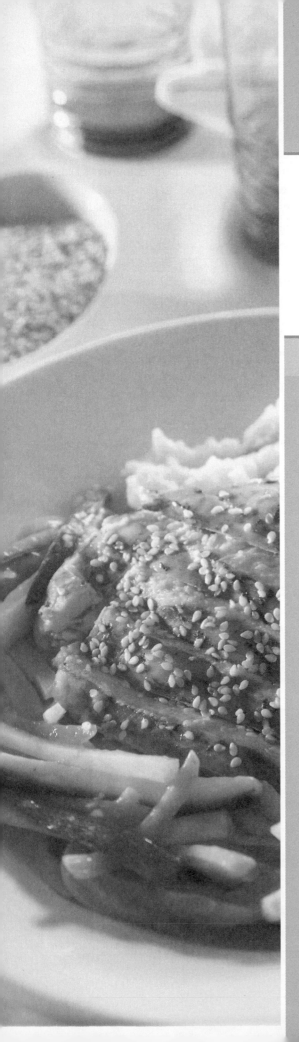

6

Vitamins

KEY CONCEPTS

- Vitamins are classified as either fat-soluble or water-soluble, based on shared properties.
- Humans must obtain vitamins from the diet to maintain good health.
- Vitamins are needed in extremely small amounts.
- Vitamins are toxic when taken in excess, especially fat-soluble vitamins.
- Each vitamin has a unique and specific function in supporting health.
- Distinct health problems are associated with the inadequate intake of each vitamin.
- Foods vary greatly in vitamin content. Consuming a variety of foods is the best way to ensure the proper consumption of each nutrient.
- Phytochemicals, found in plants, are not vitamins but may provide additional health benefits.

Vitamins are essential organic compounds that are necessary for good health and are primarily obtained through diet. If the body does not obtain the proper quantity of vitamins, poor health, physical deformities, and, in some cases, death may occur. In sufficient amounts, vitamins support growth and life.

The term vitamin is derived from *vita,* which is Latin for "life," and *amine,* which denotes that the chemical structure contains nitrogen (although, in fact, nitrogen is not a component of many vitamins). The "e" was dropped, and the name vitamin resulted.

Vitamin discovery has been a slow process, even though the association between food and the prevention and cure of disease has been known for thousands of years. In ancient Greece, Hippocrates discovered that eating liver could cure night blindness. Beginning in the early eighteenth century, individuals discovered that oranges and lemons prevented scurvy in sailors. In the Far East, researchers found that foods other than white rice were needed to prevent beriberi. At that time vitamins were not known to be the substances responsible for preventing and curing these diseases, but the groundwork for vitamin discovery was laid.

In the early 1900s Europeans conducted studies that fed purified diets of carbohydrates, protein, fat, and minerals to laboratory animals. These diets were thought to contain the only essential dietary components, yet animals failed to thrive. The results suggested that some other food element necessary for maintenance of good health was missing. Throughout the first half of the twentieth century, scientists slowly discovered each vitamin.

Although researchers established the body's need for vitamins, the specific functions of these substances were unknown. Science elucidated the functions of vitamins after their discovery, including that they work as **cofactors** with **enzymes** in many different capacities. More information on vitamins continues to be discovered even today.

Although consuming adequate amounts of vitamins is vital, not all animal species need the same vitamins. For example, dogs do not need vitamin C. Their bodies can manufacture it. Humans' bodies, on the other hand, cannot.

Thirteen vitamins are necessary for human health. They are classified into two categories—fat-soluble and water-soluble. Fat-soluble vitamins require dietary fat for absorption. Extra fat-soluble vitamins are stored in fat tissues or in the liver. Water-soluble vitamins are excreted in urine when body tissues are saturated.

The fat-soluble vitamins are A, E, D, and K; the water-soluble vitamins are C and the B complex (eight in number). This chapter will examine the structure, function, required amounts, deficiency symptoms, food sources, and stability of each vitamin. We will discuss the four fat-soluble vitamins first, followed by the nine water-soluble vitamins.

COFACTOR A chemical that activates and works with an enzyme.

ENZYME A molecule that is necessary for a chemical reaction to occur but that is not used up in the reaction.

THINK ABOUT IT

We all know that vitamins play a role in health. Can you think of any vitamin–health connections? The first that comes to mind for many people is vitamin C, which is thought to prevent colds. And of course, vitamin A is believed to benefit the eyes. Besides these connections, are there others?

As you read through the chapter, keep an open mind because what you "know" may be incorrect. Will taking vitamin C tablets in the winter really help you fight off a cold? Will eating lots of carrots enhance your eye health? To find out for yourself, read on.

CASE STUDY

Cooking for a Nursing Home

Beatrice is a line cook for a nursing home in Mississippi. She has been cooking there for 40 years. One day her supervisor, Linda, brings a complaint to Beatrice regarding overcooked, "mushy" vegetables. The complaint originated during the Department of Health's annual survey and inspection. The dietitian surveyor pointed out that excessive cooking destroys nutrients and reduces food quality. When Linda shares this information with Beatrice, the cook is shocked because she has always prepared the vegetables this way. Furthermore, she knows that some of the nursing home residents cannot chew very well.

How would you proceed if you were the supervisor overseeing meal service? How can nursing home meals be prepared to increase their nutrient content? *The resolution for this case study is presented at the end of the chapter.*

CAROTENOIDS OTHER THAN BETA-CAROTENE

With less vitamin A activity:

- **alpha-carotene**
- **beta-cryptoxanthin (orange-yellow pigment)**

With no vitamin A activity:

- **lycopene (gives a deep red color to tomatoes)**
- **lutein (yellow-green pigment)**
- **zeaxanthin (yellow-green pigment)**

CAROTENOID Any of various pigments—usually yellow to red—that are found widely in plants and animals. Carotenes are an example.

RETINOL A form of vitamin A found in foods of animal origin. Also called *preformed vitamin A*.

RETINOID Any of the different forms of vitamin A. Retinoids include retinal, retinol, and retinoic acid.

RETINOL ACTIVITY EQUIVALENT (RAE) A unit of measurement for vitamin A.

PROVITAMIN A A substance that must be converted to vitamin A before the body can use it.

BETA-CAROTENE The most abundant carotenoid and a precursor to vitamin A.

EPITHELIAL TISSUE Tissue that lines the body—both the skin on the outside and the mucous membrane on the inside.

FAT-SOLUBLE VITAMINS

Vitamin A

Hippocrates found that consuming raw liver could cure night blindness. It took another 2,000 years before anyone knew that vitamin A—plentiful in liver—is what produces this benefit. Elmer V. McCollum announced the discovery of vitamin A in 1913 while working at the University of Wisconsin (McCollum and Davis 1913). Another two decades passed before it was discovered that some plant-derived compounds, known as **carotenoids**, provide vitamin A activity (Stipanuk 2000).

Structure and Function

Vitamin A is found in the body in three active forms. **Retinol**, also called *preformed vitamin A* (Figure 6–1), is the main form of vitamin A. Retinol is found in foods of animal origin and is used as the standard for assessing biological activities of the other **retinoids**; 1 μg (read as "microgram"; equal to 1/1,000,000 gram) of retinol equals 1 **retinol activity equivalent (RAE)**. Preformed vitamin A is obtained only from animal food sources. Vegetables provide **provitamin A**. These provitamins are known as carotenoids. (But note that not all carotenoids have vitamin A activity.) **Beta-carotene**, a precursor to vitamin A, is the best known and the most potent. It occurs as an orange pigment in carrots, sweet potatoes, pumpkins, and other orange and deep green vegetables.

Vitamin A is necessary for maintaining **epithelial tissue**, gene regulation, immune function, and growth. It plays a central role in vision as well. Vitamin A helps maintain moist, healthy mucous membranes, which helps prevent respiratory infections. Without

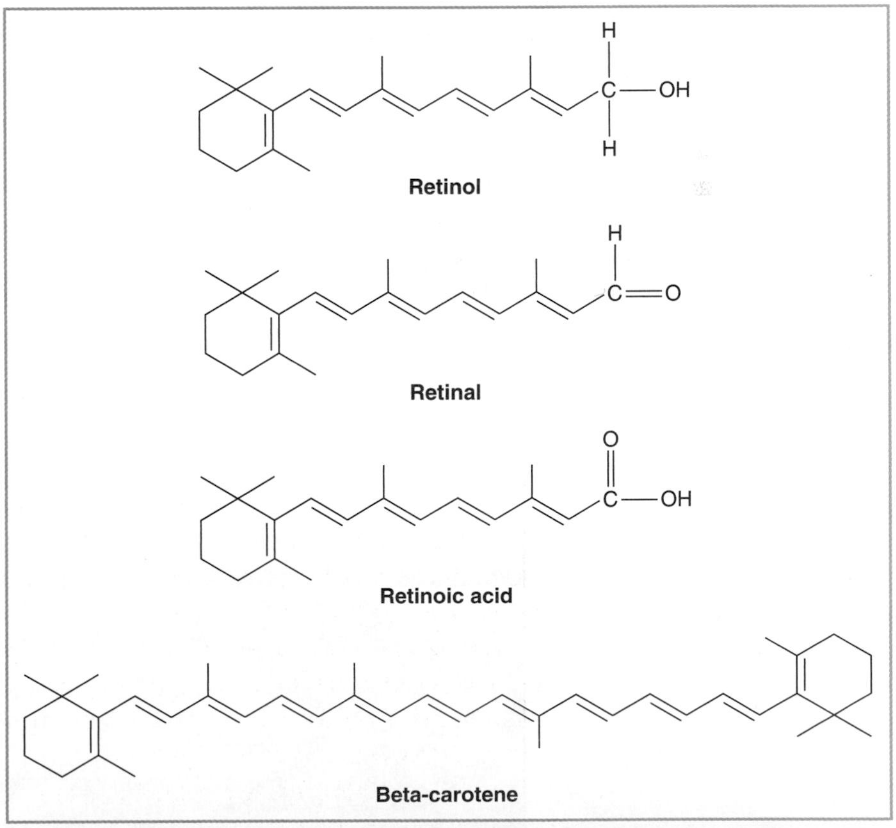

FIGURE 6–1 • STRUCTURE OF VITAMIN A

HYPERKERATOSIS Thickening of the skin's stratum corneum layer.

XEROPHTHALMIA An eye disease marked by dryness of the conjunctiva and cornea due to vitamin A deficiency.

mucus to moisten the lung's lining, the tiny hairlike structures that sweep out bacteria and foreign substances cannot perform properly. Vitamin A derivatives have been used for years to fight acne as well. A topical form of vitamin A is used as short-term treatment to lessen wrinkles in the skin. Beta-carotene, in addition to its function as provitamin A, also behaves as a mild antioxidant.

Dietary Requirement

The Recommended Dietary Allowance (RDA) for vitamin A is 900 micrograms retinol activity equivalents (RAE) per day for college-age men and 700 micrograms RAE for women. One RAE of vitamin A equals 1 microgram of retinol.

A larger intake is required if vitamin A is obtained in other forms or from vitamin precursors (Box 6–1). This is still a very small amount. For example, assume that, although the required daily intake changes slightly over time, the daily requirement of vitamin A needed during college remains constant. A college female then would need 700 micrograms RAE each day, 365 days per year, over a lifetime of 70 years. That adds up to 17.9 grams RAE, or approximately 1/2 ounce of vitamin A for a lifetime. So from birth until death, the student's required vitamin A could be stored as retinol in a half-full salt shaker. The requirement is small, but it is essential; without vitamin A, individuals cannot maintain health.

Deficiency and Toxicity

Vitamin A deficiency is rare in the United States, but this deficiency is still found in other parts of the world. Night blindness, an early deficiency symptom sometimes experienced in developing countries, is completely reversible if caught in time.

Another symptom of vitamin A deficiency is **hyperkeratosis**, a condition in which the skin becomes dry and rough. Another symptom occurs in the eye where the cells stop secreting mucus, resulting in extremely dry tissue and scarring of the cornea (outer surface). Foamy patches, known as Bitot's spots, can develop, resulting in total blindness. This process, called **xerophthalmia**, is irreversible unless it is caught in time and affects millions of children worldwide.

Vitamin A deficiency is a major cause of childhood blindness worldwide, accounting for thousands of cases per year (Institute of Medicine 2001). In certain parts of China, children receive vitamin A injections every six months to prevent blindness.

Vitamin A deficiency may occur if the nutrients that help metabolize and transport vitamin A—zinc, protein, and fat—are not included in the diet.

Vitamin A is fat-soluble and is stored in the fatty tissues of the body. Because it is stored, excess consumption is possible. Taking excessive supplements (in the range of 3,000 RAEs) of vitamin A could lead to toxicity, causing severe headaches, nausea, lethargy, skin rash, and hair loss. Very high intakes can cause death. One of the first accounts of vitamin A toxicity, however, involved a food rather than a supplement. Eskimos in

---

BOX 6–1 • APPROXIMATE EQUIVALENTS

1 retinol activity equivalent (RAE)	= 1 microgram of retinol
	= 12 micrograms dietary beta-carotene
	= 24 micrograms dietary carotenoids
	= 3.3 IU (international units)[a]

[a]International units (IU) of vitamin A are an inexact and outdated method of measuring vitamin A. Nevertheless, dietary supplement labels still list amounts in IU.

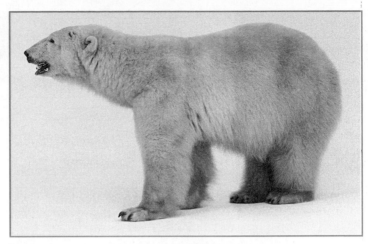

A polar bear's liver contains a toxic amount of vitamin A.
© Jerry Young

arctic regions reported that consuming polar bear liver was toxic. Yet consuming liver from walrus and other animals was not. Scientists found that walrus livers contain normal amounts of vitamin A, while polar bear livers contain large amounts. Humans who consume polar bear liver die quickly. A 6-ounce serving of polar bear liver contains over 1,000,000 RAE of vitamin A (Rodahl 1949).

Food Sources

Animal foods provide preformed vitamin A as retinol. Examples include liver, egg yolks, whole milk, milk fat products (such as butter, cream, cheeses, and ice cream), and cod liver oil. Manufacturers who sell skim milk and margarine in the United States are required to fortify them with vitamin A (Table 6–1).

The main provitamin A form is beta-carotene. It is found in plant products, such as fruits and vegetables. Beta-carotene is a yellowish-orange pigment. Generally, chlorophyll (a deep green pigment) masks beta-carotene. Green as well as orange-colored fruits and vegetables are rich in carotenoids. These include sweet potatoes, winter squash, pumpkin, carrots, cantaloupes, spinach, collard greens, turnip greens, and romaine lettuce. Fruits and vegetables that have color only in the peel, like cucumbers, or in the outer leaves, like iceberg lettuce, are not good sources of vitamin A.

Stability

Vitamin A is destroyed by oxygen. Proper care in preparing and storing food helps prevent vitamin A loss. Airtight storage containers, lids on pots, and quick preparation can help. Vitamin E acts as an antioxidant for vitamin A. Although destroyed by oxygen, vitamin A is more stable than most vitamins when heated.

Vitamin D

Vitamin D is called the sunshine vitamin because the human body converts cholesterol into vitamin D in the presence of sunlight. Rickets, caused by a lack of vitamin D, was widespread in Europe in the eighteenth century and commonly afflicted children. This may in part have been caused by much of the population moving from farms to cities, providing less exposure to sunlight. In 1920, Sir Edward Mellanby discovered that rickets was caused by a deficiency in a trace component of the diet that was found in cod liver oil (University of California, Riverside 1999).

TABLE 6–1 • FOOD SOURCES OF VITAMIN A

Food	Serving	International Units (IU)	% DVᵃ
Liver, beef (cooked)	3 oz.	27,185	545
Liver, chicken (cooked)	3 oz.	13,325	245
Egg substitute (fortified)	1/4 cup	1,300	25
Fat-free milk (fortified with vitamin A)	1 cup	500	10
Cheese, cheddar	1 oz.	284	6
Milk, whole (3.25% fat)	1 cup	249	5
Egg substitute	1/2 cup	226	5
Carrots (juice)	1/2 cup	22,600	450
Carrots (slices, boiled)	1/2 cup	13,400	270
Carrot (raw)	7 1/2 inches	8,600	175
Sweet potatoes (canned, drained, whole)	1/2 cup	7,000	140
Spinach (frozen, boiled)	1/2 cup	7,400	150
Kale (frozen, boiled)	1/2 cup	9,600	190
Vegetable soup (canned, chunky, ready-to-serve)	1 cup	5,800	115
Cantaloupe (raw)	1 cup	5,400	110
Spinach (raw)	1 cup	2,800	55
Apricots with skin (juice pack)	1/2	2,000	40
Apricot nectar (canned)	1/2 cup	1,600	35
Oatmeal, instant (fortified, plain, prepared with water)	1 packet	1,200	25
Tomato juice (canned)	6 oz.	820	15
Peaches (canned, juice pack)	2 halves	470	10
Peas (frozen, boiled)	1/2 cup	500	10
Peaches (halves or sliced, canned in water)	1/2 cup	470	10
Pepper, sweet, red (raw)	1 ring, 3 inches in diameter by 1/4-inch thick	300	6
Peach (raw)	1 medium	300	6

ᵃThe Daily Value (DV) for vitamin A is 5,000 IU (1,500 micrograms retinol).
Source: National Institutes of Health, http://www.cc.nih.gov/ccc/supplements/vita.html (accessed July 31, 2008).

Function

Vitamin D is a fat-soluble vitamin. Similar to the other fat-soluble vitamins, many compounds have varying levels of vitamin D activity. The two main forms of vitamin D are **ergocalciferol** (vitamin D_2), found in plants, and **cholecalciferol** (vitamin D_3), found in animal products. The liver and kidneys must transform either form of vitamin D obtained from food into the active form. As one might expect, a disease of these organs can cause vitamin D deficiency.

Vitamin D synthesis begins with the precursor 7-dehydrocholesterol, which the liver manufactures from cholesterol. (So despite all of the negative press that cholesterol has received, vitamin D synthesis demonstrates one of cholesterol's essential body functions.) This precursor for vitamin D is transferred to the skin, where it is irradiated by the sun's ultraviolet rays and becomes previtamin D_3 (cholecalciferol). The cholecalciferol enters the blood and travels back to the liver, where it is converted to 25-hydroxy vitamin D_3. This must then go to the kidneys for conversion to the active form 1,25-dihydroxy vitamin D_3 (calcitriol).

Vitamin D is essential for calcium utilization. It increases the absorption of calcium from food in the intestine and regulates the calcium going into and out of the bones. More recently science has demonstrated that vitamin D may affect the growth of cancerous tumors because some cancer cells have receptors for vitamin D (Leach et al. 2003). Calcitriol raises calcium levels in the body and helps prevent osteoporosis.

Dietary Requirement

The adequate intake (AI) for vitamin D for college-age males and females is 5 micrograms per day or 200 international units (IU). Earlier we noted that a salt shaker half filled with retinol would provide a lifetime supply of vitamin A. The requirement for vitamin D is even smaller. If that same shaker were filled with vitamin D, one small shake, comprising just a few grains, would fulfill a 70-year life span. This is a very small amount; yet without it, we suffer disease and deformity.

Deficiency and Toxicity

Inadequate intake of vitamin D in children can lead to **rickets**, which causes bones to soften and flare out. This condition, if untreated, produces bowed legs, knock-knee, and a distorted rib cage. Vitamin D deficiency in adults can lead to **osteomalacia**, a softening of the bones. Some antacids and some anticonvulsant drugs may contribute to vitamin D deficiency.

Toxic doses of vitamin D can cause headaches, weakness, weight loss, constipation, and calcification of soft tissue.

Food and Other Sources

Vitamin D, the precursor of the hormone 1,25-dihydroxy vitamin D_3, is technically not a vitamin because the body makes it when sunlight hits the skin. Few foods provide vitamin D. Light-skinned people can get sufficient vitamin D provided their hands, face, and arms are exposed to the sun's rays for 15 minutes a few times a week. Dark-skinned people require about three hours of sun exposure weekly to get the same amount of vitamin D from the sun (Clemens et al. 1982). (These time recommendations are based on mid-latitude sun exposure on a clear summer day.)

Many people may lack enough sun exposure to manufacture vitamin D for at least a month or two each year depending on where they live. Those residing as far north in the United States as an imaginary line connecting Baltimore, Cincinnati, Topeka, Denver, and Sacramento could be deficient. Individuals living on or above a line drawn from Boston to Milwaukee, Minneapolis, and Boise also are unlikely to receive adequate sun exposure (Tufts University Diet and Nutrition Letter 1995).

ERGOCALCIFEROL A plant form of vitamin D.

CHOLECALCIFEROL An inactive dietary form of vitamin D.

CALCITRIOL A fully activated hormone form of vitamin D.

RICKETS A disease, especially in children, caused by vitamin D deficiency and marked by a softening of the bones.

OSTEOMALACIA A disease in adults caused by vitamin D deficiency and marked by a softening of the bones.

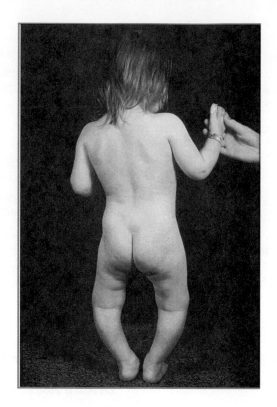

This child inflicted with rickets is showing the characteristic symptom, bowed legs.

Photo Researchers, Inc.

Relying on the sun is an imperfect method for achieving adequate vitamin D levels. Sunbathers should spread out exposure to avoid overexposure and the danger of skin cancer. Heavy clouds, smoke, or smog block ultraviolet rays from the sun that produce vitamin D. Dark-skinned people living in smoggy northern cities are more prone to rickets than are light-skinned people (Whitney and Rolfes 1996).

Ultraviolet rays from tanning lamps also stimulate vitamin D synthesis. However, the U.S. Food and Drug Administration warns that ill-filtered lamps place consumers as risk for skin cancer, burns, and damage to eyes and blood vessels (for more information, see FDA http://www.fda.gov/cdrh/tanning/).

Fatty fish and fish oil are considered good food sources of vitamin D_3, or cholecalciferol. Small amounts of vitamin D are found in eggs, butter, and liver as well. Vitamin D_2, ergocalciferol, is found in plants. Irradiation of ergocalciferol produces synthetic vitamin D (Table 6–2).

In the United States, where all milk is fortified with vitamin D (to a level of 400 IUs per quart), milk is an excellent source. Fortifying milk was a logical move, given vitamin D's role in calcium metabolism. In fact, milk is one of the best sources of calcium. Besides milk, cod liver oil is a formidable source of vitamin D, with one teaspoon providing the RDA. Individuals should avoid amounts higher than one teaspoon because too much vitamin D is toxic.

Stability

Vitamin D is stable under the influence of heat, oxygen, and alkaline substances. Opinions differ whether storage, processing, and cooking have any effect on vitamin D.

Vitamin E

Evans and Bishop discovered vitamin E in 1922 at the University of California, Berkley. They found that a substance in oil was necessary for rat reproduction. Without it, the fetus

TABLE 6-2 • FOOD SOURCES OF VITAMIN D

Food	Serving	International Units (IU)	% DVᵃ
Cod liver oil	1 Tbsp.	1,360	340
Salmon (cooked)	3 1/2 oz.	360	90
Mackerel (cooked)	3 1/2 oz.	345	90
Sardines (canned in oil, drained)	3 1/2 oz.	250	70
Tuna fish (canned in oil)	3 oz.	200	50
Milk, nonfat, reduced fat, and whole, vitamin D (fortified)	1 cup	98	25
Margarine (fortified)	1 Tbsp.	60	15
Cereal grain bars (fortified with 10% of the DV)	1 each	50	10
Pudding (prepared from mix and made with vitamin D, fortified milk)	1/2 cup	50	10
Dry cereal (vitamin D, fortified with 10%ᵇ of DV)	3/4 cup	40	8
Liver, beef (cooked)	3 1/2 oz.	30	8
Egg (vitamin D is present in the yolk)	1 whole	20	6

ᵃThe Daily Value (DV) for vitamin D is 400 IU.
ᵇOther cereals may be fortified with more or less vitamin D.
Source: National Institutes of Health, http://www.cc.nih.gov/ccc/supplements/vita.html (accessed July 31, 2008).

did not survive (Evans and Bishop 1922). This substance, labeled vitamin E, was later isolated and deemed essential for humans. Its chemical name, tocopherol, comes from the Greek root words *tokos,* meaning "birth," and *phero,* meaning "to bring forth."

Function

Vitamin E is a fat-soluble antioxidant that protects body cells from oxidative damage. An example of oxidation is when the exposed surface of a cut apple turns brown. In this case, oxygen combines with compounds in the apple's exposed area, and the fruit begins to break down. Submerging the apple in a vitamin C solution (another antioxidant) prevents oxidation, and the apple remains white.

Vitamin E performs a similar antioxidant function in the human body. It prevents oxidation damage to body cells. Vitamin E, like vitamin A, is actually a family of compounds. These compounds are called **tocopherols**, comprising alpha, beta, gamma, and delta forms. Alpha-tocopherol is the only one with any significant vitamin E activity, and thus, vitamin E content is usually stated in milligrams of alpha-tocopherol.

Vitamin E prevents oxygen from destroying vitamins C and A in the body. Sometimes manufacturers include vitamin E in processed foods containing fat. The antioxidant function of the vitamin E serves as a food preservative that prevents fat rancidity and imparts a vitamin E benefit to humans.

TOCOPHEROL Any of the different forms of vitamin E.

Vitamins **111**

Vitamin E has been the subject of many claims, especially those promoting disease cures and athletic performance. To date, however, research has not supported many of these claims. Its initial discovery as a substance necessary for reproduction in rats have given rise to fertility and sexual performance claims in humans. None of these claims have been supported by research either. There is, however, a connection between vitamin E and preventing the formation of nitrosamines (carcinogens formed from nitrites and amines).

Nitrites are naturally found in the soil, in plants, and in saliva. Sodium nitrite is a preservative added to foods, such as vacuum-packed cold cuts and canned meats, to prevent botulin formation. Botulin is the food toxin responsible for botulism. Yet nitrites can combine with amines, which occur naturally in our bodies and in food, to create carcinogenic compounds. Vitamin E may prevent this from happening.

Recent interest in vitamin E concerns its role as an antioxidant that may prevent heart disease when given in large doses (from 100 to 800 milligrams of alpha-tocopherol). Early studies showed that vitamin E could prevent the oxidation of low-density lipoprotein (LDL) cholesterol. Oxidation of LDL is linked with an increased risk of heart disease. Yet the results of large-scale studies of vitamin E with human subjects have not supported the initial findings (Blumberg and Block 1994). Short study duration may account for vitamin E's failure to reduce the risk of heart disease.

Because vitamin E is a nonspecific antioxidant, one may theorize low intakes are contributing factors in many disease states. Vitamin E has also been indicated for treatment of ulcers, wounds, scar tissue, and circulatory problems of the legs. Again, the usefulness of these treatments has not been proven.

Dietary Requirement

The RDA for vitamin E, which is based on the average polyunsaturated fat intake, is 15 milligrams alpha-tocopherol for adults. Consuming more polyunsaturated fat than average subsequently increases the body's need for vitamin E.

Deficiency and Toxicity

The average intake of vitamin E in the U.S. diet is only about half the RDA, which places a large percentage of the population at risk for chronic disease. Although fairly large doses of vitamin E, more than 50 times the RDA, have not been shown to be toxic, too much vitamin E may reduce blood clotting to an abnormally low level. Individuals taking blood thinning medication, for example, should consult a healthcare provider before taking vitamin E supplements.

Food Sources

Nuts, seeds, and oils in the form of salad dressing, cooking oil, and margarine supply most dietary polyunsaturated fat. These foods are also the richest sources of vitamin E.

Wheat germ oil is another potent source of vitamin E. Green leafy vegetables are also noteworthy sources. Whole grains contain vitamin E, whereas their refined counterparts do not (Table 6–3).

Stability

Vitamin E can be lost during food preparation and storage if it comes in contact with oxygen. To prevent losses, keep nuts, seeds, or beans whole when possible and process them only when needed. For example, incorporate whole soybeans into recipes as opposed to soy oil. The intact nut or seed preserves vitamin E content. Once whole foods are processed their vitamin E content oxidizes under oxygen exposure. In addition, store foods in airtight containers restricting oxygen and light exposure.

TABLE 6-3 • FOOD SOURCES OF VITAMIN E

Food	Serving	International Units (IU)	% DV[a]
Wheat germ oil	1 Tbsp.	20	100
Almonds (dry roasted)	1 oz.	7	40
Safflower oil	1 Tbsp.	6	30
Corn oil	1 Tbsp.	2	10
Soybean oil	1 Tbsp.	2	10
Peanuts (dry roasted)	1 oz.	2	10
Spinach (frozen)	1/2 cup	1.5	7
Mixed nuts with peanuts (oil roasted)	1 oz.	1.5	7
Mayonnaise (made with soybean oil)	1 Tbsp.	1.5	7
Broccoli (frozen, chopped, boiled)	1/2 cup	1.5	7
Dandelion greens (boiled)	1/2 cup	1	5
Pistachio nuts (dry roasted)	1 oz.	1	5
Spinach (frozen, boiled)	1/2 cup	1	5
Kiwi	1 medium fruit	1	5

[a]The Daily Value (DV) for vitamin E is 30 international units (or 20 milligrams).
Source: National Institutes of Health, http://www.cc.nih.gov/ccc/supplements/vita.html (accessed July 31, 2008).

Vitamin K

Henrich Dam, a Danish biochemist, discovered vitamin K while working on another dietary component. He fed chicks a cholesterol-free diet that was also low in fat and discovered that the chicks developed a blood disorder. When he added cholesterol back to the diet, however, this disorder remained uncured. He surmised that an additional dietary factor had been removed from the diet. His work then demonstrated that the hemorrhagic condition could be cured by adding a plant extract.

Dam continued his research, and in 1939, scientists isolated the plant component responsible for the effect. They named it vitamin K for "Koagulation." Dam received the Nobel Prize in medicine for his work on vitamin K (Dam 1934; Stipanuck 2000).

Function

PHYLLOQUINONE Vitamin K_1, a major form of vitamin K found in plant foods.

MENAQUINONE Vitamin K_2. Menaquinone is synthesized by intestinal bacterial flora.

MENADIONE Synthetic vitamin K. Menadione is soluble in water.

There are two naturally occurring forms of vitamin K, **phylloquinone** and **menaquinone.**, Phylloquinone (K_1) comes from plants, while bacteria in the intestinal tract produce menaquinone (K_2). There is also a synthetic form of vitamin K called **menadione**. Menadione has twice the biological activity as natural forms of vitamin K.

Vitamin K is necessary for blood clotting. Without vitamin K, blood would not clot. Physicians sometimes provide vitamin K injections before surgery to prevent hemorrhaging. Infants receive vitamin K immediately after birth for a similar purpose. The baby's gut is sterile in its first few days after birth. No intestinal bacteria are present to produce vitamin K until bacterial flora are established. Vitamin K is also necessary for maintaining a healthy skeleton and a healthy immune system.

Dietary Requirement

Vitamin K does not have an established RDA. An adequate intake (AI) is set at 120 micrograms for adult males and 90 micrograms for adult females.

Deficiency and Toxicity

Vitamin K deficiency results in excessive bleeding. Toxicity can occur from excessive doses of the synthetic vitamin. Symptoms of toxicity include hemolytic anemia, an accelerated breakdown of red blood cells, jaundice, and brain damage.

Food and Other Sources

Vitamin K is a fat-soluble vitamin produced naturally by plants and bacteria and synthetically in laboratories. Bacteria in the intestines that produce vitamin K supply some of the body's daily requirement. Most of the body's vitamin K, however, comes from plants in the diet. Excellent food sources of vitamin K (phylloquinone) include soybeans, cabbage, broccoli, cauliflower, and dark green leafy vegetables, such as kale. Animal products, such as pork liver and eggs, provide vitamin K as menaquinone in much smaller amounts compared with plants (Table 6–4).

An individual on a long-term antibiotic regimen may require oral vitamin K supplementation because antibiotics sometimes kill the vitamin-K-producing bacteria in the colon. People on blood-thinning medication (anticoagulants) need to watch their vitamin K intake from foods. Mineral oil and cholestyramine (a cholesterol-lowering drug) may interfere with vitamin K absorption.

TABLE 6–4 • FOOD SOURCES OF VITAMIN K			
Food	**Serving**	**Micrograms**	**% DV**[a]
Olive oil	1 Tbsp.	6.6	8
Soybean oil	1 Tbsp.	26.1	33
Canola oil	1 Tbsp.	19.7	25
Mayonnaise	1 Tbsp.	11.9	15
Broccoli (cooked, chopped)	1 cup	420	525
Kale (raw, chopped)	1 cup	547	684
Spinach (raw, chopped)	1 cup	120	150
Leaf lettuce (raw, shredded)	1 cup	118	148
Swiss chard (raw, chopped)	1 cup	299	374
Watercress (raw, chopped)	1 cup	85	106
Parsley (raw, chopped)	1 cup	324	405

[a]The Daily Value (DV) for vitamin K is 80 micrograms.
Source: Adapted from Linus Pauling Institute, http://lpi.oregonstate.edu/infocenter/vitamins/vitaminK.

Stability

Vitamin K is stable when heated but unstable under the influence of alkalis and strong acids, oxidation, and light. Therefore, cooks should never prepare green vegetables with baking soda, which is very alkaline. Although this preserves the green color of the vegetables, it destroys vitamins. Putting a lid on the cooking pot helps prevent vitamin loss from air (oxidation) and light, though it has a negative effect on color. The best strategy to preserve vitamin K in green vegetables is to cook them as quickly as possible.

WATER-SOLUBLE VITAMINS

The B Vitamins

COENZYME A molecule that attaches to an enzyme to activate or enhance the enzyme's function.

The B vitamins include thiamin, riboflavin, niacin, biotin, pantothenic acid, folate, vitamin B_6, and vitamin B_{12}. These vitamins function primarily as **coenzymes**. A coenzyme is a molecule that activates or enhances the action of an enzyme.

B vitamins were widespread in the food supply until manufacturers began processing foods. As a result, refined grain products like white flour and white rice had their B vitamins processed out. Numerous white flour products now have a few of their B vitamins replaced as a result of a U.S. government mandate in the 1940s which required refined bread and cereal products to be enriched with thiamin, riboflavin, and niacin. In 1998 folic acid was added to the enrichment process. White rice is enriched with thiamin and riboflavin but not niacin, which would make the rice yellowish.

Enrichment returns the major B vitamins needed for the utilization of carbohydrates and the prevention of deficiencies. Over time, the enrichment campaign has eradicated two vitamin B deficiency diseases: beriberi, caused by a deficiency of thiamin (vitamin B_1), and pellagra, caused by a lack of niacin (vitamin B_3). Vitamins B_6, B_{12}, pantothenic acid, and biotin are B vitamins not supplied through enrichment.

All of the B vitamins are water-soluble, and thus individuals should take care to prevent their loss during food preparation. Cooking with minimal amounts of water preserves B vitamins. Cooking liquids should be saved, and soaking should be avoided. Cooking liquids can be used again to make soups, gravies, and sauces.

Washing vegetables quickly instead of letting then stand in water helps retain their B vitamins. The use of baking soda to preserve color during cooking destroys B vitamins in vegetables, so this practice is not recommended.

Thiamin (Vitamin B_1)

Casmir Funk discovered thiamin in 1912. He found an antiberiberi vitamin in rice extracts (Funk and Dubin 1920). Other researchers looking for an antiberiberi factor found that hens given boiled polished rice instead of the usual raw husked rice developed beriberi. In addition, they found that the constituent in the raw husked rice responsible for preventing beriberi was water-soluble. Eijkman's work to combat beriberi earned him a Nobel Prize in 1929 (Liljestrand 1929).

Function

Vitamin B_1 functions as the coenzyme for thiamin pyrophosphate (TPP). It is central to the conversion of glucose to energy in energy metabolism. TPP is part of an enzyme system converting pyruvate to acetyl-Coenzyme A. Thiamin is constructed of two rings connected by a carbon atom. The bond connecting the rings is unstable in the presence of heat or alkalinity.

Dietary Requirement

The RDA for thiamin is based on total calorie intake: 0.5 milligrams per 1,000 kilocalories. That equates to 1.1 milligrams per day for adult females and 1.2 milligrams per day for adult males.

Deficiency and Toxicity

Early symptoms of a thiamin deficiency include mouth soreness and a bright red, swollen tongue. Other symptoms are fatigue, muscle weakness, and nerve damage. Because thiamin is very important in carbohydrate metabolism, a deficiency will cause decreased appetite and weight loss. Beriberi is triggered by thiamin deficiency and is associated with malnutrition.

Alcoholics commonly experience thiamin deficiency. Vitamin B therapy is a necessary part of an alcohol recovery program; however, it is not always effective. Alcohol interferes with mechanisms that regulate food intake, and alcoholics tend to eat poorly. The toxic effects of alcohol interfere with the metabolism and storage of nutrients. Malabsorption of nutrients occurs in response to alcohol ingestion, hindering thiamin metabolism. The most severe form of thiamin deficiency is **Wernicke's encephalopathy**, characterized by visual disorders, confusion, and coma (Zeman 1983).

There are no reports of thiamin toxicity. As will be seen, this is true for many of the water-soluble vitamins.

WERNICKE'S ENCEPHALOPATHY
An acute brain disease caused by thiamin deficiency and seen in alcohol abusers. Sufferers lack muscle coordination and experience confusion.

Food Sources

Major food sources of thiamin are enriched flour, pork, dried beans, and whole grains (Table 6–5). In the United States, grain products supply 42% of thiamin in the average diet, whereas meat, poultry, and fish supply almost 25%. The mean thiamin intake of the U.S. population is more than 100% of the RDA. Excess vitamin B_1 is excreted in the urine. For those cultures that consume raw fish frequently, it is noteworthy that thiamin is made unavailable by the enzyme in raw fish, thiaminase.

Stability

Thiamin is the most unstable of all of the B vitamins; however, synthetic B_1 is more stable. To prevent thiamin loss, do not soak food and cook in as little water as possible. Steaming rather than boiling is the preferred cooking method for preserving thiamin. Save cooking water for use in sauces, stocks, or gravies.

LESS COMMONLY EATEN FOODS THAT ARE RICH SOURCES OF B VITAMINS

Liver (B_1, B_2, B_3, B_6, B_{12}, folate, pantothenic acid, biotin)

Yeast (B_2, B_3, B_6, folate, pantothenic acid, biotin)

Wheat germ (B_1, B_2, B_3, B_6, folate, pantothenic acid)

Peanuts (B_1, B_3, pantothenic acid)

Soybeans (B_1, B_3, biotin)

Heart (B_2, B_{12}, biotin)

Kidney (B_1, B_{12}, biotin)

Riboflavin (Vitamin B_2)

In the early 1900s, scientists considered riboflavin and thiamin to be the same vitamin. Riboflavin was eventually isolated from vitamin B_1 (thiamin) and named vitamin B_2. Its name refers to the vitamin's yellow-green color; in Latin, *flav* means "yellow." Kuhn, Szent-György, and Wagne-Jaunegy were the first to isolate riboflavin in 1933. Kuhn later won a Nobel Prize for his work.

Function

Vitamin B_2, or riboflavin, is involved in cell respiration and the health of tissues like the lining of the esophagus. Riboflavin also helps change the amino acid tryptophan in food into niacin (B_3). Like thiamin, riboflavin also helps convert glucose to energy as part of the coenzymes flavin adenine dinucleotide (FAD) and flavin adenine mononucleotide (FMN).

TABLE 6–5 • FOOD SOURCES OF THIAMIN

Food	Serving	Milligrams	% DV[a]
Lentils (cooked)	1/2 cup	0.17	11
Peas (cooked)	1/2 cup	0.21	14
Long-grain brown rice (cooked)	1 cup	0.19	13
Long-grain white rice (enriched, cooked)	1 cup	0.26	17
Long-grain white rice (unenriched, cooked)	1 cup	0.03	2
Whole-wheat bread	1 slice	0.10	7
White bread (enriched)	1 slice	0.12	8
Fortified breakfast cereal	1 cup	0.5–2.0	33–133
Wheat germ breakfast cereal	1 cup	1.89	126
Pork (lean, cooked)	3 oz.	0.74	50
Brazil nuts	1 oz.	0.28	19
Pecans	1 oz.	0.13	9
Spinach (cooked)	1/2 cup	0.09	6
Orange	1 fruit	0.11	7
Cantaloupe	1/2 fruit	0.10	7
Milk	1 cup	0.10	7
Egg (cooked)	1 large	0.03	2

[a]The Daily Value (DV) for thiamin is 1.5 milligrams.
Source: Adapted from Linus Pauling Institute, http://lpi.oregonstate.edu/infocenter/vitamins/thiamin/.

Dietary Requirement

Like thiamin, the RDA for riboflavin is based on total calorie intake: 0.6 milligram per 1,000 kilocalories. Adult females require 1.1 milligrams per day and adult males 1.3 milligrams per day.

Deficiency and Toxicity

Riboflavin deficiency begins with fissures, or cracks, that radiate from the corners of the mouth onto the skin and can extend into the mucous membrane. This symptom is called angular **stomatitis** and is followed by **cheilosis**, painful cracks on the upper and lower lips.

Another classic symptom of riboflavin deficiency is a magenta tongue. Purplish-red in color, the tongue is sore, swollen, and glossy. Other body areas affected by riboflavin deficiency are the eyes, which feel gritty and burn or itch; the nostrils, which develop weepy, crusty lesions; and the genitalia, which develop itchy dermatitis. Riboflavin is needed for growth, and it plays a role in eye health. Inadequate riboflavin may lead to cataracts.

Like thiamin, riboflavin is quickly excreted and there are no reports of toxicity.

STOMATITIS An inflammatory mouth disease resulting from riboflavin deficiency.

CHEILOSIS An abnormal condition of the lips characterized by scaling of the mouth's surface and fissure formation in the corners.

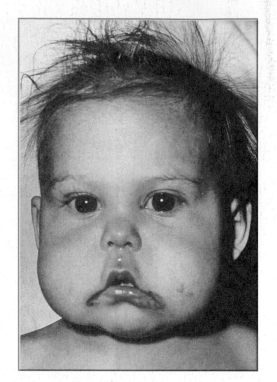

This child is suffering from a deficiency in riboflavin, displaying the typical symptoms.
Centers for Disease Control and Prevention (CDC)

Food Sources

Milk is the best source of riboflavin and provides most of the riboflavin in the American diet. Enriched and whole-grain products, meat, liver, poultry, fish, and dark leafy green vegetables provide most of the remaining riboflavin consumed (Table 6–6).

Stability

Exposure to light reduces vitamin B_2 content. Therefore, opaque containers for milk, lids on pots during cooking, and quick preparation help conserve B_2. In addition, prevention of water loss while cooking maintains vitamin content. Riboflavin is fairly stable under conditions of heat and alkalinity. Since riboflavin is water-soluble, some of it may leach from food during cooking. Avoid soaking food and cook in minimal water to preserve riboflavin content.

Niacin (Vitamin B_3)

Niacin was first isolated in 1911 from rice polishing, but researchers did not determine it to be a vitamin until 1937 when they demonstrated that niacin cured black tongue in dogs (Stipanuck 2000). One of the earliest records of pellagra was made by the Spanish physician, Casal, in 1735. Pellegra was named *mal de la rosa,* or "red sickness" because of the characteristic redness that appears around the neck. When the disease was first discovered, it was also referred to as *Casal's necklace.* Chickens with pellagra-like symptoms were cured when given niacin, the antipellagra factor (Koehn and Elvehjem 1937).

Function

Vitamin B_3, or niacin, is a coenzyme that helps produce energy in all body cells. Similar to thiamin and riboflavin, niacin functions as part of two coenzymes, nicotinamide adenine dinucleotide (NAD) and nicotinamide adenine dinucleotide phosphate (NADP), both necessary in the conversion of glucose to energy. The amino acid tryptophan is a precursor of niacin. Sixty milligrams of tryptophan convert to one milligram of niacin. Milk, which has little niacin, has enough tryptophan to prevent niacin deficiency when consumed on a regular basis.

TABLE 6-6 • FOOD SOURCES OF RIBOFLAVIN

Food	Serving	Milligrams	% DV[a]
Cereal (fortified)	1 cup	0.59 to 2.27	35–134
Milk, nonfat	1 cup	0.34	20
Cheddar cheese	1 oz.	0.11	6
Egg (cooked)	1 large	0.27	16
Almonds	1 oz.	0.24	14
Salmon (broiled)	3 oz.	0.13	8
Halibut (broiled)	3 oz.	0.08	5
Chicken (light meat, roasted)	3 oz.	0.10	6
Chicken (dark meat, roasted)	3 oz.	0.18	11
Beef (cooked)	3 oz.	0.19	11
Broccoli (boiled or steamed, chopped)	1/2 cup	0.09	5
Asparagus (boiled or steamed)	6 spears	0.13	8
Spinach (boiled or steamed)	1/2 cup	0.09	5
Bread, whole wheat	1 slice	0.07	4
Bread, white (enriched)	1 slice	0.09	5

[a]The Daily Value (DV) for riboflavin is 1.7 milligrams.
Source: Adapted from Linus Pauling Institute, http://lpi.oregonstate.edu/infocenter/vitamins/riboflavin.

NIACIN EQUIVALENT (NE) One NE equals one milligram of niacin or 60 milligrams of tryptophan.

Recommendations for niacin intake are given in **niacin equivalents (NEs)** that take into account tryptophan conversion and natural niacin.

In addition to its use as a supplement, niacin has been used as a medicine to effectively reduce very-low-density lipoprotein (VLDL) cholesterol synthesis. The high doses of niacin needed for this treatment, however, cause the objectionable side effects of flushing and itching. Physicians must monitor medicinal doses of niacin, and individuals should refrain from self-prescribing niacin.

Dietary Requirement

The RDA for niacin, as for thiamin and riboflavin, is based on the individual's total caloric intake. Generally, the allowance is 6.6 milligrams NE per 1,000 kilocalories. The RDA for adult females is 14 milligrams per day NE and 16 milligrams per day NE for adult males. Americans' niacin intake appears adequate due to their high dietary protein consumption and their use of enriched flours and grain products.

Deficiency and Toxicity

Pellagra is the disease of niacin deficiency. Its name is derived from two words: *pelle* for skin, and *agra,* which means rough. As you might expect, pellagra is characterized by red, rough skin, and the other symptoms of the disease are known as the 4 Ds—diarrhea, dermatitis, dementia, and death.

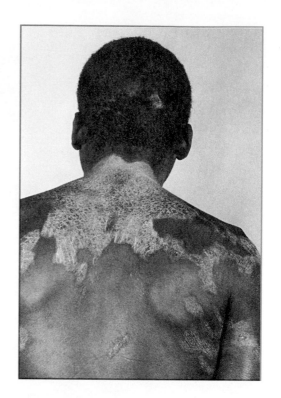

The man suffering from pellagra is displaying the typical symptoms of red, dry skin.
Photo Researchers, Inc.

Food Sources

Meat, poultry, fish, and grain products are the best sources of dietary niacin. In addition, legumes, seeds, and peanut butter are good sources (Table 6–7).

TABLE 6–7 • FOOD SOURCES OF NIACIN			
Food	Serving	Milligrams	% DV[a]
Chicken (light meat, cooked without skin)	3 oz.	10.6	53
Turkey (light meat, cooked without skin)	3 oz.	5.8	29
Beef (lean, cooked)	3 oz.	3.1	16
Salmon (cooked)	3 oz.	8.5	43
Tuna (light, packed in water)	3 oz.	11.3	57
Bread, whole wheat	1 slice	1.1	6
Cereal (unfortified)	1 cup	5–7	25–35
Cereal (fortified)	1 cup	20–27	100–135
Pasta (enriched, cooked)	1 cup	2.3	11
Peanuts (dry roasted)	1 oz.	3.8	19
Lentils (cooked)	1 cup	2.1	11
Lima beans (cooked)	1 cup	1.8	9
Coffee (brewed)	1 cup	0.5	3

[a]The Daily Value (DV) for niacin is 20 milligrams.
Source: Adapted from Linus Pauling Institute, http://lpi.oregonstate.edu/infocenter/vitamins/niacin.

Stability

Niacin is stable in the presence of oxygen and high temperatures. Yet as with the other B vitamins, some niacin may be lost during cooking due to its solubility in water. Use the cooking methods highlighted earlier to prevent leaching of the vitamin.

Pantothenic Acid (Vitamin B$_5$)

Rodger Williams discovered pantothenic acid (vitamin B$_5$) in 1933. Its name is derived from the Greek word *pantos*, which means "everywhere." This is because pantothenic acid is found in all natural foods, both plant and animal.

Structure and Function

Pantothenic acid's function, as seen with the other B vitimins, is central to the conversion of glucose to energy in the body's metabolism. It is part of the enzyme acetyl-CoA, which is the central molecule in glucose metabolism. It is also the primary component in the construction of fatty acids. Chemical reactions that produce antibodies, cholesterol, sterols, and acetylcholine, which regulates nerve tissue, all require acetyl-CoA.

Pantothenic acid is as pervasive in human tissues as it is in food. High concentrations are present in the liver and kidneys, with lesser amounts in the adrenal glands. These glands are important in the stress response and require adequate pantothenic acid to function properly.

Dietary Requirement

Pantothenic acid does not have an RDA. The Adequate Intake is 5 milligrams for adult males and females. Eating a healthful diet will supply adequate amounts of pantothenic acid, and deficiency is uncommon.

Deficiency and Toxicity

Experimentally induced deficiencies of pantothenic acid have caused irritability, restlessness, fatigue following mild exertion, alternating insomnia and sleepiness, vomiting, stomach distress, staggering gait, and tenderness of the heels and feet. Pantothenic acid treatments alleviate the "burning feet syndrome" seen in malnourished individuals. Taking supplements of pantothenic acid over the estimated requirement by even as little as 10 to 20 milligrams can cause diarrhea.

Food Sources

Liver, kidney, yeast, egg yolk, salmon, and milk are among the best sources of pantothenic acid. Whole wheat is also a good source of pantothenic acid, with 50% found in the bran. Meats, poultry, and legumes provide good amounts, whereas lesser amounts are found in fruits and vegetables (Table 6–8).

Stability

Cooking causes some pantothenic acid loss because heat readily destroys the vitamin. Canned foods therefore have less pantothenic acid because they are heated to high temperatures during the canning process. As with the other B vitamins, preventing water loss during cooking preserves pantothenic acid.

Vitamin B$_6$

Pyridoxine was first isolated by Kuhn in 1938. It was known as the antidermatitis vitamin (Kuhn 1938).

TABLE 6–8 • FOOD SOURCES OF PANTOTHENIC ACID

Food	Serving	Milligrams	% DV[a]
Fish, cod (cooked)	3 oz.	0.15	2
Tuna (canned)	3 oz.	0.18	2
Chicken (cooked)	3 oz.	0.98	1
Egg (cooked)	1 large	0.61	6
Milk	1 cup	0.79	8
Yogurt	8 oz.	1.35	14
Broccoli (steamed, chopped)	1/2 cup	0.40	4
Lentils (cooked)	1/2 cup	0.64	6
Split peas (cooked)	1/2 cup	0.59	6
Avocado, California	1 whole	1.68	17
Sweet potato (cooked)	1 medium (1/2 cup)	0.74	7
Mushrooms (raw, chopped)	1/2 cup	0.51	5
Lobster (cooked)	3 oz.	0.24	2
Bread, whole wheat	1 slice	0.16	2

[a]The Daily Value (DV) for pantothenic acid is 10 milligrams.
Source: Adapted from Linus Pauling Institute, http://lpi.oregonstate.edu/infocenter/vitamins/pa.

Function

Vitamin B_6 occurs in three forms: pyridoxine, pyridoxal, and pyridoxamine. All three forms are found in foods. Pyridoxine functions as a coenzyme in at least 50 different enzyme reactions. The most important of these reactions maintains nerve tissue and forms some of the neurotransmitters that allow nerve cells to communicate with each other. Pyridoxine also helps metabolize fatty acids.

Vitamin B_6 is also needed for the enzymes involved in the synthesis and catabolism of all amino acids. It is involved in the transformation of the amino acid tryptophan to niacin (B_3) as well as red blood cell regeneration, antibody production, insulin production, and absorption of vitamin B_{12}. Like the other B vitamins, vitamin B_6 is needed for metabolizing carbohydrates.

Some nutritionists have suggested that vitamin B_6 has a role in relieving premenstrual syndrome (PMS) symptoms; however, its effectiveness has not yet been proven. It is also used as a part of the therapy for counteracting carpal tunnel syndrome, a disorder of the hands and wrists caused by repetitive motion. Higher levels of vitamin B_6 have been related to better cognitive function (Riggs et al. 1996).

Dietary Requirement

Vitamin B_6 is necessary for protein metabolism. The National Research Council of the National Academy of Sciences, which produces the Recommended Dietary Allowances, bases the requirement for vitamin B_6 on protein intake. The RDA for B_6 is 1.3 milligrams per day for college-age males and females.

Deficiency and Toxicity

Liberal protein intake in the United States helps prevent vitamin B_6 deficiency. Deficiency is seen, however, when drugs are used that antagonize B_6 functions. Examples are alcohol, hydrazine drugs, isoniazid, penicillamine. Deficiency symptoms include depression, irritability, nausea, greasy and flaky skin, and microcytic hypochromic anemia (characterized by small, pale red blood cells).

Neurological problems develop with excess intakes of 2 to 6 grams of B_6 per day. The symptoms are numbness and tingling in the hands and feet, difficulty walking, and sharp pains in the spine and other bones. Large doses of vitamin B_6 can cause irreversible nerve damage. Use of birth control pills increases the need for vitamin B_6.

Food Sources

Most of the vitamin B_6 intake in the American diet comes from meat, poultry, fish, fruits, vegetables, and grains. Other excellent sources of B_6 include liver, kidney, peanuts, legumes, whole grains, milk products, bananas, potatoes, avocados, sunflower seeds, wheat germ, and bran. Egg is a moderate source (Table 6–9).

Stability

As with the other B vitamins, use less water while cooking and avoid high heat during food preparation to reduce loss of vitamin B_6. Up to 50% of vitamin B_6 can be lost in cooking and processing.

Folate

Function

Folate is also known as folic acid. You may have seen the term folacin, but it is no longer in use. The chemical name for folate is pteroylglutamic acid (PGA). There are many forms of folate in food, and they vary greatly in their quality.

Folate functions as a coenzyme in reactions involving the transfer of one carbon. This makes folate important in the synthesis of nucleoproteins and in blood cell production. Folate plays an essential role in making new body cells by helping to produce DNA and RNA (the cell's master plan for cell reproduction). Folate is also necessary for amino acid metabolism, and it supplies carbon and hydrogen for methyl groups needed in the metabolic process.

Folate works with vitamin B_{12} to form hemoglobin in red blood cells. In addition, folate helps convert vitamin B_{12} to one of its coenzyme forms. Vitamin B_{12}, in turn, converts folate to its active form.

Folic Acid and Birth Defects
Every year, hundreds of infants are born with the conditions of spina bifida (an open spine) and anencephaly (born without a brain). Hundreds more fetuses with birth defects of this nature (neural tube defects) are aborted. Folate has been indicated as a factor for preventing neural tube defects. Unfortunately, many women do not know they are pregnant in the early weeks—approximately 18 to 26 days after conception, a crucial time when the neural tube is closing. This tube will develop into the spinal cord. If an error occurs at the top of the tube, the child will have no brain and will die at birth. An error further down the tube results in incomplete closure of the spinal cord; children with this condition who survive may

TABLE 6–9 • FOOD SOURCES OF VITAMIN B$_6$

Food	Serving	Milligrams	% DV[a]
Ready-to-eat cereal (100% fortified)	3/4 cup	2.00	100
Potato (baked, flesh and skin)	1 medium	0.70	35
Banana (raw)	1 medium	0.68	34
Garbanzo beans (canned)	1/2 cup	0.57	30
Chicken breast (meat only, cooked)	1/2 breast	0.52	25
Ready-to-eat cereal (25% fortified)	3/4 cup	0.50	25
Oatmeal, instant (fortified)	1 packet	0.42	20
Pork loin (lean only, cooked)	3 oz.	0.42	20
Roast beef, eye of round (lean only, cooked)	3 oz.	0.32	15
Trout, rainbow (cooked)	3 oz.	0.29	15
Sunflower seeds (kernels, dry roasted)	1 oz.	0.23	10
Spinach (frozen, cooked)	1/2 cup	0.14	8
Tomato juice (canned)	6 oz.	0.20	10
Avocado (raw, sliced)	1/2 cup	0.20	10
Salmon, sockeye (cooked)	3 oz.	0.19	10
Tuna (canned in water, drained solids)	3 oz.	0.18	10
Wheat bran (crude or unprocessed)	1/4 cup	0.18	10
Peanut butter, smooth	2 Tbsp.	0.15	8
Walnuts, English/Persian	1 oz.	0.15	8
Soybeans, green (boiled, drained)	1/2 cup	0.05	2
Lima beans (frozen, cooked, drained)	1/2 cup	0.10	6

[a]The Daily Value (DV) for vitamin B$_6$ is 2.0 milligrams.
Source: National Institutes of Health, http://www.cc.nih.gov/ccc/supplements/vita.html (accessed July 31, 2008).

lack bladder and bowel control and suffer paralysis from the waist down or mental retardation.

Consuming 400 micrograms of folate daily should prevent these defects. Women who want to become pregnant should begin taking folic acid one month before conception and continue taking it throughout the first trimester. A healthful diet readily provides 400 micrograms of folate. For example, five fruits and vegetables a day supplies 400 micrograms of folate. Since most women do not consume this amount of folate from diet, food is fortified. Based on the new flour enrichment requirements established in mid-1990s, bread provides significant amounts of the daily requirement for folate (Hine 1996). Folate fortification of grains has more than doubled the mean folate intake in the United States (Bailey, Rampersaud, and Kauwell 2003).

Folic Acid and Heart Disease   Proper folate intake protects against mildly elevated **homocysteine** levels and cardiovascular disease. Homocysteine is a normal and necessary part of human chemistry. Digestion breaks protein into amino acids, one of which is methionine. When the body metabolizes methionine, it releases homocysteine into the bloodstream. Homocysteine is an amino acid used to make protein. Folic acid is needed to convert the homocysteine back to methionine. If folic acid is unavailable, too much homocysteine will be in the bloodstream, which is associated with blood vessel injury. Excess homocysteine is linked to an increased risk of coronary artery disease and stroke. This is because the injured blood vessels attract a buildup of cholesterol-containing plaque. Homocysteine also contributes to clot formation and restriction of blood flow. However, the research is inconclusive as to the effectiveness of lowering homocysteine to reduce the risk of heart disease (Margolas 1998).

Folic Acid and the Elderly   Fortification of food with folate began in January 1998, and since that time some health professionals have expressed concern that it may harm the elderly. Excess folate intake can mask vitamin B_{12} deficiency. Vitamin B_{12} absorption problems are common among the elderly. If folate is given when B_{12} is needed, the folate may cover up the symptoms of B_{12} deficiency. If the B_{12} deficiency continues to be undiagnosed, irreversible neurological damage can occur.

Accurate laboratory tests are available that screen for B_{12} deficiency by obtaining blood concentrations of the metabolite methylmalonic acid. This test does not confuse B_{12} deficiency with folate deficiency.

Dietary Requirement

The RDAs for adult males and females is 400 micrograms per day of dietary folate equivalents (DFE). The RDA for adult females increases to 500 micrograms per day during lactation and 600 micrograms per day during pregnancy.

Deficiency and Toxicity

The first symptoms of folate deficiency are fatigue, weakness, and a smooth, sore tongue, culminating in anemia. Folate deficiency impairs cell division and protein synthesis. This slows DNA synthesis, and cells lose their ability to divide, which impairs growth.

The large-cell anemia of folate deficiency is known as macrocytic or megaloblastic anemia. In this condition, the blood cells are large, malformed, and few in number. They carry insufficient hemoglobin, the body's oxygen transporter.

Food Sources

Analyzing the folate content of foods is difficult. Therefore a high percentage of folate values in the USDA nutrient database are estimated rather than measured.

Legumes are considered to be a good practical source of folate. Leafy green vegetables like spinach provide folate, and asparagus contains appreciable amounts. Other folate sources include organ meats like liver and kidney, and brewer's yeast. Lettuce, cabbage, soybeans, and wheat germ contain a form of folate that is not well absorbed by the body. Although orange juice has a form of folate that is less bioavailable, it is a popular source that contributes an important share of folate in the U.S. diet. Some fruits, such as avocados and bananas, contain folate. Meats and milk, on the other hand, are poor sources of folate. Children nursed on goat's milk formula have developed folate deficiencies (Table 6–10).

TABLE 6–10 • FOOD SOURCES OF FOLATE

Food	Serving	Micrograms	% DV[a]
Breakfast cereal (fortified)	1 cup	200–400	50–100
Orange juice (from concentrate)	6 oz.	82	21
Spinach (cooked)	1/2 cup	131	33
Asparagus (cooked)	1/2 cup (6 spears)	131	33
Lentils (cooked)	1/2 cup	179	45
Garbanzo beans (cooked)	1/2 cup	141	35
Lima beans (cooked)	1/2 cup	78	20
Bread (enriched)	1 slice	104	26
Pasta (enriched, cooked)	4 oz.	73	18
Rice (enriched, cooked)	1 cup	128	32

[a]The Daily Value (DV) for folic acid is 0.4 milligrams.

Source: Adapted from Linus Pauling Institute, http://lpi.oregonstate.edu/infocenter/vitamins/fa/ and http://www.nal.usda.gov/fnic/foodcomp/search/.

The fortification of enriched flour products, which began in 1998, makes folic acid more available. This fortification program covers foods such as breakfast cereals, cornmeal, hominy grits, breads, and pasta. Fortifying refined flour with 140 micrograms of a readily absorbable form of folic acid per 100 grams of grain supplies four times the amount of folate available in whole-grain flour. The purpose of folate fortification is to prevent neural tube defects in infants.

Stability

Heat from cooking and canning destroys a substantial amount of folate. Steaming and frying food results in 90% folate losses, whereas boiling food results in 80% losses. Simmering is one technique that may preserve folate content. After blanching vegetables, cool them quickly. Long cooling periods may result in greater folate loss.

The food service industry has studied folate retention in cook/chill production systems (Williams 1996). Reheating food after chilling it for only 24 hours at 30°C causes a 30% loss in folate content. Vitamin retention is better in conventional cooking when foods are cooked and served immediately. If foods require cooling, do so within 2 hours because longer cooling periods result in even greater folate losses.

Interaction with Drugs

Many medications interact with folate. In fact, folate is the vitamin most vulnerable to food-drug interactions. Anticancer drugs, anticonvulsives, antacids, aspirin, prednisone, and birth control pills effect folate absorption. Alcohol ingestion and smoking also interfere with folate nutrition. Smokers need 685 micrograms of folate daily to achieve a plasma folate level comparable with that of a nonsmoker consuming 200 micrograms of folate.

Vitamin B$_{12}$

Vitamin B$_{12}$ was the last of the vitamins to be discovered. In the 1920s, Minot and Murphy found that a diet of liver cured pernicious anemia. Then, about 1950, Folkers isolated crystals of vitamin B_{12}. It was not until after 1960 that Dorothy Hodgkin from Oxford determined the vitamin's exact chemical structure.

Structure and Function

Vitamin B_{12}, also called *cobalamin,* occurs in many forms, as do some other vitamins. The name cobalamin refers to the cobalt-containing corrin ring that is responsible for the vitamin's function in humans. Cobalamin is needed to preserve the protective cover around nerves. It also works with folate in red blood cell production. As with the other B vitamins, cobalamin is necessary in energy metabolism. Absorption of B_{12} requires **intrinsic factor**, a glycoprotein synthesized by the stomach.

INTRINSIC FACTOR A gastric protein required for vitamin B_{12} absorption.

Dietary Requirement

The human body's requirement for vitamin B_{12} is less than that for any other vitamin. The RDA for adult males and females is 2.4 micrograms per day. Consider the salt shaker analogy again: just a few grains worth of this vitamin fulfills a lifetime's need. Despite such a miniscule requirement, a lack of adequate B_{12} means certain death.

Deficiency and Toxicity

Lack of the intrinsic factor causes vitamin B_{12} deficiency, which will result in pernicious anemia. Appropriately named, this type of anemia is relentless and can lead to death. While iron deficiency anemia responds to increasing iron in the diet, pernicious anemia does not respond to more vitamin B_{12} in the diet.

Vitamin B_{12} deficiency manifests itself first with numbness in the extremities and then progresses to loss of muscle coordination and paralysis. Without treatment permanent nerve damage results; however, memory deficits caused by a vitamin B_{12} deficiency reverse when normal vitamin B_{12} status is restored. High doses of folic acid mask vitamin B_{12} deficiency.

Food Sources

The intestinal bacteria of humans and animals produce vitamin B_{12}. In fact, this vitamin is found only in animal products—meat, fish, poultry, milk, and eggs (Table 6–11). Strict vegetarians must obtain vitamin B_{12} via fortified cereals or other fortified foods.

Stability

As with all B vitamins, individuals should take care to prevent leaching of vitamin B_{12} into cooking liquid. Vitamin B_{12} its quite stable in the presence of heat and acid.

Biotin

Biotin was initially discovered in 1927. But because it is synthesized by intestinal bacteria, it took many years to determine its requirement in human health and become accepted as a true vitamin (IOM, 1998).

Function

The metabolism of protein, fat, and carbohydrate requires biotin.

Dietary Requirement

There is no RDA for biotin; instead, the Adequate Intake is 30 micrograms per day for adult males and females.

TABLE 6–11 • FOOD SOURCES OF VITAMIN B$_{12}$

Food	Serving	Micrograms	% DV[a]
Beef liver (cooked)	3 oz.	48	780
Breakfast cereals (100% fortified)	3/4 cup	6	100
Trout, rainbow (cooked)	3 oz.	5	85
Salmon, sockeye (cooked)	3 oz.	5	85
Beef (cooked)	3 oz.	2	30
Breakfast cereals (25% fortified)	3/4 cup	1.5	25
Haddock (cooked)	3 oz.	1	15
Clams (breaded and fried)	3/4 cup	1	15
Oysters (breaded and fried)	6	1	15
Tuna (white, canned in water)	3 oz.	1	15
Milk	1 cup	1	15
Yogurt	8 oz.	1	15
Pork (cooked)	3 oz.	0.5	10
Egg	1 large	0.5	10
American cheese	1 oz.	0.3	5
Chicken (cooked)	3 oz.	0.3	5
Cheddar cheese	1 oz.	0.3	5
Mozzarella cheese	1 oz.	0.3	5

[a]The Daily Value (DV) for vitamin B$_{12}$ is 6.0 micrograms.
Source: National Institutes of Health, http://www.cc.nih.gov/ccc/supplements/vita.html.

Deficiency and Toxicity

There are no reports of biotin toxicity, and deficiency rarely is a problem for people other than those taking antibiotics or anticonvulsants. Antibiotics destroy the intestinal bacteria that produce biotin. Apart from medication, avidin, found in raw egg whites, binds biotin and could cause deficiency if taken in large amounts.

Food Sources

Biotin is supplied in small amounts by a variety of foods. But the main source for human nutrition is from its synthesis by intestinal bacteria.

Vitamin C

In the 1700s, James Lind demonstrated that consuming citrus fruits cures scurvy. Many years later, in the 1930s, Szent-György and King isolated the chemical responsible and named it vitamin C.

TABLE 6–12 • FOOD SOURCES OF BIOTIN

Food	Serving	Micrograms	% DV[a]
Yeast, baker's active	1 packet (7 g)	14	5
Wheat bran, crude	1 oz.	14	5
Bread, whole wheat	1 slice	6	2
Egg (cooked)	1 large	25	8
Camembert cheese	1 oz.	6	2
Cheddar cheese	1 oz.	2	0.6
Liver (cooked)	3 oz.	27	9
Chicken (cooked)	3 oz.	3	1
Pork (cooked)	3 oz.	2	0.6
Salmon (cooked)	3 oz.	4	1
Avocado	1 whole	6	2
Raspberries	1 cup	2	0.6
Artichoke (cooked)	1 medium	2	0.6
Cauliflower (raw)	1 cup	4	1

[a]The Daily Value (DV) for biotin is 0.3 milligrams.

Source: Adapted from Linus Pauling Institute, http://lpi.oregonstate.edu/infocenter/vitamins/biotin/index.html.

Function

ASCORBIC ACID Vitamin C.

Vitamin C, also known as **ascorbic acid**, is an important antioxidant. In addition, it helps form collagen, the intercellular cement necessary for supporting tissues, particularly in capillaries. Cuts and wounds require extra vitamin C for healing, especially postoperatively. Vitamin C is necessary for proper immune system function and for preventing infections. Despite the folklore, studies do not support claims made for vitamin C in the prevention of colds. However, evidence suggests that very large doses of vitamin C may decrease the duration of the common cold (Hemila and Herman 1995).

Dietary Requirement

The RDA for vitamin C is 75 milligrams per day for adult females and 90 milligrams per day for adult males. People who smoke have an increased need for vitamin C—35 milligrams per day in addition to the RDA.

Deficiency and Toxicity

A mild deficiency of vitamin C causes fleeting joint pains, irritability, poor wound healing, susceptibility to infection, and easy bruising. Severe deficiency results in scurvy. Symptoms of scurvy include swollen glands, loosened teeth, anemia, and hemorrhage of blood vessels in the skin and mucous membranes. Left untreated, scurvy may result in death.

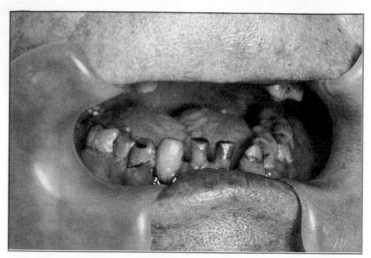

The vitamin C deficiency disease known as *scurvy* is manifested by swollen gums and loose teeth.

Photo Researchers, Inc.

Consuming large amounts of vitamin C and then drastically reducing intake can cause rebound scurvy. In other words, once the body adjusts to higher doses of vitamin C, scurvy develops with lower doses even if they meet the RDA. Newborn babies are likely to experience rebound scurvy if their mothers took large doses of vitamin C during gestation. After birth, formula provides only normal amounts of the vitamin. The sudden drop in dosage can produce infantile scurvy.

Food Sources

Orange juice is the most popular food associated with vitamin C. Kept frozen, it retains its vitamin C for up to one year. Pasteurized orange juice in a waxed container keeps well for a month. Freshly squeezed juice, tightly bottled, keeps for about three weeks. Flavor retention is a good indicator of vitamin content.

Consuming at least one food rich in vitamin C every day is a good practice because water-soluble vitamins leave the body more quickly than do fat-soluble ones. Studies have found that it is not necessary to take vitamin C daily or at every meal, but the average intake over a few days should meet the RDA. Note that vitamin C—when consumed in a meal—enhances the absorption of **nonheme iron** from foods like eggs and plant foods (Table 6–13).

Stability

Vitamin C is water-soluble. It is destroyed by baking soda, copper, and iron and is unstable at warm temperatures and when exposed to oxygen. Keep fruit juices rich in vitamin C in tightly closed jars under refrigeration. Cook vegetables quickly and without water, if possible. Microwave cooking retains most of the vitamin C in foods. Tearing or breaking vegetables, as opposed to cutting them with a knife, prevents vitamin loss because fewer of the cells are broken and less of the vitamin is exposed to oxygen. For example, tearing lettuce rather than cutting it with a knife slows the browning process. Eat fruits and vegetables raw whenever possible to maximize your vitamin C intake.

NONHEME IRON A major component of dietary iron. Nonheme iron is poorly absorbed.

WHO SHOULD TAKE FOOD SUPPLEMENTS?
- **People over the age of 50, multiple vitamins**
- **Women of childbearing age, folic acid**
- **Older adults, people with dark skin, vitamin D**
- **Vegans or strict vegetarians, vitamin B$_{12}$**

(U.S. Department of Agriculture 2005)

TABLE 6–13 • FOOD SOURCES OF VITAMIN C

Food	Serving	Milligrams	% DV[a]
Orange juice	3/4 cup	75	125
Grapefruit juice	3/4 cup	60	100
Orange	1 medium	70	117
Grapefruit	1/2 medium	44	73
Strawberries	1 cup, whole	82	137
Tomato	1 medium	23	38
Sweet red pepper (raw, chopped)	1/2 cup	141	235
Broccoli (cooked)	1/2 cup	58	97
Potato (baked)	1 medium	26	43

[a]The Daily Value (DV) for vitamin C is 60 milligrams.

Source: Adapted from Linus Pauling Institute, http://lpi.oregonstate.edu/infocenter/vitamins/vitaminC/index.html.

PSEUDOVITAMINS

Your own research may have turned up additional information about other "vitamins" or nutrients purported to be vitamins. In addition, you may have observed a media report of the same. Often this information is based on limited research or unpublished data. The following briefly lists some pseudovitamins worth noting.

Vitamin B_{17}, also known as *laetrile,* is not a true vitamin. Rather, this substance is a drug derived from apricot pits and is 6% cyanide. Laetrile has been publicized as a cancer treatment; however, this treatment lacks U.S. FDA approval.

Vitamin B_{15}, or pangamic acid, is not a true vitamin either. Extracted from apricot kernels, enthusiasts used and promoted B_{15} as a physical fitness enhancer. Valid scientific evidence is lacking to verify whether or not B_{15} improves oxygen uptake in the cells or removes lactic acid from the muscles.

Choline is included in a class of nutrients called *lypotropes*. It is manufactured by the body, which means it is a nonessential nutrient in the diet. Lypotropes are necessary for metabolic processes involved in cell proliferation and for the maintenance of tissue integrity.

PHYTOCHEMICALS

Phytochemicals are among the newest health-promoting substances found in food. At this point, however, much research remains to be done. Phytochemicals cannot be referred to as nutrients at this stage because knowledge of human requirements is lacking. Taking phytochemicals in supplement form instead of ingesting them through foods and beverages cannot be recommended at this point. Scientists do not know if isolated phytochemicals have the same health benefits as those ingested with food. However, eating plants containing phytochemicals may help prevent heart disease, cancer, and osteoporosis. The same cannot be said for supplements.

TABLE 6–14 • PARTIAL LIST OF FOODS WITH PHYTOCHEMICALS

Food	Phytochemical
Cereal grains	Phenolic compounds, flavonoids
Umbelliferous vegetables (parsley, parsnip, celery, carrot, celeriac)	Phenolic compounds, monoterpenes
Cucurbitaceous plants (squash, pumpkin, muskmelon, cantaloupe, watermelon)	Phenolic compounds, flavonoids, monoterpenes
Solanaceous vegetables (eggplant, tomato, potato, bell peppers)	Phenolic compounds, flavonoids, monoterpenes
Dark green and orange fruits and vegetables	Carotenoids
Citrus fruits	Flavonoids, monoterpenes
Wine	Flavonoids
Onions	Flavonoids, organosulfides
Garlic	Phenolic compounds; organosulfides, monoterpenes
Soybeans	Phenolic compounds, isoflavones, flavonoids
Cruciferous vegetables (cabbage, Brussels sprouts, cauliflower, kale, turnip, kohlrabi, Chinese cabbage, rutabaga, horseradish, radish)	Phenolic compounds, isothiocyanates, flavonoids, organosulfides, indoles

Some phytochemicals that are potential cancer fighters are isothiocyanates, phenolic compounds, flavonoids, indoles, monoterpenes, organosulfides, isoflavones, and carotenoids. (Remember that carotenoids are responsible for the colors found in carrots, tomatoes, beets, grapefruits, and other fruits and vegetables.) Each of these phytochemicals has many subcategories as well. For example, genistein and daidzein are two isoflavones found in soybeans.

Phytochemicals may help prevent either the initiation or progression of certain types of cancer. Soybeans contain phytochemicals found to help prevent heart disease and breast cancer, to control glucose levels in individuals with diabetes, and to relieve symptoms of menopause (Table 6–14).

A PROBLEM WITH VITAMIN SUPPLEMENTS

High intakes of both fat-soluble and water-soluble vitamins can create imbalances, and excessive amounts of certain vitamins can cause toxicity. Consuming too much of the fat-soluble vitamins A and D creates the most serious problems. Excess vitamin K usually is not a problem, except in its synthetic form, which is available only through prescription. Although the fat-soluble vitamins are more likely to cause toxicity, the water-soluble B vitamins, when taken in excess, also can pose problems.

TABLE 6–15 • SUMMARY OF FAT-SOLUBLE VITAMINS

Attribute	Vitamin A	Vitamin D	Vitamin E	Vitamin K
Technical name	Retinoic acid, retinal, and retinol	Cholecalciferol (vitamin D_3), ergocalciferol (vitamin D_2)	Alpha tocopherol	Phylloquinone (K_1) plants, menaquinone (K_2) animals
Function	Vision, skin growth, immune function, gene regulation, treatment for acne	Calcium regulation, formation of bones and teeth	Fat-soluble antioxidant	Blood clotting, bone growth, immune function
Nutrient requirement RDA or AI	RDA M 900 µg retinol activity equivalents/d F 700 µg retinol activity equivalents/d	AI M & F 5 µg/d or 200 international units (IU)	RDA M & F 15 mg alpha tocopherol	AI M 120 µg/d F 90 µg/d
Mean intake U.S. 19–30-year-olds	M 744 µg RAE/d F 530 µg RAE/d	Not available	M 9.5 mg/d F 6.7 mg/d	M 98 µg/d F 82 µg/d
Food source (other sources)	Preformed vitamin A: meats, cheese, egg yolks Provitamin: dark green and deep yellow vegetables	Fortified milk, fatty fish, egg yolk, fortified cereal (sunlight)	Nuts, seeds, and oils produced from them, salad dressing, and cooking oil	Green leafy vegetables soybeans, cauliflower, milk, eggs (intestinal bacteria)
Deficiency diseases	Night blindness, xerothalmia, hyperkeratosis (dry skin)	Rickets, osteomalacia	Overt deficiency rarely seen, risk of chronic disease	Hemorrhage (blood loss)
Tolerable upper intake level (UL)	3,000 µg/day of preformed vitamin A	50 µg/d	1,000 mg/day	None established
Stability	Unstable to oxygen	Stable to heat, oxygen, and alkali	Unstable to oxygen	Unstable to acid, alkali, oxygen

Note: M (male), F (female)

TABLE 6–16 • SUMMARY OF WATER-SOLUBLE VITAMINS

Attribute	Vitamin B_1	Vitamin B_2	Vitamin B_3	Vitamin B_6	Vitamin B_{12}
Technical name	Thiamin	Riboflavin	Niacin	Pyridoxine	Cobalamin
Function	It is part of the enzyme in energy metabolism (TPP) thiamin pyrophosphate	It is part of the enzyme in energy metabolism (FAD) flavin adenine dinucleotide	It is part of the enzyme in energy metabolism (NAD) nicotinamide adenine dinucleotide	Coenzyme in protein metabolism, part of 50 enzymes	Nerve function, blood cell formation
Nutrient requirement RDA or AI	RDA M 1.2 mg/day F 1.1 mg/day	RDA M 1.3 mg/d F 1.1 mg/d	RDA M 16 mg/d niacin equivalents (NE) F 14 mg/day (NE)	RDA M & F 1.3 mg/day	RDA M & F 2.4 µg/day
Mean intake U.S. 19–30-year-olds	M 2 mg/day F 1.2 mg/day	M 2.3 mg/d F 1.5 mg/d	M 31 mg/d F 18 mg/d	M 2.3 mg/d F 1.4 mg/d	M 5.6 µg/d F 3.5 µg/d
Food source (other sources)	Meats, fish, whole-grain and enriched breads and cereals	Milk, meat, whole-grain and enriched breads and cereals	Whole-grain and enriched breads and cereals, fish, poultry	Potato, banana, fish, poultry, beans	Liver, fish, beef, dark green and deep yellow vegetables

Note: M (male), F (female)

TABLE 6-16 • *(continued)*

Attribute	Vitamin B$_1$	Vitamin B$_2$	Vitamin B$_3$	Vitamin B$_6$	Vitamin B$_{12}$
Deficiency diseases and conditions	Beriberi: sore mouth, bright red tongue, nerve damage, decreased appetite, weight loss	Fissures that radiate from the corners of the mouth; red, swollen tongue	Pellegra; red, rough skin	Depression, nausea, flaky skin, microcytic and hypochromic anemia	Pernicious anemia
Tolerable upper intake level (UL)	None set, no reports of toxicity	None set, no reports of toxicity	35 µg/day	100 µg/day	None set No reports of toxicity
Stability	Unstable to heat, alkali, oxygen, most unstable B vitamin	Unstable to light	Stable to heat, alkali, oxygen	Unstable to high heat	Stable

Attribute	Folic Acid	Pantothenic Acid	Biotin	Vitamin C
Technical name	Pteroyl-glutamic acid	Pantothenic acid	Biotin	Ascorbic acid
Function	Blood cell production, amino acid metabolism, DNA production	Coenzyme in energy metabolism as part of acetyl-CoA	Cofactor in metabolism	Water-soluble antioxidant, collagen formation, wound healing, immune function
Nutrient requirement RDA or AI	RDA M & F 400 µg/day	AI M & F 5 mg/day	AI M & F 30 µg/day	RDA M 90 mg/d F 75 mg/d
Mean intake U.S. 19–30-year-olds	M 297 µg/d F 200 µg/d	4–7 mg/d	All ages approx. 33–35 µg/d	M 114 mg/d F 79 mg/d
Food source (other sources)	Green leafy vegetables, lentils, beans, enriched bread and cereal	Widely distributed in all foods	Liver, eggs, whole wheat (intestinal bacteria)	Citrus fruit, strawberries, sweet peppers, potatoes, broccoli
Deficiency diseases and conditions	Neural tube defects, cardiovascular disease, macrocytic anemia	Irritability, restlessness, fatigue, stomach distress	Red scaly skin around mouth and eyes and nose	Scurvy, irritability, poor wound healing, susceptibility to infection
Tolerable upper intake level (UL)	1 mg/day	None set, no reports of toxicity	None set, no reports of toxicity	2,000 mg/d
Stability	Unstable to heat	Unstable to heat		Unstable to alkali, heat, oxygen

Note: M (male), F (female)

SUMMARY

Vitamins Are Vital for Life

Vitamins are essential organic compounds that are necessary for good health and are primarily obtained through diet. If we do not consume the proper quantity of vitamins, poor health, physical deformities, and, in some cases, death may occur. In recommended amounts, vitamins support growth and life.

Thirteen vitamins are necessary for human health. These are classified into two Categories—fat-soluble and water-soluble. Fat-soluble vitamins require dietary fat for absorption. Extra fat-soluble vitamins are stored in fat tissues or in the liver. Water-soluble vitamins are excreted in urine when body tissues are saturated. The fat-soluble vitamins are A, E, D, and K. The water-soluble vitamins are C and the B complex vitamins (eight in number).

Phytochemicals are among the newest health-promoting substances found in food, but there isn't enough data to classify them as vitamins. On the other hand, eating plants containing phytochemicals may help prevent heart disease, cancer, and osteoporosis.

CASE RESOLUTION

Habits are hard to change, especially if the behavior has been practiced for 40 years. Beatrice's astonishment is normal because she probably takes her work personally. After all, we show love with food, and Beatrice has no doubt grown quite close to some residents. Moreover, Beatrice probably enjoys eating softer vegetables herself.

Linda will have a difficult time convincing Beatrice of the necessity of change, but the facts are indisputable. State regulations mandate nutritious meals for residents in long-term care. Linda should partner with the facility's registered dietitian to provide an in-service educational session to all kitchen staff on nutrient preservation and proper cooking. Together they can illustrate the benefits of eating properly cooked food versus the potential detriment of overcooked food. They can point out that every bite for an elderly person matters because the elderly have reduced appetites and chronic health conditions that have a negative impact on their dietary intake. These residents cannot afford to eat nutrient-depleted food.

REFERENCES

Bailey, L., G. Rampersaud, and G. Kauwell. 2003. Folic acid supplements and fortification affect the risk for neural tube defects, vascular disease and cancer: Evolving science. *Journal of Nutrition* 133: 1961.

Blumberg, J., and G. Block. 1994. The alpha-tocopherol, beta-carotene cancer prevention study in Finland. *Nutrition Reviews* 52 (7): 242–45.

Clemens, T. L., J. S. Adams, S. L. Henderson, and M. F. Holick. 1982. Increased skin pigment reduces the capacity of skin to synthesize vitamin D_3. *Lancet* 1: 74–76.

Dam, H. 1934. Hemorrhages in chicks reared on artificial diets: A new deficiency disease. *Nature* 133: 909–10.

Evans, H. M., and K. S. Bishop. 1922. On the existence of a hitherto unrecognized dietary factor essential for reproduction. *Science* 56: 650–51.

Food and Drug Administration. http://www.fda.gov/cdrh/tanning/ (accessed June 24, 2008).

Funk, C., and H. Dubin. 1920. A test for antiberi-beri vitamine and its practical application. *Journal of Biological Chemistry* 44: 487–98.

Hemila, H., and Z. S. Herman. 1995. Vitamin C and the common cold: A respective analysis of Chalmer's review. *Journal of the American College of Nutrition* 14: 116–23.

Hine, Jean R. 1996. What practitioners need to know about folic acid. *Journal of the American Dietetic Association* 96 (5): 451–52.

Institute of Medicine. 1998. *Dietary Reference Intakes: Thiamin, Riboflavin, Niacin, Vitamin B_6, Folate, Vitamin B_{12}, Pantothenic Acid, Biotin and Choline.* Washington, DC: National Academies Press.

Institute of Medicine. 2001. *Dietary Reference Intakes: Vitamin A, Vitamin K, Arsenic, Boron, Chromium, Copper, Iodine, Iron, Manganese, Molybdenum, Nickel, Silicon, Vanadium, and Zinc.* Washington, DC: National Academies Press.

Koehn, C. J., and C. A. Elvehjem. 1937. Further studies on the concentration of the antipellagra factor. *Journal of Biological Chemistry* (February 5): 693–99.

Kuhn, R. 1938. The Nobel Prize in Chemistry, 1938: Presentation speech. In *Nobel Lectures, Chemistry, 1922–1941.* Ed. F. W. Aston Amsterdam: Elsevier.

Leach, R., B. Pollock, J. Basler, D. Troyer, S. Naylor, and I. M. Thompson. 2003. Chemoprevention of prostate cancer: Focus on key opportunities and clinical trials. *Urologic Clinics of North America* 30 (2): 227–37.

Lichtenstein, A. 1943. Nobel Prize in Physiology, 1943: Presentation speech. In *Les Prix Nobel.*

Liljestrand, G. 1929. Nobel Prize in Physiology or Medicine, 1929: Presentation speech. In *Les Prix Nobel.*

Margolas, Simeon. 1998. Coronary artery disease in diabetes. Continuing education lecture for dietitians at Johns Hopkins University, March 18.

McCollum, E. V., and M. Davis. 1913. The necessity of certain lipins in the diet during growth. *Journal of Biological Chemistry* 15: 167–75.

Riggs, K., A. Spiro III, K. Tucker, and D. Rush. 1996. Relations of vitamin B_{12}, vitamin B_6, folate, and homocysteine to cognitive performance in the normative aging study. *American Journal of Clinical Nutrition* 63: 306–14.

Rodahl, K. 1949. Toxicity of polar bear liver. *Nature* 164: 530.

Stipanuk, M. H. 2000. *Biochemical and physiological aspects of human nutrition.* Philadelphia: W. B. Saunders.

Tufts University Diet and Nutrition Letter. 1995. 13 (5): 1.

University of California, Riverside. 1999. History of vitamin D. http://vitamind.ucr.edu/history.html (accessed July 31, 2008).

U.S. Department of Agriculture. 2005. *Dietary Guidelines for Americans,* 6th ed. Washington, DC: U.S. Government Printing Office.

Whitney, E., and S. Rolfes. 1996. *Understanding Nutrition,* 7th ed. Minneapolis: West.

Williams, Peter G. 1996. Vitamin retention in cook/chill and cook/hot hold for hospital foodservice. *Journal of the American Dietetic Association* 96 (5): 490–96.

Wolf, G. 2001. History of nutrition. *Journal of Nutrition* 131: 1647–50.

Zeman, Frances J. 1983. *Clinical nutrition and dietetics.* Lexington, MA: Collamore Press.

REVIEW QUESTIONS

1. How would a low-fat diet affect vitamin A nutrition?
2. What environmental factors are important in vitamin D nutrition?
3. Which vitamins are antioxidants? What diseases do these protect against?
4. Which two serious deficiency diseases has enrichment of bread helped to eliminate?
5. List some fruits and vegetables that supply the daily requirement of vitamin C in one serving.
6. Explain which B vitamins are involved in energy metabolism.
7. Lack of which vitamin produces pernicious anemia?
8. What are the deficiency diseases associated with thiamin and niacin?
9. What nutrients are added to processed flour in enrichment?

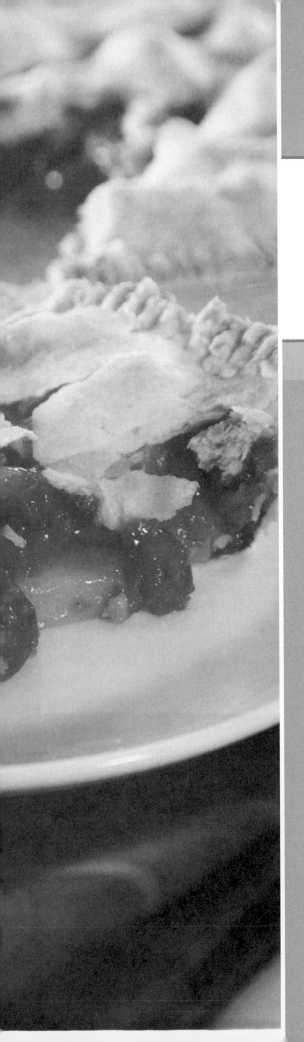

7

Minerals

KEY CONCEPTS

- Macrominerals are required in large quantities.
- Microminerals are required in small quantities.
- Minerals maintain health.
- Mineral deficiencies are common in certain regions of the world.
- Excess mineral intake is toxic.
- Foods vary in mineral content.

Minerals are inorganic elements that play an important role in maintaining good health. They help regulate body processes and provide structure for body tissues. Minerals occur naturally in food sources, and they are absorbed through the stomach and the intestines directly into the bloodstream for transportation to cells. Some excess minerals are excreted via urine, stool, and sweat, while others attach to body proteins for storage and later use.

High intake of some minerals over long periods of time can be harmful. Excess dietary intake is unlikely with a balanced diet containing a variety of foods. Mineral supplements can provide toxic doses and should be used with caution.

Macrominerals, or major minerals, are essential minerals needed in the greatest amount (more than 100 milligrams a day). These include calcium, phosphorus, magnesium, sulfur, and the electrolytes potassium, sodium, and chloride. Electrolytes regulate the movement of fluid into and out of all cells, and they transmit nerve or electrical impulses.

Microminerals are also essential but are needed only in trace amounts (under 100 milligrams a day). These include chromium, copper, fluoride, iodine, iron, manganese, molybdenum, selenium, and zinc. Scientists have evaluated microminerals for their health benefits, and Recommended Dietary Allowances (RDAs) or Adequate Intakes (AIs) have been established.

There are additional minerals for which nutritional science has not been able to determine a specific need. Examples include vanadium and boron, which are available in a well-balanced diet of whole foods (not overly processed). Nickel deficiencies are known to harm the liver and other organs. Silicon and tin have known functions in animals, but more work is needed before requirements can be established. Mercury, silver, barium, cadmium, and arsenic are elements that future nutrition research may address.

THINK ABOUT IT

When you eat fish, do you wonder whether it is contaminated with mercury? Perhaps you have seen reports on the nightly news or have read about this subject in a newsmagazine or newspaper. Have you altered your consumption of some or all types of fish because of these stories? Apart from following news reports, how else do you keep current in this area?

CASE STUDY

A Chef's Dilemma with Fish

Chef Vivian Krowse at New Castle's upscale assisted-living and adult day care facility specializes in preparing fish and seafood delicacies. Before moving to New Castle, she spent a year after culinary school studying with an esteemed chef at his popular seafood restaurant in San Francisco. In fact, Chef Vivian was raised partly on her family's fishing boat. Their primary catch was swordfish.

With all that history and experience under her belt, few are as talented as Chef Vivian when it comes to swordfish preparation. Individuals residing in the New Castle facility where the chef works look forward to the weekly fresh seafood dinners. In fact, they marvel at how creative the swordfish is each week.

The facility's medical director alerted Chef Vivian of the mercury content in certain fish, particularly swordfish. Mercury is particularly harmful if consumed excessively by women who may become pregnant, pregnant women, breast-feeding mothers, and young children.

What should Chef Vivian do to the menu, if anything, at her facility? *The resolution for this case study is presented at the end of the chapter.*

MAJOR MINERALS (MACROMINERALS)

The macrominerals are essential minerals needed in amounts greater than 100 milligrams a day. These include calcium, phosphorus, magnesium, sulfur, and the electrolytes potassium, sodium, and chloride.

Calcium

Function

Calcium's main function in the body is making, repairing, and maintaining bones and teeth. This process, called *mineralization*, involves combining calcium and phosphorus to create

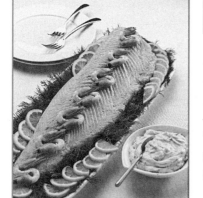

When eating seafood like salmon, do you worry whether it is contaminated with mercury?
Edward Allwright © Dorling Kindersley

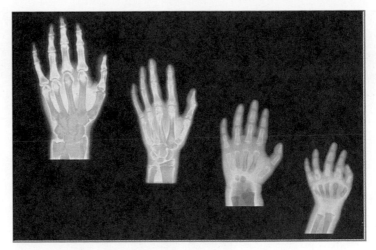

Progressive bone growth in a human hand.
Photo Researchers, Inc.

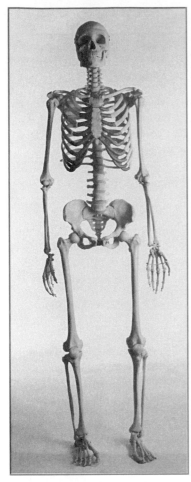

Most of the calcium in the human body is found in bones and teeth.
© *Dorling Kindersley*

TETANY A painful condition characterized by muscle spasms due to inadequate blood calcium levels.

PARATHYROID HORMONE A hormone, produced by the parathyroid gland, that regulates calcium balance.

CALCITONIN A hormone of the thyroid gland that counterbalances parathyroid hormone. Calcitonin lowers excessively high levels of blood calcium.

the calcium phosphate deposited in bone protein matrix. The skeleton contains 99% of the body's total calcium.

Calcium also binds with protein for other vital functions, such as blood clotting and muscle contraction, and it helps release neurotransmitters in the brain and activate digestive enzymes. Excess blood calcium leads to respiratory or cardiac failure, while too little results in **tetany**, a condition marked by muscle spasms. Proper muscle contraction of the heart depends on calcium contained in fluid around heart cells.

Hormones regulate calcium balance. When blood calcium levels are too low, the body releases **parathyroid hormone**, extracting calcium from bones. On the other hand, when blood calcium levels are high, **calcitonin** decreases the release of calcium from the bone, reducing blood levels of calcium.

Dietary Requirement

Adequate Intake (AI) for calcium is 1,300 milligrams for children ages 9 to 18 and 1,000 milligrams for adults 19 to 50 years. Adults ages 51 and older require 1,200 milligrams daily to prevent osteoporosis, a condition in which bones become brittle and fragile. Calcium absorption decreases in people over age 60. Oddly enough, the requirement for calcium does not increase during pregnancy and remains at 1,000 milligrams of calcium daily for women ages 19 to 50 who are pregnant or breast-feeding (Institute of Medicine 1997).

The AI for calcium is set higher than the actual calcium requirement because of the high protein and phosphorus content of the American diet (caused by the high consumption of meat). Urinary excretion of calcium is increased by this type of diet. For individuals living in countries where meat is not a primary part of the diet and phosphorus intake is low compared to the U.S. diet, daily calcium intakes between 400 and 500 milligrams do not lead to calcium deficiencies.

The Tolerable Upper Intake Level (UL) for all life-stage groups, except infants, is 2,500 milligrams per day.

Food Sources

Milk and milk products like cheese and yogurt are the richest food sources of calcium. In areas of the world where milk is not a prominent food, soy products (tofu and miso), edible seaweed, oysters, and small fish with soft edible bones like sardines provide calcium.

Soybeans and other legumes and dark green leafy vegetables, particularly collard greens, turnip greens, mustard greens, and kale, are high in calcium. Vegetable sources of calcium are less bioavailable, however, than calcium from animal sources.

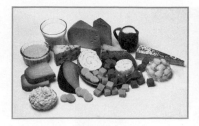

Dairy and dairy products are rich sources of calcium.
© *Dorling Kindersley*

Food	Serving	Milligrams
TABLE 7–1 • FOOD SOURCES OF CALCIUM		
Plain yogurt, nonfat (13 g protein)	8-oz.	450
Pasteurized processed Swiss cheese	2 oz.	440
Plain yogurt, low-fat (12 g protein/8 oz.)	8-oz.	410
Fortified ready-to-eat cereals (various)	1 oz.	230–1,000
Soy beverage (calcium fortified)	1 cup	370
Sardines, Atlantic (in oil, drained)	3 oz.	320
Provolone cheese	1.5 oz.	320
Muenster cheese	1.5 oz.	300
1% low-fat milk	1 cup	290
Tofu (firm, prepared with nigari)	1/2 cup	250
2% reduced-fat milk	1 cup	280
Reduced-fat chocolate milk (2%)	1 cup	280
Pink salmon (canned, with bone)	3 oz.	180
Collard greens (cooked from frozen)	1/2 cup	170

Source: National Institute of Health, http://ods.od.nih.gov/factsheets/calcium.asp (accessed July 31, 2008).

BIOAVAILABILITY The degree to which a nutrient can be absorbed and used for physiological activity.

A nutrient's chemical form, plus the presence of other nutrients in certain amounts in a food source, affect the absorption rate of that nutrient during digestion. This is referred to as **bioavailability**. For example, oxalic acid in spinach binds 95% of calcium so that it cannot be absorbed. Beet greens and chocolate contain oxalic acid. Calcium in these foods is poorly absorbed. In addition, foods high in dietary fiber, phytic acid (found in wheat bran), and phosphates (found in brown rice) decrease calcium absorption. Yeast inactivates phytic acid, so baked goods made from whole-wheat flour and raised with yeast do not hinder calcium absorption.

Food rather than supplements is the preferred source for calcium. Refer to Table 7–1 for calcium-rich food sources.

Note that products made mostly from milk fat, such as cream cheese and butter, are not good sources of calcium.

Deficiency and Toxicity

Osteoporosis has become a major problem in recent times. Since people are living longer, there will be a corresponding increase in the number of osteoporosis cases in the future. Women are more susceptible than men—although men are not totally immune—and Caucasian women more so than African-American women. Women with small bones and a fair complexion are at greater risk for osteoporosis than are bigger boned, darker complexioned women.

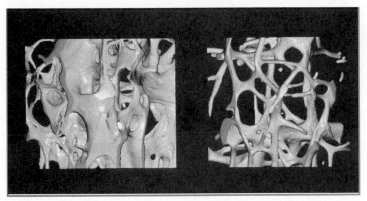

This displays the reduced amount of bone seen in osteoporosis.
Photo Researchers, Inc.

Consuming adequate calcium and vitamin D in early years and performing weight-bearing exercises are the ideal measures to take to prevent osteoporosis. Estrogen replacement is another measure available for women. This therapy is given under medical supervision.

The popularity of calcium supplements has engendered much research. Calcium carbonate, calcium acetate, calcium citrate, calcium gluconate, and calcium lactate are different forms of calcium supplements. The calcium content of supplements varies (Figure 7–1). For example, calcium carbonate is 40% calcium, whereas calcium gluconate is 9% calcium. The amount of calcium in a supplement is listed as elemental calcium on the label.

Calcium citrate is the best calcium supplement and is better absorbed than the others. Furthermore, taking calcium citrate supplements with meals increases absorption.

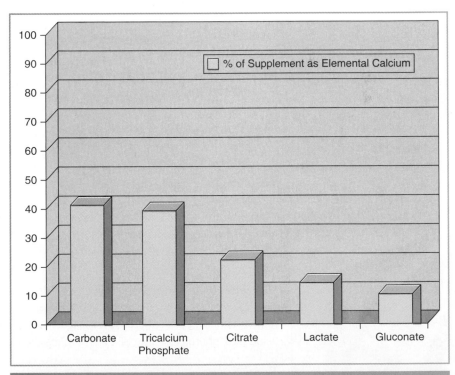

FIGURE 7–1 • CALCIUM CONTENT OF SUPPLEMENTS
Source: Office of Dietary Supplements. 2004. *Dietary Supplement Fact Sheet: Calcium.* Bethesda, MD: National Institutes of Health.

Lactose also assists with absorption of calcium from milk. An 8-ounce glass of milk provides 290 milligrams of calcium. The calcium citrate in fortified fruit juices also appears to be readily absorbed.

Calcium supplements sometimes have side effects. Some calcium supplements reduce iron absorption, which could interfere with nutritional status. Calcium carbonate, the key component of oyster shell supplements and some antacids, may cause constipation.

A calcium pill must dissolve in the stomach to provide benefit; however, not all supplements dissolve properly. To test whether a particular supplement will dissolve, submerge it in 6 ounces of vinegar. Stir every few minutes. Avoid taking pills that remain hard and intact in the vinegar (Women's Health Watch 1995). Also, never use dolomite and bone meal as a calcium supplement; these may be contaminated with lead.

Phosphorus

Function

All foods contain phosphorus, which is necessary for energy production. Moreover, all body cells contain phosphorus. Most of the body's phosphorus is bound with magnesium and calcium in bones and teeth to provide strength and rigidity. The remaining phosphorus is found in cells and body fluids.

PHOSPHORYLATE To undergo a chemical reaction that adds a phosphate group.

The body needs phosphorus to convert sugar into energy for the body. B vitamins that act as enzymes in carbohydrate metabolism are **phosphorylated**, which means that they require phosphorus. RNA and DNA, carriers of the genetic code, are phosphorylated as well. Some lipids (fats) like lecithin combine with phosphorus and then become part of all cells. Other fats are connected to phosphorus for transportation through the blood. Besides this, phosphorus is involved in body **pH** regulation. Blood needs to be at a neutral pH, neither too acidic nor too alkaline.

pH A measure of acidity and alkalinity.

Phosphorus is also the main vehicle for transferring energy throughout the body. When carbohydrates are digested, the energy contained in their chemical bonds is transferred to the bonds in **adenosine triphosphate (ATP)**. ATP travels throughout the body, distributing energy where it is needed.

ADENOSINE TRIPHOSPHATE (ATP) An energy source for cellular reactions.

Ideally, phosphorus should be in a 1:1 ratio with calcium. Excessive amounts of phosphorus upset this balance. For instance, if soda routinely replaces milk as the beverage of choice, the balance is at risk and osteoporosis cases may increase (Institute of Medicine 1997).

Dietary Requirement

The RDA for phosphorus is the same for males and females: 1,250 milligrams per day for children 9 to 18 years and 700 milligrams per day for adults ages 19 and older. The upper limit (UL) is set at 4,000 milligrams per day for males and females 9 to 70 years of age (Institute of Medicine 1997). Absorption efficiency varies with the phosphorus source and the dietary ratio of calcium to phosphorus. Vitamin D, considered as a hormone, also stimulates phosphorus absorption. Other hormones, particularly parathormone (also called *parathyroid hormone*), influence blood phosphorus regulation. The kidneys play a major role in regulating phosphorus levels, so some patients with insufficient kidney function develop phosphorus toxicity, called *hyperphosphatemia*.

Food Sources

Adequate protein intake ensures adequate phosphorus intake. This is because phosphorus is a component of DNA, RNA, and ATP, so it is abundant in all foods containing protein (Table 7–2).

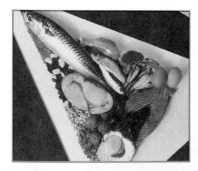

Phosphorus is found in abundance in foods high in protein.
Andrew Whittuck © Dorling Kindersley

TABLE 7–2 • FOOD SOURCES OF PHOSPHORUS

Food	Serving	Milligrams
Milk, skim	8 oz.	247
Yogurt, plain nonfat	8 oz.	383
Cheese, mozarella (part skim)	1 oz.	131
Egg (cooked)	1 large	104
Beef (cooked)	3 oz.	173
Chicken (cooked)	3 oz.	155
Turkey (cooked)	3 oz.	173
Fish, halibut (cooked)	3 oz.	242
Fish, salmon (cooked)	3 oz.	252
Bread, whole wheat	1 slice	64
Bread, enriched white	1 slice	24
Carbonated cola drink	12 oz.	44
Almonds	1 oz.	139
Peanuts	1 oz.	101
Lentils (cooked)	1/2 cup	356

Source: Adapted from Linus Pauling Institute, http://lpi.oregonstate.edu/infocenter/minerals/phosphorus.

Deficiency and Toxicity

Phosphorus is abundant, so deficiency rarely occurs. There are no reports of phosphorus toxicity due to overconsumption in the diet. But as stated earlier, if it is consumed in excess, the calcium/phosphorus ratio may be thrown off, increasing the risk of disease.

Magnesium

Function

The body needs magnesium to efficiently use amino acids in protein formation. Magnesium also acts with many enzyme systems, particularly in carbohydrate metabolism. Extracellular magnesium—or magnesium outside the cell—is important in neuromuscular transmission. Recent reports show magnesium can reduce symptoms of migraine headaches and depression.

About 60% of the body's magnesium is contained in the bones. Soft tissues contain more magnesium than calcium. When the body receives too much magnesium from food, it absorbs less. When it does not obtain enough, more is absorbed. Little magnesium is held in the blood, so a blood test is not a good indicator of the body's magnesium levels.

Dietary Requirement

The body needs about 200 milligrams of magnesium daily. Magnesium is only 30% to 40% absorbed, so RDAs are 400 milligrams per day for men 19 to 30 years of age and 310 milligrams per day for women 19 to 30 years.

Deficiency and Toxicity

Magnesium deficiency produces **vasodilation** and hyperirritability, which have led to convulsions and death in experimental animals. In humans, magnesium deficiency is rarely related to poor dietary intake. Diuretic use, alcoholism, and medical conditions that lead to urinary losses are more likely causes of a magnesium deficit. Severe magnesium deficiency stemming from these conditions also causes calcium deficiency. Calcium deficiency, in turn, creates magnesium deficiency.

Muscle twitching, tremors, numbness, and tingling are early symptoms of magnesium deficiency. Muscle weakness, convulsions, depression, delirium, and irregular heartbeat follow. Magnesium is important for proper cardiovascular function. After all, the heart is a muscle. Epidemiological data show a greater incidence of heart attacks and stroke in areas with soft water. This may be related to lower amounts of magnesium in the water.

Magnesium toxicity has not been seen from its natural occurrence in food but can occur with supplementation. Individuals with kidney failure may experience magnesium toxicity.

Food Sources

Nuts, especially cashews and almonds, are a good source of magnesium (Table 7–3). Whole grains provide much more magnesium than do refined grains. Vegetables containing chlorophyll also contain magnesium in moderate amounts. Protein foods like soybeans and other legumes provide magnesium, while flesh foods provide smaller amounts. In general, dairy products and most fruits are poor sources of magnesium. Hard water contains significant amounts of magnesium.

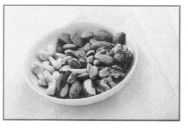

Nuts are a good source of magnesium.

Ruth Jenkinson © Dorling Kindersley

Sodium

Function

Sodium is found in the fluid surrounding the cells and is one of the most important minerals in the body. Along with potassium and chloride, it forms the body's electrolytes. An electrolyte is an element with a positive or negative charge that helps regulate water. In addition, sodium helps regulate acid/base balance, osmotic pressure, and neuromuscular transmission of nerve impulses, and it facilitates intestinal nutrient absorption.

Dietary Requirement

Average daily sodium intake in the United States ranges from 6,000 to 10,000 milligrams. There is no RDA for sodium. The AI for men and women ages 9 to 50 is 1,500 milligrams per day, and the UL is 2,300 milligrams per day. Sodium is pervasive in the American diet, so achieving adequate intake of this nutrient is effortless.

The body may require additional sodium when heat or exercise leads to a loss of body water. Drinking 1/3 teaspoon of table salt dissolved in a quart of water safely replaces the sodium lost in a 5- to 10-pound water loss. Measure body water loss by weighing before and after exertion. A pickle or a few potato chips with lemonade or fruit juice is the most practical way to recoup sweat losses since the average person does not enjoy drinking salt water. Salt tablets can cause dehydration and should not be taken unless prescribed by a doctor.

Deficiency and Toxicity

Sodium deficiency can cause cardiac arrest, convulsions, collapse, and heat exhaustion. In humans with normal kidney and heart function, 90% of sodium is excreted through the kidneys. Vomiting and diarrhea, especially in children, the frail, and the elderly, can cause large sodium losses, which might require medical attention. Dehydration and disturbance of the body's acid/base balance can lead to death.

TABLE 7–3 • FOOD SOURCES OF MAGNESIUM

Nuts (Small Size or Chopped)	Milligrams	Grains (Cooked)	Milligrams
Almonds	420	Wheat germ	239
Cashews	356	Bran	366
Peanuts	760	Whole-wheat flour	166
Black walnuts	253	All-purpose flour	26
Hazelnuts (filberts)	327	Whole-wheat macaroni	42
Pistachios	166	Enriched-flour macaroni	25
Pecans	138	Oatmeal	56
English walnuts	203	Pearl barley	34
Fresh coconut	26	Wild rice	52
Chestnuts	47	Brown rice	84
		White rice	25
		Millet	106
		Cornmeal	22
Legumes (Cooked)	**Milligrams**	**Vegetables**	
Pinto beans	47	Although green vegetables are a known source of magnesium, the amounts of magnesium vary widely depending on whether the vegetable is fresh, frozen, or canned.	
Soybeans	148		
Split peas	70		
Lima beans	58		
Lentils	72		
Garbanzo beans	79		

Note: Serving size is 1 cup.

Sodium toxicity occurs only if large amounts of sodium and insufficient fluids are taken. It also can occur when a person has medical problems that create fluid retention, inhibiting proper sodium excretion.

Hypertension (high blood pressure) is the most common health problem linked with sodium, which is a concern for many Americans. Hypertension has no symptoms at first; years later, a person can become short of breath, develop heart irregularities, suffer a stroke, or have a heart attack with little warning. Epidemiological evidence suggests that in cultures with low salt intake, hypertension is rare. On the other hand, hypertension is common in cultures with high salt intake. Genetics predisposes a person to hypertension, however, so not everyone with a high salt intake becomes hypertensive.

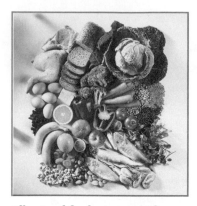

All natural foods contain sodium.
Jules Seimes © Dorling Kindersley

The events that can lead to high blood pressure are as follows: A high concentration of sodium in the blood causes water to enter the blood vessel to dilute the sodium. The heart then works harder to pump this extra fluid resulting in increased blood pressure.

Food Sources

All natural foods contain sodium, and extra dietary sodium comes from food additives (Table 7–4). Of the natural foods, fruits and oils have the least amount of sodium. Vegetables, grains, flesh foods, and milk contain a bit more sodium.

Cheese, a concentrate of milk, has a very high sodium content, and it has added salt as well. Processed cheese has even more sodium than natural cheese. Some over-the-counter and prescription drugs also contain sodium.

The greatest addition of dietary sodium comes from the use of table salt to season foods. Table salt, chemically called *sodium chloride*, contains about 40% sodium. Soy sauce also contains a lot of sodium. Monosodium glutamate (MSG), a natural flavor enhancer, contains substantial amounts of sodium too. Leavening agents—baking soda and baking powder—contribute to food sodium levels (Box 7–1).

TABLE 7–4 • SODIUM CONTENT OF FRESH AND PROCESSED FOODS	
Food	**Milligrams**
Fresh Foods	
Fresh meat, poultry, fish	30 mg/oz.
Milk	120 mg/cup
Natural (hard) cheeses	300 mg/oz.
Vegetables	9 mg/1/2 cup
Fruits	2 mg/1/2 cup
Grains and bread	5 mg/1/2 cup or slice
Fats and oils	Trace
Sugar	Trace
Processed Foods	
Cold cuts and hot dogs	500 mg/oz.
Processed cheeses	500–600 mg/oz.
Sauerkraut	1,000 mg/cup
Some processed cereals	Over 200 mg/oz.
Potato chips	1,000 mg/3 oz.
Some commercial breads	Over 100 mg/oz.
Some commercial salad dressings and condiments	Over 200 mg/Tbsp.
Salted butter	50 mg/teaspoon

BOX 7–1 • MILLIGRAMS OF SODIUM IN CONDIMENTS PER TEASPOON

Each teaspoon of salt adds 2,300 mg.
Each teaspoon of soy sauce adds 1,000 mg.
Each teaspoon of monosodium glutamate adds 500 mg.
Each teaspoon of baking powder adds 500 mg.
Each teaspoon of baking soda adds 1,000 mg.

Commercially processed foods often contain high amounts of sodium in the form of preservatives. Preservatives extend a food product's shelf life by preventing spoilage and by protecting color, texture, and flavor. Sodium-containing preservatives include the following:

sodium acetate
sodium alginate
sodium aluminum sulfate
sodium benzoate
sodium bicarbonate
sodium calcium alginate
sodium citrate
sodium d-acetate
sodium erythorbate
sodium nitrate
sodium nitrite
sodium propionate
sodium sorbate
sodium stearyl fumarate
dioctyl sodium sulfosuccinate
disodium guanylate
disodium inosinate
MSG

Canned soups and vegetables, factory-made puddings, frozen dinners, bouillons, and dehydrated soups can contain hundreds of milligrams of sodium in a single serving. In general, except for maraschino cherries and some dried fruits, canned fruits are one of the few processed foods that are low in sodium.

Potassium

Function

Potassium and sodium have interrelated roles and some similar functions, except that potassium operates inside the cell and sodium functions outside it. These electrolytes regulate normal water balance, conduction and transmission of nerve impulses, muscle contractions, heart action, and some enzyme system functions. Through excretion and conservation, healthy kidneys help maintain steady levels of potassium and sodium.

Dietary Requirement

There is no RDA for potassium. The AI is set at 4,700 milligrams per day for men and women 18 years and older (Institute of Medicine 2004). In rare cases, individuals who sweat profusely (in sports activities or in physical labor in hot climates, for example) may need more potassium. The kidneys' ability to conserve potassium in these conditions may negate any additional need. There is no established UL for potassium.

Deficiency and Toxicity

Potassium deficiency is rarely caused by dietary factors, except in cases of starvation. Health problems, such as diarrhea, vomiting, burns, injury, and surgery, are more likely than diet to create potassium losses. For example, diuretic medications that eliminate sodium and thus reduce blood pressure can also remove large amounts of potassium through urine. These diuretics are referred to as potassium wasting. Doctors routinely prescribe potassium supplements to patients on potassium-wasting diuretics, and dietitians instruct patients to consume high-potassium foods in conjunction with their diuretic therapy.

Concentrated potassium supplements can injure the intestinal lining unless taken with adequate fluid. Excessive potassium in the blood can lead to death. Individuals whose heart does not pump correctly or whose kidneys fail to excrete properly should limit dietary potassium. A dietitian can plan a low-potassium diet when necessary (Institute of Medicine 2004).

High blood pressure treatment usually involves decreasing dietary sodium, or salt. Another lesser-known measure to help control hypertension is to increase potassium intake. Foods with the least sodium and the most potassium are fresh fruits and vegetables, which do not contain preservatives or added salt. Potatoes, oranges, bananas, tomatoes, cantaloupes, and broccoli, when eaten in appropriate quantity to replace higher-calorie foods, will result in weight loss that also lowers high blood pressure.

Food Sources

All natural foods, except oils, contain potassium. Fruits and vegetables provide the most potassium, followed closely by milk and meats (Box 7–2). Whole grains contain more potassium than do refined grains. Some medications and some salt substitutes also contain potassium. Sometimes consumers, especially those with heart or kidney disease, are counseled to avoid salt substitutes because they contain potassium. In the place of salt substitutes for individuals on a low-sodium diet who cannot consume the extra potassium, they can easily add flavor to food by adding herbs and spices. Processed foods contain potassium in the form of additives that help stabilize and preserve commercially produced food products.

Chloride

Function

Although the element chlorine is a poisonous gas, its ionic form, chloride, is a required nutrient. Chloride's main function is to maintain the acid/base balance of the body and osmotic pressure. **Osmotic pressure** is the regulation of fluid flow into and out of body cells.

Chloride is one of the body's three mineral electrolytes. The other two—sodium and potassium—were discussed earlier.

OSMOTIC PRESSURE The regulation of water movement within the body's cells.

BOX 7–2 • POTASSIUM CONTENT OF NATURAL FOODS

200 TO 300 MILLIGRAMS

Apricots, 2 to 3

Pork, 3 oz.

Lima beans, 1/2 cup

Lentils, 1/2 cup

Cantaloupe, 1/4

Tuna, 3 oz.

Avocado, 1/4

Raisins, 3 Tbsp.

Broccoli, 1/2 cup

300 TO 400 MILLIGRAMS

Chicken, 3 oz.

Milk, 1 cup

Sweet potato, large

Bamboo shoots, 1/2 cup

Lamb, 3 oz.

Orange, medium size

400 TO 500 MILLIGRAMS

Winter squash, 1/2 cup

Watermelon, 5-inch by 8-inch wedge

Salmon, 1/2 cup

Grapefruit juice, 1 cup

500 TO 600 MILLIGRAMS

Prune juice, 1 cup

Tomato juice, 1 cup

Orange juice, 1 cup

Sardines, 8

Potato with skin, medium

Halibut, 3 oz.

Banana, medium or large

Dates, 10

Electrolytes help transmit nerve impulses and signals (Figure 7–2). Chloride binds with both sodium and potassium. It also forms part of the hydrochloric acid in the stomach, which is used for food digestion and nutrient absorption.

Dietary Requirement

There is no RDA for chloride. AI is set at 2,300 milligrams per day for young adults, while the UL is 3,500 milligrams per day (Institute of Medicine 2004).

Deficiency and Toxicity

Although sodium is recognized as the mineral most closely related to high blood pressure, one study of hospitalized patients showed that sodium citrate did not raise blood pressure

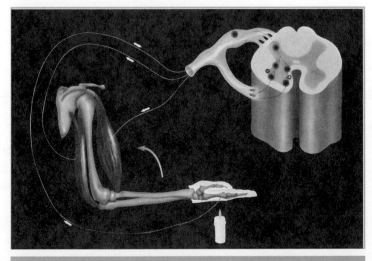

FIGURE 7–2 • HUMAN NERVOUS SYSTEM
Source: Photo Researchers, Inc.

in the same way as sodium chloride (Kurtz et al. 1987). Therefore, we may theorize that the chloride component of table salt plays a role in hypertension. More study, however, is needed to confirm or to refute this.

Chloride deficiency is unlikely unless dehydration results from excessive sweating, diarrhea, or vomiting. These processes deplete body chloride content as well as sodium. Normal food and beverage intake will replenish chloride. Severe dehydration requires hospitalization and treatment with intravenous fluids.

Food Sources

Table salt is a large dietary source of chloride. One-fourth teaspoon of salt contains 750 milligrams of chloride. Many processed foods, such as frozen meals, canned foods, snacks, cereals, dairy products, and lunch meats, contain chloride from salt.

Sulfur

Function

Sulfur is an important constituent of many body tissues and enzyme systems. The sulfur from sulfur dioxide, which maintains the color of dried fruit, is unavailable to the body.

Dietary Requirement

There is no Dietary Reference Intake (DRI) for sulfur.

Food Sources

Most sulfur in the diet comes from organic sources. Sulfur is found in all flesh foods, milk, eggs, and vegetables of the cabbage family (cabbage, cauliflower, broccoli, and Brussels sprouts), as well as in legumes and nuts.

TRACE MINERALS (MICROMINERALS)

Microminerals are essential nutrients but are needed only in trace amounts (under 100 milligrams a day). These include chromium, copper, fluoride, iodine, iron, manganese, molybdenum, selenium, and zinc.

Iron

Function

HEMOGLOBIN An iron-containing pigment made of protein that transports oxygen in the blood.

The body uses iron mainly to manufacture **hemoglobin** in red blood cells. Hemoglobin transports oxygen to every cell and carries carbon dioxide from cells to the lungs. The carbon dioxide is a waste product that is exhaled through respiration. The four beadlike disks in Figure 7–3 contain the iron pigment, heme, and these transport oxygen throughout the body. Hemoglobin is made in the bone marrow from an iron-containing pigment called *hematin* and a protein called *globin*. Copper and cobalt are also necessary in the process of hemoglobin formation.

MYOGLOBIN A muscle protein that contains oxygen.

Iron is also an essential component of **myoglobin**, which is a receptor and storage point for some of the oxygen in muscles. Iron is stored in the liver, spleen, and bone marrow as ferritin and hemosiderin.

Iron is also part of many enzymes. Too little or too much iron can increase susceptibility to infections. Iron is needed by neutrophils and lymphocytes, blood cells that fight

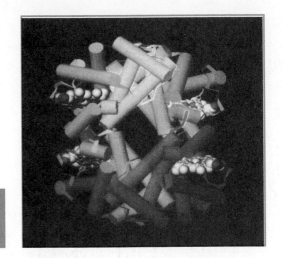

FIGURE 7–3 • REPRESENTATION OF THE IRON PIGMENT, HEME
Source: Photo Researchers, Inc.

infection, for good immunity; but large doses of supplemental iron hasten bacterial growth. Iron supplements can also interfere with copper absorption.

Dietary Requirement

The RDA for iron takes into account the fact that iron is lost in feces, urine, and sweat at the rate of 1 milligram per day. Because only one-tenth of dietary iron is absorbed, allowances are set much higher than the loss: 8 milligrams per day for men, and 18 milligrams per day for women in the reproductive years, 19 to 50 years of age, to cover iron losses in the menstrual flow. Following the reproductive years, for women over 50 years of age, the requirement for women drops to only 8 milligrams of iron daily.

Deficiency and Toxicity

Iron deficiency is common in women and is the most common deficiency worldwide. The usual symptoms are pallor, weakness, headache, palpitations, and persistent lethargy. Iron is of great importance during pregnancy, and iron supplements are often necessary. Many women are iron deficient even before pregnancy, which creates a bigger dilemma. Infants need iron from their mothers before birth to accumulate a five-month supply.

An infant's early diet is breast milk, which is low in iron. But the infant's body absorbs this iron five times more efficiently than iron from cow's milk. An infant would have adequate iron nutrition provided that the mother's body stored enough iron during pregnancy and the infant is breast-fed. Most baby formulas are iron fortified to prevent iron deficiency anemia. Many toddlers and school-age children do not get enough iron-rich foods, however. Iron deficiency affects a child's ability to learn and defend against infection. Laboratory tests can check for iron deficiency anemia. The test most commonly performed measures blood hemoglobin levels.

HEMOCHROMATOSIS A genetic disease, seen mostly in men, that is characterized by iron overload.

The hereditary disorder **hemochromatosis** causes uncontrolled iron absorption in the liver, skin, pancreas, and joints, which leads to multiorgan failure and early death from iron toxicity. The UL for men and women 14 years and older is 45 milligrams per day.

Enrichment and fortification of grain foods have greatly reduced iron deficiency anemia in the United States. Supplements for women and infants have reduced anemia even further. Despite these improvements, iron deficiency is still common; and although the iron levels of many women and children are not low enough to be classified as anemia, they are still below normal. It is unknown if mild shortages of iron are harmful. Continued research needs to be done in this area.

BOX 7–3 • FOODS HIGH IN HEME IRON

Clams	Dark-meat poultry
Oysters	Light-meat poultry
Liver	Tuna
Beef	Sardines
Pork	Salmon
Lamb	Whitefish

Food Sources

HEME IRON Iron from foods of animal origin. Heme iron is absorbed more readily than nonheme iron.

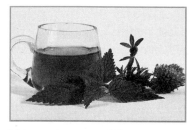

The tannin in tea inhibits iron absorption.
Steve Gorton © Dorling Kindersley

There are two types of dietary iron: **heme iron** and nonheme iron. Heme iron is obtained from animal sources and is about 15% to 30% assimilated. For example, iron in meat, poultry, and fish is heme iron, which comes from myoglobin and hemoglobin. Box 7–3 lists sources of heme iron. Iron obtained from nonanimal sources is nonheme iron (Box 7–4), which is absorbed at the rate of 3% to 8% (some sources state ranges from 2% to 20%).

Vitamin C facilitates iron absorption when present at the time of iron intake. For example, orange juice enhances iron absorption from a meal containing sweet potatoes and beef tenderloin. The sweet potatoes contain nonheme iron; the orange juice contains nonheme iron and vitamin C; and the beef tenderloin contains both heme iron and nonheme iron. The orange juice will enhance the absorption of nonheme iron in the meat, and the meat will enhance the absorption of iron from the juice. This example demonstrates clearly why all foods can and should fit into a healthy diet. Variety improves overall nutritional intake.

While vitamin C aids absorption, other substances block it. The tannin in tea, for instance, inhibits iron absorption by binding nonheme iron. Iced tea is a popular American beverage; thus, many people are affected by this interaction. Heme iron is absorbed by a different mechanism, so its assimilation is unaffected by tea.

There are other iron detractors besides tannins. Polyphenols in coffee inhibit iron absorption. Oxalic acid in spinach, rhubarb, and chocolate; phytates in whole grains and soybeans; and phosvitin in egg yolks all bind iron. The preservative EDTA and antacids, if consumed in large amounts, also inhibit iron absorption.

BOX 7–4 • FOODS HIGH IN NONHEME IRON

Egg yolk	Peaches
Dark green leafy vegetables	Grapes and raisins
Legumes	Plums and prunes
Nuts	Figs
Sweet potatoes	Dates
Peas	Brewer's yeast
Carrots	Blackstrap molasses
Broccoli	Enriched grains
Watermelon	Whole grains
Apricots	

Note: Breakfast cereals are sometimes fortified to deliver the entire RDA of iron in one serving.

Zinc

Function

Zinc is needed for healthy skin, hair, and nails, so a sizable amount of this mineral is found in these structures. Twenty percent of the body's total zinc is found in the skin alone. Most zinc in the body is bound to enzymes. At least 40 different enzyme systems require zinc.

Zinc appears to play a major role in the synthesis of nucleic acids, including DNA and RNA, and in protein synthesis. Wound healing also requires zinc. No good method is yet available for assessing body stores of zinc.

Dietary Requirement

The RDA for zinc is 11 milligrams per day for adult males and pregnant women, and 8 milligrams for nonpregnant adult women. Zinc absorption averages about 40%. Women require additional zinc during pregnancy and lactation. Children 1 to 8 years old need from 3 to 5 milligrams of zinc daily and may lack adequate intake if they eat refined cereals. In general, zinc intake is proportional to protein intake. Seafood and meat are the commonly eaten foods that contain the highest amounts of natural zinc.

Deficiency and Toxicity

Because meat and seafood are the highest sources of zinc, strict vegetarians are at risk for zinc deficiency; but this deficiency is rare. Zinc deficiencies usually arise from genetic defects, disease, or burns. Deficiency results in a rash on the face and limbs, poor growth, loss of taste and smell, loss of hair, infertility, loss of sexual function in males, poor wound healing, and depression. Zinc deficiency is also associated with a lessened insulin response to glucose. Moreover, zinc deficiency may affect immunity because the immune system requires zinc.

Zinc toxicity is uncommon because dietary excess is unlikely. In addition, the body has a very efficient mechanism for regulating zinc levels. An exorbitant zinc intake, such as 10 times the RDA, could interfere with copper and iron absorption. Therefore, the UL is about 4 times the RDA at 40 milligrams per day for adult men and women. Excess zinc is also thought to impair the immune response, and it affects some liver enzyme activities in animals.

Populations that eat high amounts of unleavened whole-grain bread may develop zinc deficiency because fiber and phytates bind zinc. This deficiency, however, occurs only in areas with marginal overall nutrition.

High calcium and phosphate intake decreases zinc absorption. Zinc losses occur mainly in stool, sweat, and during menstruation.

Food Sources

Oysters are the best food source of zinc. Herring is the next-best source. Besides oysters and herring, other good food sources of zinc are milk, meat, eggs, seeds, whole grains, and brewer's yeast (Box 7–5). Human milk contains the most bioavailable form of zinc. Cereals lose zinc during the milling process. Zinc bioavailability from beef is about four times greater than that from high-fiber cereals.

Iodine

Function

Iodine is needed to produce **thyroxin**, a hormone made in the thyroid gland. Nearly all of the body's iodine is located in this gland. Thyroxin regulates body heat and influences

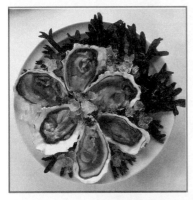

Oysters are a good source of zinc.
Clive Streeter © Dorling Kindersley

THYROXIN A hormone, produced by the thyroid gland, that is responsible for the rate of metabolism.

BOX 7–5 • FOODS HIGH IN ZINC

Oysters	Fish
Herring	Shellfish
Liver	Nuts
Beef	Sesame seeds
Pork	Milk
Lamb	Hard cheeses
Poultry	

protein synthesis, cell metabolism, and basal metabolic rate. Thyroxin also keeps connective tissues healthy and promotes physical and mental development.

Dietary Requirement

The RDA for iodine is set at 150 micrograms per day for adults. Infants and children, however, need less. Average iodine intake is usually well above the required amount because of most people's liberal use of iodized salt.

Deficiency and Toxicity

Iodine deficiency (less than 50 micrograms daily) causes the thyroid gland to enlarge so that it can use all available iodine. This enlargement, called a *goiter*, causes the thyroid gland to protrude visibly from the neck. Goiters are common in Africa, Asia, and South America. In certain areas of Africa where iodine deficiency is epidemic, whole populations have massive goiters that hang onto the chest.

Thyroxin insufficiency causes people to feel sluggish, tired, and cold and to gain weight. Iodine deficiency during the first three weeks of pregnancy can result in the birth of a child who is a dwarf and mentally deficient. This condition is called *cretinism*. Excessive iodine (25 to 70 times the RDA) leads to high levels of thyroxin as well as thyroid enlargement, impaired glucose tolerance, and heart failure. Excessive iodine intake can also

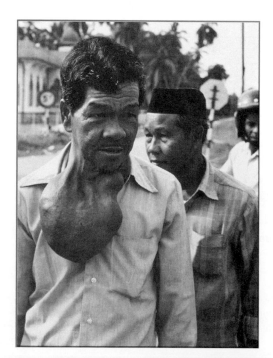

This man has a goiter.
Pearson Education/PH College

cause hypothyroidism, which results in a slowed metabolic rate and listlessness because the thyroid gland stops producing thyroxin. The UL for iodine is less than 10 times the RDA at 1,100 micrograms daily for adults.

Allergies to iodine can produce a rash that appears as a raised sore over the skin, nasal congestion, or asthmatic symptoms. People who are allergic to iodine must avoid foods like kelp, dried seaweed, and shellfish.

Food Sources

Iodine is found in the ocean; therefore, saltwater fish is an excellent source. Iodine also reaches the soil from rain that comes from evaporated ocean water. Thus, land near the ocean and land once covered by the sea are rich in iodine. Foods grown in these iodine-rich soils and food products from animals feeding on this land are natural sources of iodine.

The U.S. diet may contain extra iodine introduced by the iodine sanitizers used on utensils and processing equipment employed in food manufacturing. Certain food colors and dough conditioners also contain iodine. The introduction of iodized salt in 1924 was an important health intervention that eliminated goiter in the United States. Today, salt is available with or without iodine.

Selenium

Function

Selenium's main function is protecting cell membranes from oxidative damage. Selenium is part of glutathione peroxidase, an enzyme that neutralizes hydrogen peroxide. Hydrogen peroxide is a by-product of metabolism and can damage cellular membranes. Selenium binds to a blood protein carrier and defends against oxidants. Selenium also plays a role in electron transfer function and protects against cadmium and mercury toxicity.

Dietary Requirement

The RDA for selenium is 55 micrograms for adults.

Deficiency and Toxicity

Excess selenium is toxic. Cattle that graze in pastures with high concentrations of selenium develop hair loss, long-bone joint erosion that causes lameness, blindness, and liver disease. Animals sometimes die from selenium toxicity. Humans develop problems with intakes of only 10 times the RDA. Therefore, the UL is set at 400 micrograms per day for adults. Liver failure caused by selenium toxicity can lead to death.

Selenium deficiency is a problem in regions of China where the soil lacks selenium. Children who ingest less than 38 micrograms of selenium daily develop Keshan disease, which is characterized by heart failure. Kaschin–Beck disease is another regional human disease in China characterized by degeneration in the arm and leg joints.

New research on cancer and selenium has led to conflicting opinions. Several studies discount the role of selenium deficiency as a cause of cancer. Although cancer patients have lower selenium levels, this is possibly a consequence, not a cause, of the cancer. Thus a firm conclusion on the role of selenium in cancer risk is not justified at present.

The FDA has limited trials of selenium to 200 micrograms because of its toxicity. Selenium toxicity, however, is dependent on other factors, even if the selenium is from dietary sources. For example, some Japanese, known to consume large amounts of fish, ingest more than 700 micrograms of selenium daily without toxic results. In animal studies, researchers have used 20 to 60 times the nutritional requirement of selenium, without toxicity, to demonstrate its effect against cancer.

Food Sources

Seafood, meat, liver, and kidney are rich food sources of selenium. Rice and whole grains contain varying amounts of selenium depending on the soil content where the plants were grown. Fruits and vegetables are generally considered poor sources of selenium, but tomatoes and cabbage have the highest levels among vegetables. Limited data exist regarding the amount of selenium in processed and refined foods. Milling, however, causes loss of selenium in grains.

Copper

Function

An important function of copper is its role as a catalyst in hemoglobin formation. Hemoglobin is necessary for carrying oxygen to the body's tissues, so copper deficiency could be one cause of anemia. Another aspect of copper's relationship to iron is its presence in ceruloplasmin, which transports stored iron. Copper is also necessary for the oxidation of ferrous iron (Fe^{2+}) to ferric iron (Fe^{3+}), the precursor of circulating iron called *transferrin*.

Copper influences iron absorption and movement from the liver and other tissue stores. Copper-containing enzymes like tyrosine (tyrosinase + copper) become dopa, which becomes melanin. Melanin is necessary for color, especially in hair. Dopa, with copper, becomes norepinephrine, a hormone and neurotransmitter that delivers chemical messages within the body as part of central nervous system function.

Copper is a constituent of the elastic connective tissue protein elastin. Moreover, copper is involved in the formation of myelin, the material that covers nerve fibers. Copper also acts as part of enzymes that make cross-links in bone matrix, hair, and blood vessels. Furthermore, copper is important in respiration, acts as an antioxidant, and protects cells.

Dietary Requirement

The RDA for copper is 900 micrograms daily for adults.

Deficiency and Toxicity

Copper deficiency can cause anemia, osteoporosis, depigmentation of skin and hair, and weakness of elastic tissue in the blood vessels and the central nervous system. Central nervous system abnormalities include apnea (difficulty breathing), hypotonia (loss of muscle tone), and psychomotor retardation.

Copper deficiency occasionally is seen in children whose diet mainly consists of milk. While a nutritious beverage, milk is low in copper. Infants born with an inherited defect in copper absorption do not respond to copper supplementation. This disease, called *Menkes' syndrome*, prevents copper absorption into the tissues. Menkes' syndrome results in death in about four to five years.

Excess copper can cause restlessness, insomnia, and elevated blood pressure. It also competes with other minerals in absorption. Evidence indicates that some psychiatric symptoms result from copper toxicity as well.

Food Sources

Oysters are one of the richest food sources of copper (3,623 milligrams in a 100-gram portion), followed by liver (2,450 milligrams of copper per 100 grams). Dry beans contain a substantial amount of copper as well (960 milligrams per 100 grams). Nuts, peas, whole rye and wheat, and avocados also contain very high levels of copper compared to other foods. The UL for copper is 10,000 micrograms for adults. Copper cooking utensils and water pipes are also a source of copper in the diet.

Manganese

Function

Manganese works together with enzymes in the carbohydrate, protein, and lipid metabolism pathways. Therefore, it facilitates energy production. The average human body has 20 milligrams of manganese, distributed primarily in bone and glands. In addition, manganese is an essential ingredient of spinal disks.

Dietary Requirement

The DRI for manganese is an AI of 2.3 milligrams per day for adult males and 1.8 milligrams per day for adult females.

Deficiency and Toxicity

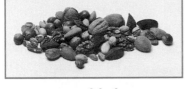

Nuts are some of the best sources for manganese.
Gary Ombler © Dorling Kindersley

There are no blood tests to determine manganese levels. Instead, pathologists test tissue that is dried, ashed, and prepared with acid. Manganese deficiency has not been identified in humans. In animals, manganese deficiency causes malformations of the young, and it lowers animal immunity. Taking iron and calcium inordinately may decrease manganese absorption.

Manganese toxicity is rare and results only from dust or fumes from industry. Toxicity causes brain disease and nervous system disorders. The UL for manganese is 11 milligrams per day for adults.

Food Sources

The manganese content of plant sources depends on the soil where the plant grew. The best sources of manganese are whole grains, nuts, and legumes. Tea and cloves also contain manganese. Blueberries are the best source in the fruit category. Dairy, meat, and fish, however, are poor sources.

Fluoride

Function

Fluoride is necessary for bone and tooth development. When bones and teeth are mineralized, the calcium and phosphorus form a crystal called *hydroxyapatite*. Then fluoride

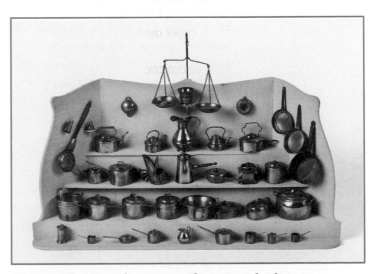

Copper cookware can be a source of copper in the diet.
© Judith Miller/Dorling Kindersley/Pook and Pook

replaces portions of the hydroxyapatite crystal, forming fluorapatite, which makes bones and teeth stronger. The great benefit of fluoride is that it prevents tooth decay.

The National Institute of Dental Research has recommended fluoridation of public water supplies. Tooth decay rates have dropped over 50% in the past 20 years because of fluoride added to water supplies. One part fluoride per 1 million parts water is ideal to provide protection against dental cavities. Some areas have naturally high fluoride content in the water. Crown calcification occurs if fluoride reaches this level.

Dietary Requirement

The DRI set as an AI for fluoride is 4 milligrams per day for men and 3 milligrams per day for women. The average diet provides 1.0 to 1.5 milligrams of fluoride for adults and 0.4 to 1.1 milligrams of fluoride for children 1 to 12 years of age if water containing 1 ppm fluoride is ingested in the adequate quantity of 4 cups per day.

Dentists recommend a 1-milligram daily dietary fluoride supplement for individuals who have a nonfluoridated water supply. Applying a 2% sodium fluoride solution directly to children's teeth is also effective in preventing dental cavities. Babies need 0.01 to 0.5 milligram of fluoride per day to maintain dental health.

Breast milk does not provide adequate fluoride to an infant regardless of the mother's intake. A cup of water a day in addition to mother's milk provides an infant adequate fluoride if the water supply contains 1 ppm fluoride. Check with your local water department to see if fluoride is added to the water supply in your area. Otherwise, a prescription supplement is in order for the infant. Many commercial baby formulas also contain fluoride as an additive.

Application of fluoride directly to teeth by the dentist should start at age 3 and continue until age 18. Fluoride should be applied twice a year to prevent tooth decay.

MOTTLING Pitting and white spotting of the tooth enamel.

Some people argue against water fluoridation because a fine line exists between the amount of fluoride that prevents tooth decay and the amount that causes **mottling**. According to one study, 1% of the population using water at the standard concentration of 1 ppm fluoride has at least two mottled teeth. Mottling, which is the appearance of paper-white opaque areas on the teeth, is not dangerous, although it is disfiguring.

Deficiency and Toxicity

Overt fluoride deficiency does not occur in humans because fluoride is present in all water, plants, and animals. The main adverse effects of excessive intake are seen in the teeth and bones. Excess fluoride causes mottling, paper-white opaque areas on the teeth. At fluoride levels of 1.8 ppm, brown stains begin to appear on teeth. Mottling is also proportional to temperature and humidity. Allergic reactions, usually hives, caused by normal concentrations of fluoride in fluoridated water and toothpaste are alleviated when the fluoride is discontinued. The UL for fluoride for both men and women is 10 milligrams per day.

Research published in the *Journal of Public Health Dentistry* states that the negative effects attributed to fluoridation are uncontrolled observations and are not based on clinical trials. The article shows that mortality rates and other health statistics in fluoridated and nonfluoridated communities are similar (Newbrun 1996).

Some health professionals have employed fluoride therapy in osteoporosis treatment, but there is no convincing evidence that it is beneficial. In some studies spinal bone mass increased with fluoride treatment, while in others bones fractured more often. Another point against the use of fluoride in the treatment of osteoporosis is that bone diseases are prevalent in areas with very high fluoride levels (7 ppm).

Food Sources

Water is the major source of fluoride today. The water used to prepare food will greatly influence dietary fluoride content. Fluoride intake can vary from 1 to 4 milligrams per day, depending on the water supply. The water used in commercial food processing can also increase dietary fluoride content. Where food is grown and animals graze is more important than the type of food in determining fluoride levels.

Chromium

Function

Chromium combines with nicotinic acid and amino acids in the body to form a complex called *glucose tolerance factor*. This factor helps insulin attach to cell membranes, aiding cells with glucose uptake. Chromium stimulates fatty acid and cholesterol synthesis and may help prevent cardiovascular disease as well as diabetes. An adequate dietary intake of chromium improves glucose tolerance factor, cholesterol, triglyceride, and HDL levels.

Dietary Requirement

The DRI for chromium, set as an AI, is 35 micrograms per day for men 19 to 50 years of age and 25 micrograms per day for women of the same age. Some data show that the typical American diet lacks adequate chromium, but other evidence supports the theory that individuals with less than the recommended intake do not have a chromium imbalance. Only 1% to 2% of chromium intake is available, however, so urinary chromium levels are poor indicators of chromium status. Most chromium is lost in stool.

Chromium is the only one heavy metal whose levels in body tissue continually decrease throughout life. Hair, for example, contains 990 ppm of chromium at birth and 440 ppm at age 3. And analysis of adult hair for chromium is inaccurate because of environmental contaminants. So the best way to check chromium levels is to look for diabetes-like symptoms. If these symptoms lessen with the addition of chromium to the diet, there is a chromium deficiency.

Deficiency and Toxicity

Chromium toxicity is not found in humans, and thus, no UL is set for chromium. In animals, toxicity is associated with lung tumors. Studies on human runners show that chromium losses in the urine are increased after running. Physical traumas produce the same finding (National Research Council 1990).

Food Sources

Of all the foods, brewer's yeast provides the most chromium, but it is seldom eaten. Spices have a high chromium content, but they are taken in such minute quantities that their chromium contributions are negligible.

Mushrooms are a good source of chromium, but are not a regular part of most diets. Oysters, liver, and other organ meats, rich sources of many nutrients, are also an excellent source of chromium. Eggs, meat, raisins, nuts, some beer, wines, whole grains, bran, seafood, and chicken are also sources of chromium. If the skin is eaten, potatoes provide more chromium than most vegetables.

A nonfood source of chromium is stainless steel cookware that leaches chromium into food in the presence of acid, such as tomato, vinegar, molasses, or citrus juice. It is unknown whether the body can use chromium from cookware. Furthermore, the amount of chromium in food tends to decrease with commercial processing.

Molybdenum

Function

Molybdenum functions as part of the enzymes sulfite oxidase and xanthine oxidase, which are involved in chemical reactions.

Dietary Requirement

The RDA for molybdenum is 45 micrograms per day for both adult men and women.

Deficiency and Toxicity

The UL for molybdenum is 2,000 micrograms per day for adults. Excess molybdenum may decrease the body's copper levels, and molybdenum toxicity is possible. Using over-the-counter molybdenum supplements is not recommended because imbalances and excesses could result.

The importance of molybdenum for humans was demonstrated in a case study of a patient who developed a molybdenum deficiency after eight months of intravenous feeding. The deficiency symptoms included severe headaches, night blindness, nausea, vomiting, edema, lethargy, disorientation, and coma; all these symptoms reversed with 300 micrograms of molybdenum. Lack of the sulfite oxidase enzyme, which contains molybdenum, results in severe nervous system problems, as described in this case history (Johnson 1980).

Molybdenum helps degrade soil nitrates. The nitrate concentrations are higher in plants when the soil is molybdenum deficient. When these plants are eaten, their nitrates are converted into nitrosamines, which are known carcinogens. Besides having fewer carcinogens, food grown in soil with molybdenum fertilizer contains more vitamin C.

Food Sources

The best food sources of molybdenum are legumes, followed by grains, leafy vegetables, liver, kidney, and spleen. Fruits, berries, and most root or stem vegetables contain some molybdenum. Brewer's yeast is also a source. The molybdenum content of food depends on where it was grown because soil is an important contributing factor.

OTHER MICRONUTRIENTS

Several other minerals may be essential to good health. Because the potential requirement for these minerals is so small, it is difficult to determine if they are essential.

Boron

Boron may help prevent osteoporosis because it aids the body in retaining calcium, magnesium, and phosphorus in bone. Involved in brain function, low intakes of boron affect alertness. Plant foods, especially beet greens, broccoli, nuts, and all noncitrus fruits, contain boron. Signs of boron toxicity include poor appetite and the resulting weight loss. A UL of 20 milligrams per day has been established.

Vanadium

Even though research has been ongoing for the past four decades, scientists still do not know enough about how vanadium works or how much is needed; therefore, health professionals cannot declare vanadium an essential nutrient. So far, research proves that some animal species develop problems with vanadium-deficient diets. Vanadium appears

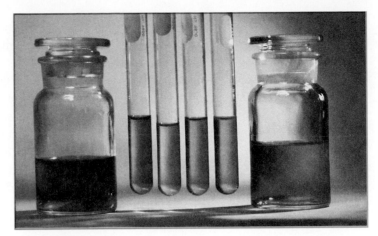

Vanadium at different oxidation states.
Pearson Education/PH College

to affect bone development in goats and the repair of tooth tissue in guinea pigs and rats. Studies have shown that vanadium regulates glucose metabolism in rats in a way similar to insulin, and vanadate, another form of vanadium, reverses diabetes in rats. Human studies show that vanadium lowers endogenous cholesterol production in healthy young men but not in older men or in those with hypercholesterolemia or heart disease.

Vanadium occurs in tiny amounts in natural food. Giving very large doses of vanadium to humans has illustrated some of its effects, but the mechanism by which vanadium works is unknown.

The best food sources of vanadium are black pepper, dill seed, parsley, mushrooms, and shellfish. Smaller amounts are found in fruits, vegetables, fats, and oils.

The total amount of vanadium in the body is about 100 micrograms, found mainly inside the cells. The daily intake of vanadium is low in comparison to other trace minerals and averages about 20 micrograms. Ten to 100 micrograms probably constitutes a safe intake. Large amounts—22.5 milligrams—from supplements can cause cramps and diarrhea. Some reports show that elevated vanadium levels are associated with manic depression. Drugs used to treat this disorder are effective in reducing vanadate. High vitamin C intake is helpful as well.

Vanadium is used to make steel for automobile parts and for aircraft engines. It is used in the rubber, plastic, and ceramics industries and found in crude petroleum deposits as well. Excess vanadium in the environment is a serious problem. In some industrial environments, exposure to vanadium is chronic and high levels are inhaled, causing lung irritation, chest pain, coughing, wheezing, runny nose, and sore throat.

Everyone is exposed to vanadium to some degree. It exists in low levels in air, water, and food. Breathing air near an industry that burns fuel oil exposes one to vanadium oxide. Waste sites and landfills containing vanadium contaminate air and drinking water. Unfortunately, the Agency for Toxic Substances and the Disease Registry do not know the health effects in people who ingest vanadium. High vanadium levels in drinking water given to pregnant animals, however, have resulted in minor birth defects. The carcinogenicity of vanadium is unknown. Laboratory analysis can measure vanadium in urine and blood, but such tests cannot determine whether harmful health effects will occur. People who have high vanadium exposure may develop a green-colored tongue.

The Occupational Safety and Health Administration (OSHA) has set an exposure limit of 0.05 milligrams per cubic meter for vanadium pentoxide dust and 0.1 milligram per cubic meter for vanadium pentoxide fumes in workplace air for an 8-hour workday in a 40-hour work week. The UL for vanadium is 1.8 milligrams per day for adults.

Aluminum

There is no nutritional requirement for aluminum. It is included in this section because of its possible role in dementia.

Individuals have suggested that aluminum may cause Alzheimer's disease, but the bulk of the scientific evidence suggests this is unlikely. Aluminum toxicity as a result of a high concentration of aluminum in the water used to prepare dialysate does cause dementia in dialysis patients. The aluminum accumulation seen in Alzheimer's patients may be the result of a defect rather than a cause of the disease. However, there are more Alzheimer's cases in areas of England and Wales where drinking water has high levels of aluminum. Some of those municipal water supplies contain as much as 2 to 4 milligrams of aluminum per liter.

Aluminum-containing foods include pickles, artificial creamers, and dry mixes. Aluminum additives keep moisture out of packaged mixes. In pickles, aluminum imparts a crisp texture. Ingestion of aluminum in foods ranges from 3 to 5 milligrams daily. According to the National Research Council, there is no reliable evidence that aluminum is carcinogenic.

Mercury

We ingest mercury, in the form of methyl mercury, primarily through fish and seafood. Fish heavily contaminated with mercury can cause severe poisoning with resulting neurological and kidney problems. In nature, mercury is found in very low concentrations. Occupational exposure is mainly through inhalation. Safe levels and regulations have been established. Visit the U.S. Food and Drug Administration Web site (http://www.fda.gov) to determine current recommendations for fish consumption.

Arsenic

Tiny amounts of arsenic, a known poison, may be essential for health. This is a matter for future research, however. Arsenic is widespread in nature, but arsenic in food may derive from pesticide residue. According to estimates, daily intakes of arsenic in the United States range from 10 to 130 micrograms, and serious health consequences have not been observed. On the other hand, studies of countries with high levels of arsenic in well water yield reports of skin and lung cancer.

Cadmium

Cadmium may have a biological role in humans. That role, however, currently remains unknown. Cadmium exists in the body in trace amounts but does not appear to be an essential nutrient. It is found in minute amounts in food. Higher amounts are found in beef liver and kidney. Plant uptake depends on the cadmium content of the soil in which the plants are grown. Because cadmium is toxic at certain levels, researchers are evaluating crop fertilization as a possible source of cadmium. Soil pH is also a factor in plant uptake of cadmium.

Cigarette smoke contains cadmium, and increased cadmium levels are found in the lung tissue of lung cancer patients. In some studies, cadmium levels in food and drinking water correlate with the incidence of prostate and other cancers. The association may be a result rather than a cause of the cancers, however. Although cadmium is a possible cancer concern, findings are insufficient to establish a relationship between cadmium and high blood pressure. Exposure to cadmium can cause kidney and bone disease, however.

Lead

In the past, the canning industry used lead-soldered cans, which contributed to lead contamination. Lead-free cans are now in use and have eliminated the main source of lead in foods. Dust particles from lead paint, chipped paint, and soil are the main causes of lead contamination today. Blood lead levels greater than 20 micrograms per deciliter in children are dangerous and cause anemia, learning disabilities, and behavior problems.

SUMMARY

The Strength of Minerals

Minerals are inorganic elements that play an important role in maintaining good health. They help regulate body processes and provide structure for body tissues. Minerals are obtained from food sources. They are absorbed in the stomach and through the intestines, where they may pass directly into the bloodstream for transportation to cells. Some excess minerals are excreted via urine, stool, and sweat, while others attach to body proteins for storage and later use.

Macrominerals, or major minerals, are essential minerals needed in large amounts (more than 100 milligrams a day). These include calcium, phosphorus, magnesium, sulfur, and the electrolytes potassium, sodium, and chloride. Electrolytes regulate fluid movement into and out of body cells, and they help transmit nerve or electrical impulses.

Microminerals are needed in trace amounts (under 100 milligrams a day) and are also essential. These include chromium, copper, fluoride, iodine, iron, manganese, molybdenum, selenium, and zinc. Scientists have evaluated microminerals for their health benefits, and Recommended Dietary Allowances (RDAs) or Adequate Intakes (AIs) have been established.

CASE RESOLUTION

Residents of an assisted-living program are usually active seniors who need only minor assistance with daily activities. Adult day care programs provide daytime supervision of functionally or cognitively impaired adults who may need interaction with health professionals as well as stimulation. Neither population is likely to bear children or breast-feed; therefore, restricting potentially high-mercury foods is unnecessary. In addition, the cardiovascular benefit of fish outweighs any risk for this population. Chef Vivian should discuss this with the medical director and should continue with her swordfish meals as planned. In the event that New Castle receives a younger female resident, the facility should reevaluate the potential risks associated with mercury.

REFERENCES

Institute of Medicine. 1997. *Dietary Reference Intakes for Calcium, Phosphorus, Magnesium, Vitamin D, and Fluoride.* Washington, DC: National Academies Press.

Institute of Medicine. 2004. *Dietary Reference Intakes for Water, Potassium, Sodium, Chloride, and Sulfate.* Washington, DC: National Academies Press.

Johnson, J. 1980. *The Molybdenum Cofactor Common to Nitrate Reductions, Xanthine Dehydrogenase and Sulfite Oxidase.* New York: Pergamon Press.

Kurtz, T., A. Hamoudi, S. Al-Bander, and R. Curtis. 1987. "Salt-sensitive" essential hypertension in men—Is the sodium ion alone important? *New England Journal of Medicine* 317: 1043–48.

National Research Council. 1990. *Diet and Health.* Washington, DC: National Academies Press.

Newbrun, E. 1996. The fluoridation war: A scientific dispute or a religious argument? *Journal of Public Health Dentistry* 56 (5): 246–52.

Women's Health Watch. 1995. *Harvard Health Letter* (March).

1. Name the minerals that play a major role in bone health.
2. Name two minerals that play a role in insulin production.
3. Name the macrominerals.
4. Which minerals have no established safe intake level?
5. What is an electrolyte?
6. What are the main food sources for calcium?
7. What are the main food sources for sodium?
8. What is the major function of iron?
9. What mineral is most necessary for thyroid function?
10. What mineral is necessary for proper immune function?
11. List the minerals that function as electrolytes.
12. List good sources of iodine and potassium.

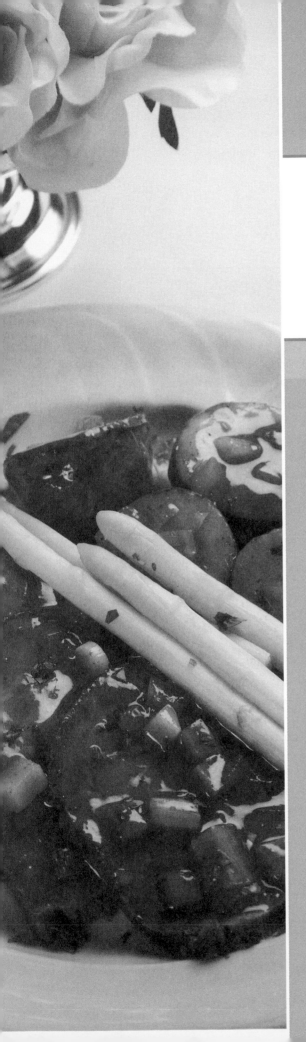

8

Health and Diet

KEY CONCEPTS

- A correlation exists between health and diet in many common ailments and degenerative diseases.
- Positive lifestyle changes reduce the risk for degenerative disease.
- Risk factors for osteoporosis include gender, age, weight, ethnicity, and exercise.
- Many determinants affect calcium absorption, including diet composition and current calcium status.
- Improving diet diminishes the risk for heart disease, cancer, diabetes, and obesity.
- Antioxidants from food partially counteract cancer-causing free radicals in the body.

Current research is revealing the relationship between health and diet. Diet is not merely a way of losing weight but should be an intelligent selection of what we should eat each day. Scientists and doctors are beginning to find connections between the food we eat and the health of our bodies. Remaining abreast of these findings will inform our decision making, enabling us to modify personal lifestyles and eating habits to ensure a long, healthy life.

Enough of a correlation exists between diet and health to suggest the importance of learning some ways in which lifestyle impacts health. As research in the field of nutrition science continues to verify its findings, the dependence of health on diet will become increasingly evident. In the meantime, there are some commonly accepted connections between diet and disease worth noting. This chapter will discuss these connections.

THINK ABOUT IT

Think about the last time you visited your personal physician. Did you leave with a prescription for medication? You probably did. We value medication because it has proven to be an important component of disease treatment, and we have come to rely on the convenience of taking a pill. But are there other ways, albeit slightly more challenging and involved, to improve health and treat disease?

Reflect on your view of diet as a therapy for disease. Have you practiced any form of diet therapy to promote wellness or to improve your health during sickness? Consider a time in your life, if any, when food was your only form of therapy.

CASE STUDY

Pureed Production 101

Mrs. Hernandez placed an advertisement in the local paper for a chef to prepare meals for her husband, who was recovering from a stroke. The stroke left Mr. Hernandez with a severe swallowing problem, requiring him to eat pureed food. In the six-week period following the stroke, Mr. Hernandez lost 15 pounds. Several factors contributed to this weight loss, but chief among them was the baby food he received while hospitalized. The fact that it looked like green mush did not help one bit.

Roger is a personal chef catering to special needs. He has experience modifying menus to make them low-sodium and low-fat. And he knows this type of diet is appropriate for someone with cardiovascular disease. What advice can you offer Roger when he goes on the interview? *The resolution for this case study is presented at the end of the chapter.*

DIET AND AGING

DENTITION A set of teeth.

OLFACTORY Relating to the sense of smell.

Although we cannot stop the aging process, we can postpone or lessen some of aging's ill health effects through proper nutrition. Research has demonstrated that diet plays a role in the development of many of today's chronic health maladies, including osteoporosis, diabetes, and heart disease. Undoubtedly, food impacts health.

The diet of elderly people tends to be nutritionally deficient because these individuals require fewer calories. So the elderly must eat nutrient-dense food to obtain all of the essential nutrients. In addition to their limited caloric intake, a large percentage of the elderly population suffers from a general loss of appetite. Physical changes also contribute to this age-related appetite reduction. For instance, the loss of natural teeth interferes with chewing, which limits the selection of foods that the elderly can consume. Without proper **dentition**, most of these individuals can eat only soft or pureed foods (Sharkey et al. 2002). Producing appetizing pureed food is a challenge to food service workers. Furthermore, deterioration of the **olfactory** neurons and taste buds results in a reduction of taste information to the brain (Schiffman 2000).

There are many ways in which chefs can help elderly people overcome these difficulties. For example, culinary professionals can produce healthful and tasty soups and stews that the elderly can enjoy. Selecting naturally tender meats like slow-roasted beef tenderloin, poultry, and fish helps those with a chewing impediment. Spices and fresh herbs compensate for a diminished sense of smell. Chefs who employ proper ingredients stimulate the five basic taste sensations of bitter, sweet, sour, peppery, and salty

The Administration on Aging (AoA) provides information for the elderly. To learn more about issues the elderly face and for more information related to aging, visit the Administration on Aging at http://www.aoa.dhhs.gov.

(although salt intake is usually restricted for those with high blood pressure). Chefs may also make food enticing with visual appeal. Colorful foods with a variety of color, tastes, and textures, when presented attractively, excite elderly senses more than do large portions or fancy foods.

OSTEOPOROSIS

OSTEOPOROSIS Disease in which the bones deteriorate, becoming weak and porous.

Osteoporosis results when bone cell loss or breakdown occurs faster than bone cell production. This condition makes bones porous and weak. Fractures happen more easily, and the spinal vertebrae can collapse, causing the slightly humped appearance associated with those who have severe osteoporosis.

Children, teenagers, and adults should consume proper amounts of calcium because it is the main bone-building material. Vitamins D and K, magnesium, zinc, fluoride, and boron are also needed for healthy bones. Building strong bones in the developing years is most important because some bone loss is normal after reaching adulthood. Storing more calcium in the skeleton early in life lessens the effect of bone loss later in life.

The long bones in the limbs reach their peak mass by ages 20 to 25; bone loss starts in them gradually from that time forward. The soft bones in the back continue to increase in density for another 10 years, possibly to age 40, before they begin to lose calcium (Teegarden et al. 1999). In light of this fact, adequate calcium consumption early in life up through the late teens and early twenties is critical. Attending to diet in these early years can provide great benefit later in life.

Other factors influence osteoporosis development. Low amounts of the hormone estrogen may cause osteoporosis. A lack of estrogen may affect the absorption rate of calcium, which then affects bone cell replacement. Women who have reached **menopause** or who have had their ovaries removed experience difficulty maintaining appropriate estrogen levels. Although the treatment now is controversial, these individuals can take estrogen during and after menopause. The stronger the bones are in youth, the more they will hold up to estrogen depletion and short-term deficiencies of calcium and other nutrients.

MENOPAUSE Period in a woman's life when menstruation naturally ceases.

A balanced diet together with weight-bearing exercise, both in childhood and throughout life, helps prevent osteoporosis and other bone diseases. Milk and all milk products are naturally rich in calcium. Dried beans and peas, tofu that has been processed

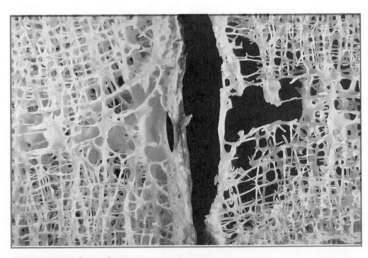

Osteoporosis bone loss.
Peter Arnold, Inc.

with calcium carbonate (be sure to check the label), edible fish bones from sardines and anchovies, juices fortified with calcium, and dark green leafy vegetables are excellent sources of calcium and other necessary bone-building nutrients.

Vitamin D ensures the proper absorption of calcium into the human body, but it is not easily obtained through food. Generally humans obtain vitamin D through sunlight exposure or through fortified foods. Milk, for example, is fortified with vitamin D because it is also a good source of calcium. Oily fish and egg yolks also contain vitamin D.

As mentioned in Chapter 3, many people are deficient in the enzyme lactase, which breaks down lactose in milk and milk products. This deficiency leads to the condition known as lactose intolerance. Lactase tablets and milk with added lactase enable lactose-intolerant individuals to enjoy the taste and nutritional benefits of dairy products. Lactose-intolerant individuals who avoid fortified milk and milk products must obtain calcium and vitamin D from other sources.

DIABETES

Diabetes is a chronic genetic disease that can affect both the young and the elderly. After eating a meal, blood sugar normally raises and then returns to normal levels after a few hours. But for people with diabetes this is not the case. Their blood sugar levels remain elevated and do not return to normal (Figure 8–1). Two forms, type 1 (insulin-dependent diabetes mellitus [IDDM]) and type 2 (non-insulin-dependent diabetes mellitus [NIDDM]), affect people in different ways, but both reduce the body's ability to use glucose as an energy source.

Insulin is the hormone that transports glucose into the cells so it can be used for energy. Diabetics don't produce insulin, cannot produce enough insulin, or have insulin receptors on the cells that do not function properly, so they require either insulin (IDDM) or medications that make their bodies produce more insulin (NIDDM). Individually planned diets, exercise, and medication help balance insulin production and glucose utilization. This treatment combination also aids in weight loss.

People with IDDM require prescription doses of insulin to keep their systems balanced. Their bodies may never be able to supply the right amount of insulin. People with NIDDM (adult-onset diabetes) usually can control symptoms through exercise, diet, and oral hypoglycemic agents (OHAs). However, they also may require injected doses of insulin depending on established treatment goals.

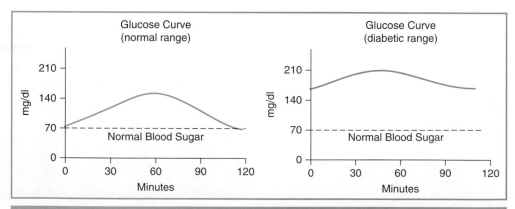

FIGURE 8-1 • COMPARISON OF BLOOD SUGAR

Occurrences of NIDDM are on the rise in America. As the U.S. population ages, more people are becoming susceptible because of lack of exercise and an increase in obesity. Due to the rise in childhood obesity, diabetes is being found more frequently in children as young as 6 or 7 years of age. Excessive fat, in itself, may interfere with the body's ability to use naturally produced insulin.

Elderly diabetics may find it difficult to eat a proper diet and attain enough exercise. Sometimes they may require care from a registered dietitian. Dietitians can design meal plans based on a person's age and particular health problem. For most adults with diabetes, this usually means a low-fat, controlled-carbohydrate, high-fiber diet to help maintain normal body weight and to ensure adequate nutrition. Diabetes, if it is not controlled, can lead to long-term complications such as cardiovascular disease, blindness, kidney failure, and nervous system disorders. If left untreated, diabetes may impair circulation in the extremities, resulting in loss of fingers, toes, and feet through gangrene and subsequent amputation. Treatment of diabetes is a team effort. A registered dietitian and a physician should work together to help increase quality of life and prolong occurrence of these complications.

THE AMERICAN DIABETES ASSOCIATION

The American Diabetes Association provides information to consumers and health professionals as well as funding for research. Visit http://www.diabetes.org for meal tips, recipes, and ideas for living healthfully with diabetes.

HEART DISEASE

The American Heart Association (AHA) estimates that more than 64 million Americans have some form of cardiovascular disease (American Heart Association 2003). Risk factors include heredity, age, gender (premenopausal women have a lower risk than do men and older women), cigarette smoking, diet, and sedentary lifestyle. Diabetes and high blood pressure also can lead to heart disease.

Poor diets include excessive saturated and trans fat and cholesterol, which promote obesity and the buildup of fatty deposits in coronary arteries (Figure 8–2). A heart-healthy diet is the same balanced diet that protects against cancer, adult-onset diabetes, and obesity; it is low in fat, high in fiber, and features plentiful fruits, whole grains, and vegetables daily. Prudent dietary practices ideally begin in childhood. Atherosclerosis, or clogging of the arteries by fatty deposits, may begin in early childhood and can continue throughout life. Some parents are of the mistaken belief that plump children are healthy children. Although children need more calories than adults, the calories should come from a balanced diet and not one heavily laden with fatty or high-sugar foods. Other common myths permeate childhood dietary practices; examples include the belief that children will not drink water because they prefer soda and the notion that kids dislike vegetables. Instead of soda, offer children a single daily serving of 100% fruit juice along with low-fat milk and water. Offer vegetables, especially "new" ones, on at least 10 or more occasions; some children willingly accept vegetables only after they have been presented several times.

Particularly healthful foods for adults and children include all fruits and vegetables, especially those high in vitamin C, beta-carotene, and other antioxidants. Vitamin E may impact heart health and is found in eggs, wheat germ, nuts, seeds, and dark green leafy vegetables.

The omega-3 fatty acids found in cold-water fish species like salmon, herring, and trout reduce blood's tendency to clot. Certain types of fish should be consumed in moderation due to their methyl mercury content. The free flow of blood helps prevent many forms of heart disease and strokes caused by blood clots. Balance and moderation are still prudent, however, because overconsumption of blood-thinning nutrients is possible. Hemorrhagic stroke, for example, is worsened by extreme blood-thinning regimens that include superfluous vitamin E or fish oil. Individuals should avoid excessive consumption of these supplements and take them only with a health professional's guidance. Natural food sources of vitamin E and omega-3 fatty acids are safer choices.

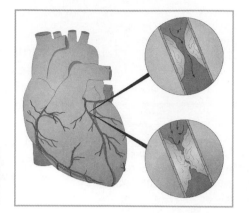

FIGURE 8-2 • PLAQUE BUILDUP IN CORONARY ARTERY
Source: Photo Researchers, Inc.

You will find mountains of useful information at the American Heart Association (AHA) Web site (http://www.americanheart.org). This site has many heart-healthy recipes. Whether you know someone with heart disease or just want to keep your own cardiovascular system in good health, the AHA can help.

In addition to vitamin E's possible benefit, oat bran, pectin, many fruits, dried beans, peas, and other foods containing soluble fiber also help to lower cholesterol in the blood and regulate glucose absorption (Stevens et al. 2002).

CANCER

There is no cure for cancer, but ample evidence suggests a correlation between eating certain foods and cancer risk reduction. Such anticancer foods contain high amounts of antioxidants, or positively charged molecules, that attract negatively charged free radicals. This neutralizing marriage renders free radicals harmless, and they are excreted through normal bodily functions.

Cancer is partially the result of too many free radicals in the body. These are harmful end products of natural bodily processes, such as using oxygen to help convert food to energy. The natural enzymes that protect healthy cells usually protect against free radical damage. But too many free radicals or other forms of oxidative damage (such as tobacco smoke, ultraviolet sun rays, pollution, and automobile exhaust) may cause cancer. Proper diet helps balance the free radicals with the antioxidants that counteract them.

The body's immune system tries to eliminate the damage caused by free radicals by seeking out and destroying decaying body cells, much as it does to invading bacteria and viruses. But as the body ages, it becomes more susceptible to free radical damage. Instances of degenerative damage increase. The results may be slight skin blemishes, liver disease, tumor growth, and cancer.

The major antioxidants are vitamins C and E, beta-carotene (the precursor for vitamin A), and selenium. The first three may be found in fruits and vegetables; selenium is found in Brazil nuts, beef, poultry, seafood, whole-grain products, eggs, and rice. Moreover, scientists have recently identified phytochemicals in many fruits and vegetables that perform as antioxidants as well.

Cancer is also associated with certain types of dietary fat (American Cancer Society 2002). As fat in the diet increases, so does the incidence of certain types of cancer. Some of the most prevalent cancers in the United States are associated with increased dietary fat.

A lack of dietary fiber increases the risk of colon cancer (American Cancer Society 2002). As stated in Chapter 3, fiber exercises the intestinal muscle and helps it maintain an ideal shape.

Antioxidants, fat, and fiber are not the only dietary factors that have an impact on cancer. Recent epidemiological evidence links higher vitamin D intake with reduced incidence of cancer.

Current research suggests that vitamin D may reduce the risk of cancer, although the results are not conclusive. A dilemma arises from the fact that vitamin D is difficult to

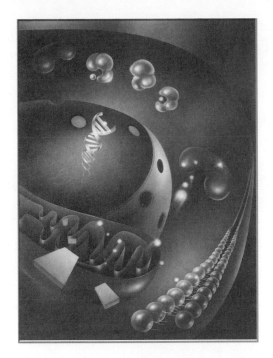

Small free radicals are captured by the large antioxidants.
Phototake NYC

The National Institutes of Health has a branch devoted to cancer research and information. Visit the National Cancer Institute Web site (http://www. nci.nih.gov).

obtain through diet alone. Many people dislike fatty fish, and most of the world's population is intolerant to milk and dairy products, both of which are major food sources of vitamin D. The other major source of vitamin D is exposure of the skin to the sun's ultraviolet rays. But how can we obtain enough sun exposure to produce adequate vitamin D without initiating skin cancer? Several studies are under way to examine this relationship. The current position is that approximately 15 minutes of sun exposure a few times each week may help an individual achieve adequate vitamin D status. Just remember not to overdo it.

ARTHRITIS

Arthritis, represented by more than 100 disorders, affects one in seven Americans. It is characterized by inflammation of the joints, stiffness, swelling, and pain and leaves individuals with some measure of disability and dysfunction. Certain nutrients may prevent or alleviate arthritis symptoms.

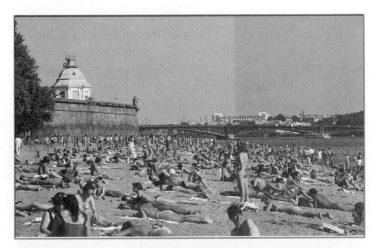

A delicate balance exists between the benefits of sunbathing for vitamin D exposure and its dangers in triggering skin cancers.
Demetrio Carrasco © Dorling Kindersley

For information on the major forms of arthritis and the science of its treatment, go to the Arthritis Foundation Web site at http://www.arthritis.org.

Omega-3 fatty acids, found in fatty cold-water fish, may help reduce inflammation (Simopoulos 2002). Some doctors recommend two or three servings of fatty cold-water fish weekly to help supply the omega-3 fatty acids. Excessive amounts of omega-3 fats, however, are not recommended as they may lead to internal bleeding if taken with certain medications that thin the blood. In addition to fish oil, capsaicin (pronounced "cap-say-uh-sin"), found in capsicum peppers and in concentrated forms in the hot varieties of peppers, also reduces inflammation when rubbed on inflamed joints.

HIGH BLOOD PRESSURE (HYPERTENSION)

When the heart muscle contracts, it distributes blood to every cell of the body. The blood, as it circulates through the body's arteries, exerts pressure against arterial walls referred to as blood pressure. **Systolic** pressure, denoted by the top number in blood pressure notation, is the pressure on arterial walls when the heart contracts. Normal systolic pressure is about 120 millimeters of mercury (mm Hg). **Diastolic** pressure, indicated by the bottom number, is the pressure on the arteries when the heart is at rest. Optimal diastolic pressure is less than 80 mm Hg. Both numbers are typically written together as follows: 120/80 mm Hg (Table 8–1).

SYSTOLIC Refers to pressure within the arteries when the heart contracts.

DIASTOLIC Refers to pressure within the arteries when the heart relaxes.

Narrowing or hardening of the arteries raises blood pressure and increases the risk for stroke and heart disease. Stress, diabetes, obesity, smoking, excessive alcohol consumption, and sedentary lifestyles contribute to hypertension. Salt also raises blood pressure in those who already suffer from hypertension. However, not everyone is salt sensitive. Since we cannot easily determine who is salt sensitive and who is not, it is wise for everyone to limit excess salt.

The American Heart Association (AHA) has hypertension covered from A to Z. Visit its Web site at http://www.americanheart.org.

Salt allows the body to retain water for proper fluid balance. So reducing salt subsequently eliminates water from the body. But if blood pressure is too high when this happens, blood pressure is also lowered.

Dietary means of controlling high blood pressure include keeping fat intake low to maintain a healthy body weight and restricting salt intake to 2,300 milligrams per day or less. High-potassium foods, such as fruits and vegetables, also help control blood pressure

Category	Systolic[a] (mm Hg)[b]		Diastolic[a] (mm Hg)[b]	Result
Normal	Less than 120	*and*	Less than 80	Good for you!
Prehypertension	120–139	*or*	80–89	Your blood pressure could be a problem. Make changes in what you eat and drink, be physically active, and lose extra weight. If you also have diabetes, see your doctor.
Hypertension	140 or higher	*or*	90 or higher	You have high blood pressure. Ask your doctor or nurse how to control it.

TABLE 8–1 • BLOOD PRESSURE LEVELS FOR ADULTS

[a]If systolic and diastolic pressures fall into different categories, overall status is the higher category.
[b]Millimeters of mercury.
Source: U.S. Department of Health and Human Services and National Institutes of Health National Heart, Lung, and Blood Institute. 2003. *The Seventh Report of the Joint National Committee on Prevention, Detection, Evaluation, and Treatment of High Blood Pressure.* NIH Publication No. 03-5230. Washington, DC: NIH.

by eliminating sodium from the body (Akita et al. 2003) and help replace some of the nutrients leached out by medications.

The National Heart, Lung, and Blood Institute has published guidelines to control high blood pressure, *Dietary Approaches to Stop Hypertension* (DASH) (Table 8–2). The DASH diet, replete with fruits and vegetables, also encourages the consumption of low-fat dairy, nuts, fish, poultry, and whole grains (Moore et al. 2001). The DASH diet lowers blood pressure

TABLE 8–2 • DASH DIET

The DASH Eating Plan shown below is based on 2,000 calories a day. The number of daily servings in a food group may vary from those listed, depending on your caloric needs. Use this chart to help you plan your menus or take it with you when you go to the store.

Food Group	Daily Servings (except as noted)	Serving Sizes	Examples and Notes	Significance of Each Food Group to the Dash Eating Plan
Grains and grain products	7–8	1 slice bread 1 oz. dry cereal[a] 1/2 cup cooked rice, pasta, or cereal	Whole-wheat bread, English muffin, pita bread, bagel, cereals, grits, oatmeal, crackers, unsalted pretzels, popcorn	Major sources of energy and fiber
Vegetables	4–5	1 cup raw leafy vegetable 1/2 cup cooked vegetable 6 oz. vegetable juice	Tomatoes, potatoes, carrots, green peas, squash, broccoli, turnip greens, collards, kale, spinach, artichokes, green beans, lima beans, sweet potatoes	Rich sources of potassium, magnesium, and fiber
Fruits	4–5	6 oz. fruit juice 1 medium fruit 1/4 cup dried fruit 1/2 cup fresh, frozen, or canned fruit	Apricots, bananas, dates, grapes, oranges, orange juice, grapefruit, grapefruit juice, mangoes, melons, peaches, pineapples, prunes, raisins, strawberries, tangerines	Important sources of potassium, magnesium, and fiber
Low-fat or fat-free dairy foods	2–3	8 oz. milk 1 cup yogurt 1 1/2 oz. cheese	Fat-free (skim) or low-fat (1%) milk, fat-free or low-fat buttermilk, fat-free or low-fat regular or frozen yogurt, low-fat and fat-free cheese	Major sources of calcium and protein
Meats, poultry, and fish	2 or less	3 oz. cooked meats, poultry, or fish	Select only lean; trim away visible fat; broil, roast, or boil, instead of frying; remove skin from poultry	Rich sources of protein and magnesium
Nuts, seeds, and dry beans	4–5 per week	1/3 cup or 1 1/2 oz. nuts 2 Tbsp. of 1/2 oz. seeds 1/3 cup cooked dry beans, peas	Almonds, filberts, mixed nuts, peanuts, walnuts, sunflower seeds, kidney beans, lentils	Rich sources of energy, magnesium, potassium, protein, and fiber
Fats and oils[b]	2–3	1 tsp. soft margarine 1 Tbsp. low-fat mayonnaise 2 Tbsp. light salad dressing 1 tsp. vegetable oil	Soft margarine, low-fat mayonnaise, light salad dressing, vegetable oil (such as olive, corn, canola, or safflower)	DASH has 27% of calories as fat, including fat in or added to foods
Sweets	5 per week	1 Tbsp. sugar 1 Tbsp. jelly or jam 1/2 oz. jelly beans 8 oz. lemonade	Maple syrup, sugar, jelly, jam, fruit-flavored gelatin, jelly beans, hard candy, fruit punch, sorbet ices	Sweets should be low in fat

[a]Equals 1/2–1 1/4 cups, depending on cereal type. Check the product's Nutrition Facts label.

[b]Fat content changes serving counts for fats and oils. For example, 1 Tbsp. of regular salad dressing equals 1 serving; 1 Tbsp. of a low-fat dressing equals 1/2 serving; 1 Tbsp. of a fat-free dressing equals 0 servings.

Source: U.S. Department of Health and Human Services and National Institutes of Health National Heart, Lung, and Blood Institute. 2003. *The Seventh Report of the Joint National Committee on Prevention, Detection, Evaluation, and Treatment of High Blood Pressure*; NIH Publication No. 03-5230. Washington DC: NIH.

DIURETIC A substance that increases urine output.

primarily by **diuretic** effects, but its benefits also come from its high potassium and antioxidant content (Akita et al. 2003). Participating in regular physical activity and stress-relieving activities, avoiding tobacco, and reducing alcohol intake also foster healthy blood pressure.

DIET AND SKIN CARE

Dermatology is a highly specialized field. To learn more about it, visit the American Academy of Dermatology public resource Web site at http://www.aad.org/public.

The skin is the largest organ of the body, and its health is an unmistakable indication of the body's health (Purba et al. 2001). Clear, glowing skin reflects good health, whereas dry and brittle skin may indicate poor diet. Vitamin A and zinc are essential for producing new skin cells to replace those lost naturally each day. Vitamin C is necessary for the development of collagen fibers that provide the skin's structure. Fresh vegetables and fruits, particularly citrus fruits, contribute vitamins A and C to the diet. Meat provides zinc.

SUMMARY

There is a strong relationship between health and diet. It is important for students in the culinary arts to stay abreast of the current research so that they may be able to provide the most delicious as well as nutritious meals to their patrons and make wise decisions about their personal lives. How well we progress through the aging process is profoundly affected by the diet and lifestyle choices we make. The major diseases in the United States—heart disease, cancer, diabetes and hypertension—are all greatly influenced by our dietary choices. Choosing a healthy diet rich in fruits, vegetables, whole grains, and protein foods will ensure we have the best chance at a life dominated by wellness and not disease.

CASE RESOLUTION

Pureed food looks like slop and mush if it is handled improperly. Expecting someone to willingly eat this is unrealistic. But attractive presentation makes a world of difference. Pureed food should be molded or shaped to resemble the actual food. For example, chefs can pour pureed pork chop into a pork-chop-shaped mold. This helps increase patient/customer acceptance and nutrient intake. Roger must discuss this option with Mrs. Hernandez and make arrangements to purchase the molds, which are available in the shapes of various meats, fruits, and vegetables.

REFERENCES

Akita, S., F. M. Sacks, L. P. Svetkey, P. R. Conlin, and G. Kimura. 2003. Effects of the Dietary Approaches to Stop Hypertension (DASH) diet on the pressure-natriuresis relationship. *Hypertension* 42: 8–13.

American Cancer Society. 2002. *Nutrition and Cancer.* http://www.cancer.org/downloads/PRO/nutrition.pdf.

American Heart Association. 2003. *Heart Disease and Stroke Statistics—2004 Update.* Dallas, TX: American Heart Association.

Moore, T. J., P. R. Conlin, J. Ard, and L. P. Svetsky. 2001. DASH (Dietary Approaches to Stop Hypertension) diet is effective treatment for stage 1 isolated systolic hypertension. *Hypertension* 38: 155–58.

Purba, M. B., A. Kouris-Blazos, N. Wattanapenpaiboon, W. Lukito, E. Rothenberg, B. Steen, and M. L. Wahlqvist. 2001. Can skin wrinkling in a site that has received limited sun exposure be used as a marker of health status and biological age? *Age and Aging* 30: 227–34.

Rumsfield, J. A., and D. P. West. 1991. Topical capsaicin in dermatologic and peripheral pain disorders. *Annals of Pharmacotherapy* 25: 381–87.

Schiffman, S. S. 2000. Intensification of sensory properties of foods for the elderly. *Journal of Nutrition* 130: 927S–30S.

Sharkey, J. R., L. G. Branch, N. Zohoori, C. Giuliani, J. Busby-Whitehead, and P. S. Haines. 2002. Inadequate nutrient intakes among homebound elderly and their correlation with individual characteristics and health-related factors. *American Journal of Clinical Nutrition* 76: 1435–45.

Simopoulos, A. P. 2002. Omega-3 fatty acids in inflammation and autoimmune diseases. *Journal of the American College of Nutrition* 21: 495–505.

Stevens, J., K. Ahn, Juhaeri, D. Houston, L. Steffan, and D. Couper. 2002. Dietary fiber intake and glycemic index and incidence of diabetes in African-American and white adults: The ARIC study. *Diabetes Care* 25: 1715–21

Teegarden, D., R. M. Lyle, W. R. Proulx, C. Johnston, and C. M. Weaver. 1999. Previous milk consumption is associated with greater bone density in young women. *American Journal of Clinical Nutrition* 69: 1014–17.

REVIEW QUESTIONS

1. Nutrition mitigates a number of diseases associated with aging. Name four of these diseases.

2. What can chefs do to encourage proper eating habits in the elderly?

3. How does osteoporosis develop, and why does this disease affect mostly women?

4. What are the best food sources of vitamin D, and why is it added to many milk products?

5. What is insulin, and what function does it perform in the human body?

6. What are the risk factors that may contribute to heart disease, and which are diet related?

7. How does food containing omega-3 fatty acids reduce the risk of heart disease and stroke?

8. Which foods contain large amounts of antioxidants? What are the benefits of antioxidants?

9. Why are the elderly more susceptible to cancer?

10. Why are arthritis patients treated with omega-3 fatty acids and capsicum peppers?

11. What is the suggested daily sodium intake for good health?

12. When does sodium consumption become a health concern?

13. Create a one-day meal plan for an adult on the DASH diet.

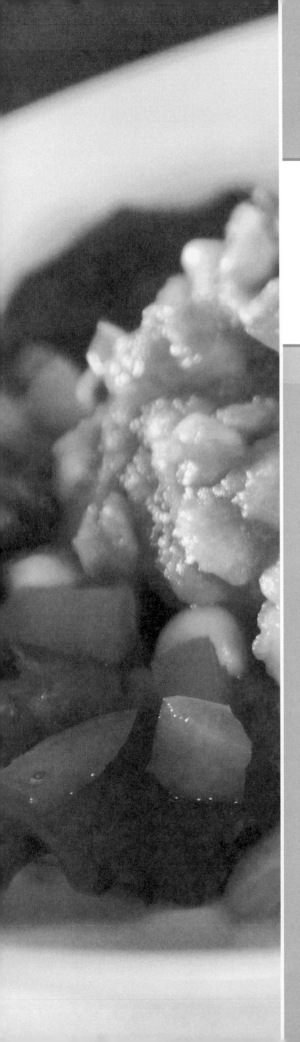

9

Weight Control

KEY CONCEPTS

- Obesity is increasing in the United States and is reaching epidemic proportions.
- Obesity is a major health problem.
- The cause of obesity is multifactorial.
- Successful obesity treatment has been elusive.
- Obesity incidence remains unimproved despite the many weight-reduction diets on the market.
- Balancing individual caloric needs with exercise is the overall solution to obesity. Individuals, however, must incorporate specific changes appropriate to their lifestyles.

Obesity is one of the biggest health problems facing Americans today. A few extra pounds do not seem to cause any harm. Obesity, however, increases the risk of multiple health conditions, including gallbladder and heart disease, cancer, and type 2 diabetes, and contributes to thousands of deaths in the United States each year (Surgeon General 2004).

Weight management is obviously a subject of concern for millions of Americans, as evidenced by the many diets (Weight Watchers, South Beach, and Atkins), televised exercise programs, and home exercise videos on the market today, and science has documented obesity's multiple and elusive causes. Nevertheless, as modern civilization becomes increasingly prosperous and mechanized, Americans are becoming less physically active than their ancestors. In addition, the availability of food, especially fast food, provides Americans many opportunities to overindulge in food and dining pleasures.

The best defense against overweight and obesity is to eat sensibly and exercise regularly. A large weight loss is unnecessary to obtain a health benefit; even modest weight loss reduces blood cholesterol levels and mortality due to heart disease (American Heart Association 2004).

THINK ABOUT IT

Why do we react differently to people with certain health conditions? For example, why do we think it is okay for someone to have high cholesterol but completely unacceptable to be obese? Certainly that individual with high cholesterol must have inherited the condition, while the obese person has a character flaw involving reduced willpower, right?

Think about your own reactions to different health conditions. Have you ever had negative thoughts about someone with high cholesterol? What about someone who is obese? Why?

CASE STUDY

Ice-Cream Cart

Franklin is the executive chef for Cole's Foodservice, a contract management company running the food service at Wheelan Nursing Facility. Each Wednesday, Franklin personally delivers a special dessert cart to the residents of Wheelan. Franklin's cart contains all the best premium ice creams plus every topping imaginable. And, of course, the residents love it!

Franklin's brother, a doctor at Wheelan, has pointed out that many of the residents are gaining weight and suffering from weight-related health conditions, such as diabetes and hypertension. Wheelan's medical staff wish to improve the residents' health and improve their dietary intake. But Franklin cannot bear eliminating his special ice-cream service. He knows how much the residents enjoy the sweet treat as well as the social interaction with each other. What should Franklin do? Eliminate the ice cream, or devise a substitute? *The resolution for this case study is presented at the end of the chapter.*

PREVALENCE OF OBESITY

Obesity is increasing in the United States and in other countries at a disturbing rate (Figure 9–1). Not only are 50% of adults in the United States overweight, but, more importantly, one-third are obese. Worldwide, 300 million people are clinically obese (World Health Organization 2003). The World Health Organization defines obesity as having a body mass index (BMI) of 30 or greater (World Health Organization 2004). Others define obesity as a percentage over the desirable weight.

The U.S. population has one of the highest BMIs in the world, but many other countries are experiencing this problem as well (World Health Organization 2004). According to the Centers for Disease Control and Prevention, 44 million Americans were considered obese in 2001, and this number is steadily rising.

Obesity in the United States is more prevalent in African-American and Hispanic populations as well as in middle-age adults (Centers for Disease Control, 2006), with over 50% of adult African-American females being obese. Many other developed countries are also experiencing an increase in obesity, although not as high as the United States, including the United Kingdom, Russia, and Greece. The occurrence of obesity in island nations is

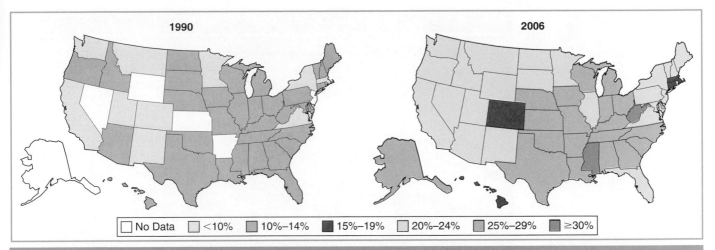

FIGURE 9–1 • OBESITY TRENDS* AMONG U.S. ADULTS
*BMI ≥ 30, or about 30 pounds overweight for 5′4″ person
Source: Centers for Disease Control. *Behavior Risk Factor Surveillance System, 2006.* http://www.cc.gov?nccdphp/dnpa/obesity/trend/maps/
obesity_trebds_2006.ppt (accessed June 15, 2008).

PANDEMIC An epidemic that covers a vast geography.

even more striking: 43% of females in French Polynesia and 66% in American Samoa are obese (Box 9–1 and Box 9–2).

The World Health Organization attributes this **pandemic** to increased industrialization, urbanization, and mechanization worldwide and the resulting diet and lifestyle changes. Specifically, people are consuming more fat and calories in their diets, and their lifestyles are more sedentary. In developing countries, obesity and chronic undernutrition often occur simultaneously in the same population (World Health Organization 2002).

BOX 9–1 • PERCENT OF OBESE ADULT FEMALES BY COUNTRY

3% Philippines	17% Austria	25% Argentina
5% Switzerland	17% France	26% Czech Republic
6% Thailand	18% New Zealand	28% Greece
8% Malaysia	18% Australia	29% S. Africa
9% Italy	19% Yugoslavia	30% Iran
10% Norway	19% Finland	31% Jamaica
10% Brazil	20% Saudi Arabia	34% Bahrain
11% Netherlands	20% Germany	34% United States
12% Canada	21% Portugal	36% Curaçao
12% Sweden	21% Colombia	36% Malta
13% Saudi Arabia	23% Romania	40% Lebanon
13% Belgium	23% Scotland	40% Trinidad and Tobago
14% Spain	23% Chile	41% Kuwait
15% Iceland	23% England	43% French Polynesia
15% Denmark	25% Russia	66% American Samoa
16% Ireland	25% Mexico	74.3% Samoa (urban areas)
16% Slovakia		

Source: World Health Organization. 2003. Food and agriculture organization expert consultation on diet, nutrition and the prevention of chronic diseases. http://www.who.int/hpr/NPH/docs/who_fao_expert_report.pdf.

BOX 9–2 • PERCENT OF OBESE ADULT MALES BY COUNTRY

2% Philippines	14% Portugal	20% Finland
2% Tunisia	14% Belgium	21% Lebanon
5% Malaysia	14.7% Israel	21% England
5% Singapore	15% Mexico	21% Colombia
6% Switzerland	15% Denmark	22% Malta
7% Jamaica	15% New Zealand	23% Bahrain
9% Latvia	17% Romania	26% Brazil
9% S. Africa	18% Hungary	28% United States
9% Italy	18% Uruguay	28% Argentina
10% Russia	18% Germany	29% Greece
10% Spain	18% Australia	32% Kuwait
10% Sweden	19% Curacao	35% French Polynesia
10% Iran	19% Iceland	36% Panama
11% Lithuania	20% Trinidad and	64% American Samoa
11% Netherlands	Tobago	
12% Austria	20% Ireland	
12% France	20% Scotland	

Source: World Health Organization. 2003. Food and agriculture organization expert consultation on diet, nutrition and the prevention of chronic diseases. http://www.who.int/hpr/NPH/docs/who_fao_expert_report.pdf.

CAUSES OF OBESITY

The cause of obesity has been hard to pin down. Although no single cause of obesity has been found, many factors influence its prevalence. In the United States and other developed nations, the dramatic increase in obesity coincides with certain lifestyle changes, such as sedentary routines. Technology and other modern conveniences have made people less active than in times past. Computers, cell phones, drive-through restaurants, household appliances, the Internet, and TV remote controls have decreased physical activity. People who walked more frequently in the past now mostly use their cars, even for short trips to the store.

Increased availability, variety, and quantity of food have added to the problem. In the United States, food is readily available in almost any location. Individuals can purchase food not only in grocery stores but also in clothing stores, gas stations, vending machines, and fast-food restaurants. This increased availability has had a remarkable effect on Americans' eating habits. Over the past several decades, the proportion of total food dollars spent on food away from home has doubled (Lin and Frazao 1999). Now Americans spend about half of their food dollars away from home (Figure 9–2).

More available food has led to an increase in per capita food consumption. In the past, fast food was eaten only occasionally, so it was not a problem; however, as consumption of fast food has grown, so has the obesity epidemic.

Not only has fast-food consumption increased in terms of meals consumed per person, but portions have also become significantly larger since the introduction of fast-food chains. Increased portions mean that more calories are consumed when dining at a fast-food restaurant. The typical serving size of fast-food burgers, French fries, and beverages today is more than twice what it was in the past (Young and Nestle 2003).

Prosperity may also contribute to increased obesity in developed nations. Although all nations experience obesity, more affluent countries are more likely to have obesity problems

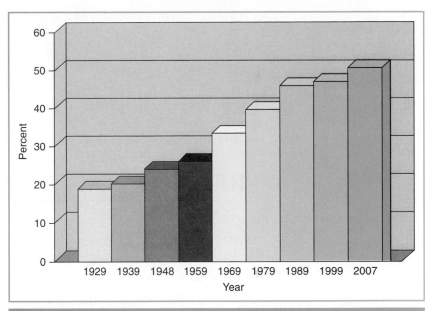

FIGURE 9–2 • AWAY-FROM-HOME FOOD EXPENDITURES AS A SHARE OF TOTAL U.S. FOOD EXPENDITURES
Source: Economic Research Service, United States Department of Agriculture. 2008. Food away from home as a percentage of expenditures. http://www.ers.usda.gov/Briefing/CPIFoodAndExpenditures/Data/table1.htm (accessed June 24, 2008).

because their citizens can consume more calories if they wish. Residents can purchase more costly convenience foods as well as dine out more often.

ILL EFFECTS OF OBESITY

Excess weight creates a burden on the body that leads to disease, especially when the individual is two to three times heavier than their "normal" weight. Obesity increases risk factors that can lead to heart disease, such as elevated blood levels of low-density lipoprotein (LDL) cholesterol (the unhealthy form). Hypertension, which damages coronary vessels and causes heart disease, is also associated with obesity. Furthermore, hypertension can cause stroke and kidney disease.

Health experts advise modest weight reduction to combat these ill effects. A weight loss of as little as 5% can lower blood cholesterol and blood pressure. Decreasing BMI as little as 0.5 kilograms per square meters has been shown to reduce LDL cholesterol, triglycerides, insulin resistance, and both systolic and diastolic blood pressure (Reinehr and Andler 2004).

Moreover, excess body fat facilitates development of other undesirable health conditions or worsens existing ones. The resulting diseases combine to produce billions of dollars of expenses for developed nations. The United States spends more per capita on healthcare than does any other country (Anderson et al. 2003). Obesity and conditions caused or aggravated by obesity have been thought to be responsible for 100,000 to 400,000 deaths annually (Pi-Sunyer 1993; Moskowitz 2004; Flegal et al. 2005).

Obesity is also a risk factor for diabetes in those who are genetically prone. Diabetes, in turn, can lead to heart disease, blindness, and neuropathies. Obese individuals suffer from osteoarthritis and gout more often than does the general population. People who are overweight are at particular risk for osteoarthritis of the knees and hands (Foran et al. 2004). Gallbladder disease is more prevalent in obese people, and obesity appears to be a risk factor for certain cancers in men (Steinbach et al. 1994).

The location of excess body fat is a factor in terms of disease development. Heart disease and diabetes, for example, are associated with surplus fat in the abdominal area (Vega 2004). Fat on the hips and thighs, however, does not correlate with an increased risk of heart disease and diabetes.

Obesity not only has an ill effect on physical health but also may impact an individual socially, professionally, and emotionally. The obese may experience discrimination socially and on the job. In a recent study, obese children rated the quality of their lives lower than did children with cancer (Schwimer, Burwinkle, and Varni 2003).

TREATMENT FOR OBESITY

Dieting has been the standard treatment for obesity for many years. The media present consumers with myriad weight-loss diets that they may follow. Physicians recommend diets for patients who require weight loss. Exercise is often added to calorie-restricted diets in weight-loss regimens to enhance the outcome. Other treatments for obesity include diet pills, behavior modification, bariatric surgery, and medication. All of these measures have resulted in minimal long-term success.

Although weight-loss diets abound and diet books are best sellers, frequently weight loss is only temporary. Most dieters regain their weight within five years. Failure to stay slim leads to guilt and repeated efforts at dieting. Some individuals turn to highly restrictive diets with unreasonable requirements. Many of these dieters fail in the long run due to the off-putting nature of these programs.

Food abounds in our society, so it is not easy to resist the vast array of culinary delights. Depriving oneself of food through fad dieting often yields disappointing results. Although fad weight-loss diets are not effective, there are some beneficial dietary practices that all diet proponents agree on. Incorporating these common suggestions into a lifestyle change may be part of the answer. These suggestions are discussed later in the chapter in the section on the National Weight Control Registry.

COMPARING WEIGHT-LOSS DIETS

The various weight-loss diets can appear conflicting and misleading. But these diets contain some common components that can be included as part of a lifestyle change. All of the theories behind these diets contain some truth. We will examine these in this section.

The popular high-protein diets (e.g., Atkins, Zone, Carbohydrate Addict's, Protein Power, SugarBusters!) are all based on a similar theory: Today's common medical problems—cardiovascular disease, diabetes, and cancer—are caused or exacerbated by elevated blood glucose levels or insulin resistance. In its broadest sense, the theory states that frequent consumption of refined carbohydrates and sugars causes a rapid increase in blood glucose levels. In response, the body releases more insulin, allowing sugar utilization and conversion to fat. Refined carbohydrates are used quickly, resulting in a fairly rapid decrease in blood sugar (hypoglycemia), which brings on hunger and subsequent consumption of more carbohydrate. The detrimental cycle continues (Atkins 1991) (Figure 9–3).

High insulin levels (hyperinsulinemia) for prolonged periods can result in insulin resistance. This means that even more insulin production is needed for the same amount of carbohydrate consumed. Eventually the insulin's reduced effectiveness plus the elevated blood glucose levels cause type 2 diabetes. In contrast, the high-carbohydrate, low-fat diet theories (U.S. Department of Agriculture, American Dietetic Association, American Heart Association, Pritikin, and Ornish) focus on reducing dietary saturated and total fat content to reduce cholesterol levels

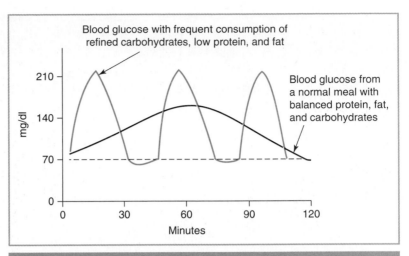

FIGURE 9–3 • GLUCOSE CURVE SHOWING THE NEGATIVE EFFECT OF REFINED CARBOHYDRATE FOODS

and to decrease the risk of heart disease (Pritikin 1990). Yet both Pritikin and Atkins agree that a healthful diet limits consumption of sugars and refined carbohydrates. Thus limiting refined carbohydrates as part of a healthy lifestyle would be a good way to attain a normal body weight.

Not only do most of the popular diet book authors agree on this point, but most nutrition authorities do as well (Table 9–1). The USDA recommends that Americans limit their intake of added sugar. My Pyramid describes a healthy diet as one that is low in added sugars. Despite all these recommendations, the U.S. food supply currently provides 34 teaspoons of sugar per person each day (Putnam, Kantor, and Allshouse 2000). Clearly Americans are consuming much more added sugar than recommended.

Another point of agreement is that Americans need to consume more vegetables. The USDA recommends at least five to nine servings of vegetables each day. Vegetables provide many vitamins and minerals that the body requires. For example, vitamin C, a potent antioxidant, is found in green peppers, red peppers, broccoli, and kale. Antioxidants like vitamin C protect against free-radical damage and provide numerous other benefits (Shils et al. 1999). Pritikin's low-fat diet plan emphasizes plant-based foods, recommending a daily consumption of seven vegetable servings (Pritikin 1990). Dr. Atkins recommends similar amounts of low-glycemic vegetables on his "maintenance" diet (Atkins 1999). Although most agree that eating fruits and vegetables promotes good health, only "1 in 5 children eat the recommended 5 or more servings of fruits and vegetables each day, and nearly one quarter of all vegetables eaten by children and adolescents are French fries" (Kreb-Smith et al. 1996). Also, adding fruits and vegetables to a healthy lifestyle would be another great way to attain a normal body weight.

Yet another point of agreement is that physical activity is key to achieving and maintaining a healthy body weight. Physical activity helps individuals attain energy balance and prevents obesity (Rippe and Hess 1998). According to the Surgeon General's call to action, regular physical activity helps prevent heart disease, controls cholesterol levels and diabetes, slows bone loss, and helps reduce anxiety and depression (Department of Health and Human Services 1996).

The Dietary Guidelines for Americans advocate physical activity each day (U.S. Department of Agriculture 2000). In addition, the National Academy of Sciences has recommended one hour total activity every day (National Academy of Sciences 2002). Both Dr. Atkins and Pritikin offer similar recommendations in their books. Despite consistent pronouncements supporting physical activity, however, only 25% of Americans meet exercise recommendations (National Academy of Sciences 2002). In fact, many Americans are so inactive that some health authorities have declared the inactivity to be an epidemic (Rippe and Hess 1998).

TABLE 9–1 • DIETARY RECOMMENDATIONS BY GOVERNMENTAL AUTHORITIES AND VARIOUS POPULAR DIET AUTHORS

General Recommendations	Atkins	Zone	Protein Power	CHO[a] Addict	New Pyramid	USDA Pyramid	Pritikin	Ornish
Eat a higher-protein diet	Yes	Yes	Yes	Yes	No	No	No	No
Eat a high-carbohydrate diet	No	No	No	No	No	Yes	Yes	Yes
Eat a low-fat diet	No	Yes	No	No	No	Yes	Yes	Yes
Eat plenty of fruits	No	No	No	No	Yes	Yes	Yes	Yes
Get adequate fluids	Yes	Yes	Yes	Yes	Yes	Yes	Yes	Yes
Get adequate fiber	Yes	Yes	Yes	Yes	Yes	Yes	Yes	Yes
Eat plenty of nonstarchy vegetables	Yes	Yes	Yes	Yes	Yes	Yes	Yes	Yes
Eat plenty of starchy vegetables	No	No	No	No	No	Yes	Yes	Yes
Limit or avoid sweets and refined sugars	Yes	Yes	Yes	Yes	Yes	Yes	Yes	Yes
Limit refined grains like white bread, pasta, and refined cereals	Yes	Yes	Yes	Yes	Yes	Yes	Yes	Yes
Eat plenty of whole grains	No	No	No	No	Yes	Yes	Yes	Yes
Exercise for health and prevention of obesity	Yes	Yes	Yes	Yes	Yes	Yes	Yes	Yes

[a]CHO = Carbohydrate

In short, the majority of nutrition authorities and popular diets agree that decreasing the consumption of refined carbohydrates and increasing vegetable consumption and exercise are good recommendations. Simply implementing these behaviors as lifestyle changes would make the U.S. diet healthier and reduce Americans' risk of disease.

Weight-loss diets seem to fail due to a basic flaw in their logic. All diets are successful for a period of time if they limit calories. But merely dieting for only a specified period of time is doomed to failure. Dieters who stay on their diets only until they lose a certain amount of weight or for a limited period of time with no maintenance plan except to go back to their initial eating pattern are certain to fail. Returning to the pattern that caused the weight gain in the first place will certainly cause the weight to come back. Only making a permanent lifestyle change will result in a permanent change in weight.

Although no single weight-loss program has had great success, some individuals have succeeded at losing excess weight and keeping it off. The National Weight Control Registry (NWCR), founded in 1994, has inventoried common practices of people who have succeeded at weight management. The NWCR comprises over 3,000 individuals who have lost at least 10% of their initial weight and kept it off for at least one year. The average weight loss of the group is 30 kilograms over an average of five and one–half years. Researchers discovered the following common behaviors: a low-fat, high-carbohydrate diet; frequent self-monitoring of body weight and food intake; and high levels of regular physical activity. Registry subjects averaged approximately one hour of moderate-intensity activity each day.

BALANCING ENERGY INTAKE AND EXPENDITURE

The key to maintaining a healthy weight is to balance energy intake and expenditure. We will look first at controlling intake and then at increasing energy expenditure. To determine energy need, a dietitian assesses the individual's nutritional status. A nutrition assessment includes the individual's current weight and ideal body weight as well as other factors, such as diet history, food preferences, and laboratory values (if available).

Determining Normal Weight

The old method of assessing weight was to compare weight to Metropolitan Insurance weight charts. This is rarely done today. Individualized formulas are now used for determining healthy body weight (Box 9–3). The most common method is to use body mass index (BMI). The Dietary Guidelines for Americans recommend a BMI of 19 to 25 kilograms per square meters for adults under 35 years and a BMI of 21 to 27 kilograms per square meters for adults over the age of 35. A BMI that exceeds the recommendation but is less than 30 kilograms per square meters is considered overweight, and a BMI over 30 kilograms per square meters is considered obese. Box 9–3 shows how to determine BMI.

Achieving an ideal body weight, however, is probably an unrealistic goal for people who are extremely obese. In these cases, health professionals should establish reasonable, attainable goals and direct the individuals to lose the weight gradually. A reasonable weight-loss goal is 5% to 10% of current body weight.

The methods shown thus far consider only total weight without differentiating between fat and muscle. Thus they may produce inaccurate results. The composition of the weight is more important than the total amount of weight. Other methods provide

---

BOX 9–3 • THREE WEIGHT FORMULAS FOR ADULTS

1. Height in inches × wrist in inches = _____ divided by 3 = _____
   (*Note:* Wrist and ankle measurements are not influenced by body fat and are accurate sites for measuring frame size.)
2. *Men:* 106 pounds for the first 60 inches + 6 pounds for each inch over 60 inches.
   Women: 100 pounds for the first 60 inches + 5 pounds for each inch over 60 inches.
   For both sexes:
   Add 10 pounds for large frame.
   Subtract 10 pounds for small frame.
   Subtract 1 pound for each year under 25.
3. Body mass index (Desirable 22.4)
   a. 1 kilogram = 2.2 pounds (determine kilograms by dividing pounds by 2.2)
   b. height in inches × 0.0254 = height in meters
   c. Square your height in meters
   d. Divide weight in kilograms by your height in square meters.

Sources: Formula 1: Dr. Roger Sherwin, Professor of Epidemiology. University of Maryland School of Medicine.

Formula 2: Hartmann, P., and E. Bell, *Nutrition for the Athlete, Sports Medicine for the Primary Care Physician*, East Norwalk, CT: Appleton-Century-Crofts, 1984, p. 108.

Formula 3: Nutrient Data Laboratory, Agricultural Research Service, Beltsville Human Nutrition Research Center, 4700 River Road, Unit 89, FDA. http://www.fda.gov/search.html

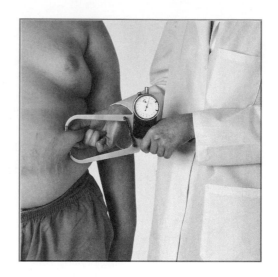

Calipers may be used to measure body fat.
© *Dorling Kindersley*

BIOELECTRIC IMPEDANCE ANALYSIS (BIA) Lean body mass measurement; measures the electrical resistance of the body to an imperceptible flow of electricity through its tissues.

more accurate results because they assess weight by its components, breaking it down into body fat and lean body mass.

The least expensive of these methods utilizes skinfold calipers to determine body fat percentage. Skinfold calipers measure the thickness of fat in millimeters.

An inexpensive and widely available "high-tech" method for assessing weight is **bioelectric impedance analysis (BIA)** (sometimes called *bioelectrical impedance*).

Some health spas, gyms and healthcare facilities use BIA, which is performed with an instrument that looks somewhat like an electrocardiograph. Electrodes are applied to the top of the feet and the back of the hands. A computer printout tells the individual his or her body proportions of lean tissue, fat, and water.

The gold standard for determining proper weight and body composition is underwater weighing. With this method individuals are weighed underwater. Freestanding weight is compared to underwater weight, and percentage body fat is determined.

Whatever method is used, if the results indicate that the individual is overweight or underweight, the individual should change his or her lifestyle in a way that balances energy intake and output. The next section discusses making this determination.

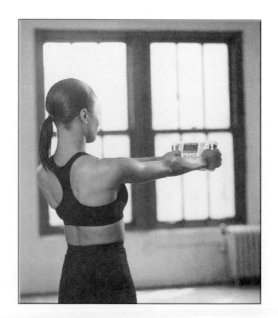

Bioelectric impedance machines are used to determine body fat percentage.
Phototake NYC

BOX 9–4 • CALORIE REQUIREMENT FORMULAS FOR ADULTS

FORMULA 1

The Harris Benedict equation:

Men: 66.47 + 13.75 (weight in kilograms) + 5.0 (height in centimeters) − 6.76 (age)

Women: 65.10 + 9.56 (weight in kilograms) + 1.85 (height in centimeters) − 4.68 (age)

(This formula is for basal calories. Add 5%–20% for activity, or multiply by 1.3.)

FORMULA 2

For sedentary individuals, 25 to 30 cal/kg

For moderately active individuals, 30 to 35 cal/kg

For very active individuals, 35 to 40 cal/kg

Adjust for age:

    For individuals ages 35 to 45, 94% of calories

    For individuals ages 45 to 55, 92% of calories

    For individuals over age 55, 89% of calories

DETERMINING CALORIE NEED

Basal calorie requirements and physical activity levels dictate calorie needs. Basal calorie needs are determined by age, muscle mass, and overall body weight. The amount of food we eat does not necessarily match what we require. Calorie requirement formulas exist to assist professionals in determining calorie need (Box 9–4).

After the calorie level is determined, an individual can use it as a guide for dietary intake. But it is only a guide, not a hard rule requiring strict compliance. After all, counting calories has not proven to be a successful weight-loss strategy.

For example, consider a person who normally eats 4,000 calories daily and attempts a 1,200-calorie diet. This extreme calorie deficit will probably bring about misery, and the individual will discontinue the diet. On the other hand, eliminating only 500 calories for a total of 3,500 calories each day would minimize the pain of dieting. As a result, weight loss progresses slowly and successfully. Incorporating permanent small changes into the diet is always a better solution than counting calories or severely restricting calories. Making healthy food substitutions is also a good strategy for triumphing over excess weight.

MAKING HEALTHY FOOD CHOICES AND SUBSTITUTIONS

Rich desserts and sweet beverages provide many calories because they contain large amounts of fat and sugar. Dieters usually consider sweets and desserts to be "off limits." Thus some of them experience guilt after eating sweets. They feel they have failed to stay on their diet because they gave in to their "sweet tooth." They think, "I've blown it anyway, so I might as well eat this whole box of cookies." This self-destructive thinking often begins in childhood, when parents use food as a reward or a punishment (for example, a child is told she can have cake for completing homework).

There is nothing wrong with eating dessert in moderation; sweets do not cause any disease or obesity by themselves. An occasional small portion of dessert will provide a dieter the satisfaction of eating something delicious while staying on a weight-loss program.

Many healthful substitutions can be made in traditional recipes in ways that reduce calories yet maintain flavor. This is extremely important when preparing high-calorie,

TABLE 9–2 • FOOD SUBSTITUTIONS

Replace	With	Reduction in Fat Grams
1 cup whole milk	1 cup skim milk	8
1/2 cup ice cream	1/2 cup ice milk	6
1/2 cup sour cream	1/2 cup low-fat yogurt	20
1 oz. cream cheese	1 oz. fat-free cream cheese	9
3 oz. prime rib	3 oz. round steak	6
3 oz. fried chicken	3 oz. chicken without skin	12
3 oz. tuna in oil	3 oz. tuna in water	7
1 oz. corn chips	1 cup popcorn	11

Note: An extensive list of food substitutions may be found at http://www.foodsubs.com.

high-fat recipes. Using skim milk in pudding recipes, for example, lowers calorie content while preserving overall taste. Preparing pancakes with fresh fruit imparts additional sweetness, which cuts down on the pancake syrup.

In short, a diet should feature enough variety and flexibility that one can follow it permanently. Furthermore, individuals should be encouraged to view healthy eating more as a lifestyle than a diet since diets are routinely started and stopped in an on-again, off-again cycle. Obesity is caused mostly by the unhealthy habits of eating too much food and too much fat and sugar. Making healthier food choices is fundamental to promoting and sustaining health (Table 9–2).

MODIFYING BEHAVIOR

Behavior modification is another approach to weight loss. This involves carefully analyzing activities that lead to eating and forming a plan of action to change patterns that trigger overindulgence. Professional guidance from a dietitian or psychologist may help.

By keeping careful records of what foods are consumed and when, the obese person can disrupt activity that leads to overeating by substituting another activity. The individual avoids bingeing by planning eating behavior ahead of time, such as before attending celebrations and social situations involving food. Behavior modification works with those who are unaware of their unhealthy eating habits.

ENVIRONMENTAL FACTORS

Environmental factors can influence food consumption but often are ignored as possible obesity contributors. Two influential factors, visibility and convenience, impact how much we eat. One study found that people eat more when savory snacks are in sight and within reach. This research examined office workers and assessed their consumption of pretzels placed in three locations over a period of four days. Containers of 30 pretzels were placed either on top of the desk (visible and convenient), in a desk drawer (not visible and convenient),

THE PEN AND PAPER DIET

If you are overweight and want to lose those extra pounds, just write down everything that you eat. Keep a 3– by 5–inch card or a small notepad and a pen in your pocket. Then every time you sit down to eat, simply record the foods and portions (for example, 1 bowl of cereal, 1 sandwich, 2 cookies, or 8 oz. of milk). You don't need to track calories, points, or fat grams. The more consistently you do this, the greater the effect will be.

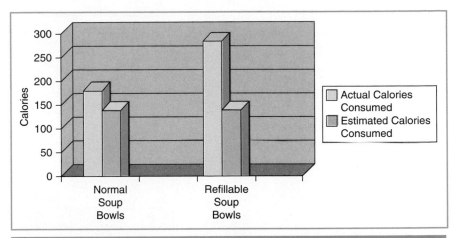

FIGURE 9-4 • REFILLABLE SOUP BOWLS INCREASE CONSUMPTION, BUT
NOT PERCEPTION OF CONSUMPTION (OUNCES)
Source: Wansink, B., J. E. Painter, and J. North. 2005. Bottomless bowls: Why visual
cues of portion size may influence intake. *Obesity Research* 13 (1): 93–100.

or two meters away, which required the workers to leave their desks (not visible and
inconvenient). Data showed a significant decrease ($p \leq 0.001$) in consumption of 34%
when the pretzels were in the drawer (invisible) instead of on the desk (visible). A significant decrease ($p \leq 0.001$) in consumption of 30% was found when subjects had to get
up from their desks (inconvenient) as compared to when the pretzels were in the desks
(convenient) (Painter and North 2003).

The most important element in changing behavior may simply be to be aware of what
one is eating. In one study, subjects lost track of how much soup they were eating because
the bowls were being filled from a tube under the table and never ran dry. The subjects
consumed almost twice as much soup when they lost track of their soup intake (Wansink,
Painter, and North 2005) (Figure 9–4).

Consumers can become more aware of dietary intake by recording what they
eat. Documenting what one eats all day builds awareness. This awareness enables
individuals to discern the barriers that cause them to overeat and to make appropriate
changes.

Boutelle assessed the weight change in 57 subjects for six weeks over a holiday season. Half of the subjects self-monitored their dietary intake, and the other half did not. The
group that tracked the foods they ate lost weight before, during, and after the holiday season, while the control group that did not track their intake gained weight (Figure 9–5)
(Boutelle et al. 1999).

Baker and Kirschenbaum found that consistency of self-monitoring was also important. They assessed the weight change in 38 subjects during three holiday weeks and
seven nonholiday weeks. The sample was split into four quartiles based on the participants' self-monitoring consistency. Only those who were very inconsistent in self-monitoring food intake gained weight during the nonholiday weeks. Everyone gained weight during
the holiday weeks except for those who were the most consistent in self-monitoring food intake (Figure 9–6) (Baker and Kirschenbaum 1998).

Self-monitoring of dietary intake is an essential component for promoting dietary
change. Keeping accurate records of diet has been found to improve control over food intake
in individuals trying to lose weight. Tracking dietary intake may be especially important for
people who work in the food industry and the culinary arts, where food is available most of the
time. Sampling the cooking can become a way of life for a chef. And anyone who samples

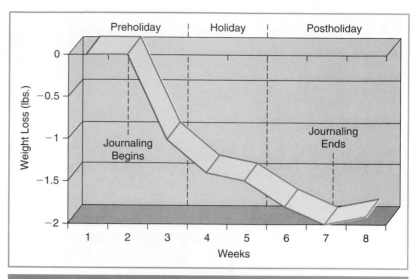

FIGURE 9–5 • WEIGHT LOSS DURING SELF-MONITORING
DIETARY INTAKE
Source: Adapted from Boutelle, K. N., D. S. Kirschenbaum, R. C. Baker, and M.
E. Mitchell. 1999. How can obese weight controllers minimize weight gain during
the high risk holiday season? By self-monitoring very consistently. *Health Psychology* 18 (4): 364–68.

food all day could lose track of the amount of food consumed. Recording food items and portion amounts consumed is an easy and effective way of preventing this from happening.

Another method for tracking and moderating consumption is to buy food in individual serving bags or pouches. Consider a time when you did not do this: For example, maybe you have watched a movie with a family-size bag of chips or cookies as your companion. When the movie ended, you discovered the bag completely empty, and you realized to your horror that you ate the entire bag. Eating from a large container in this manner can

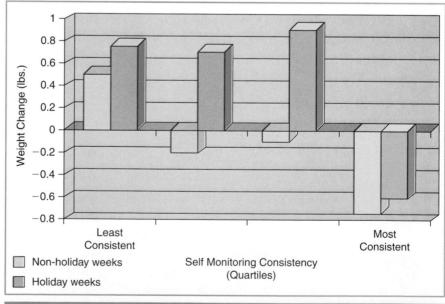

FIGURE 9–6 • WEIGHT LOSS WITH CONSISTENCY OF SELF-MONITORING
FOOD INTAKE
Source: Baker, R. C., and D. S. Kirschenbaum. 1998. Weight control during the holidays:
Highly consistent self-monitoring as a potentially useful coping mechanism. *Health Psychology* 17: 367–70.

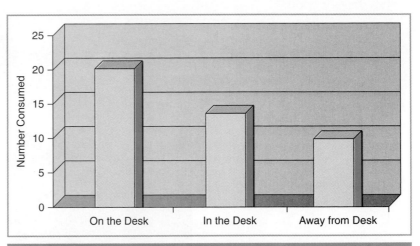

FIGURE 9–7 • AVERAGE NUMBER OF CANDY KISSES CONSUMED BY CONDITION
Source: Painter, J. E., and J. North. 2003. Effects of visibility and convenience on snack food consumption. *Journal of the American Dietetic Association* 103 (9): A-81.

cause you to lose track of the amount of food consumed. Buying food in single-portion containers, however, or portioning out a serving from a large container helps consumers track food volume. That way, the consumer must make a conscious decision to return to get a second or third portion.

Other techniques also contribute to successful long-term weight control. These include eating more slowly, chewing longer, and taking small bites of food (Painter and North 2002).

Nutrition scientists have obtained comparable results in a similar study utilizing candy kisses. Consumption decreased by approximately one-third when the candy was out of sight and two-thirds when it was out of sight and inconvenient (Figure 9–7) (Painter, Wansink, and Hieggelke 2002). Understanding this relationship of visibility and proximity to total food consumption helps nutrition professionals counsel overweight individuals to place calorie-dense food inconveniently out of view.

EXERCISE AND WEIGHT CONTROL

BASAL METABOLIC RATE (BMR) The level of energy required to support body activities while at rest following a fasting period.

Fad diets fail partially because dieting decreases muscle mass with a corresponding reduction in metabolism. A slowed metabolism burns fewer calories, causing the dieter to gain weight. In fact, **basal metabolic rate** may remain suppressed for years after the dieter goes off a severely calorie-restricted diet. To keep their metabolic rate up while dieting, individuals must maintain muscle mass with exercise. Exercising increases metabolism by building muscle mass, which burns more calories than does fat tissue. Note that calorie utilization varies with the type of exercise. Note also that not all dieters can perform exercise safely. Furthermore, some may require supervision and coaching from a certified personal trainer. By partnering with certified fitness trainers, dieters who want to exercise can avoid unnecessary injury and maximize benefit.

GROUPS THAT PROVIDE TRAINER CERTIFICATION

The American College of Sports Medicine (http://www.acsm.org/certification/index.htm)

American Council on Exercise (http://www.acefitness.org)

Regular exercise provides other benefits besides weight loss. These include increased high-density lipoprotein (HDL) cholesterol ("good" cholesterol), decreased LDL cholesterol ("bad" cholesterol), decreased blood pressure, increased glucose tolerance, and decreased risk of cardiovascular disease.

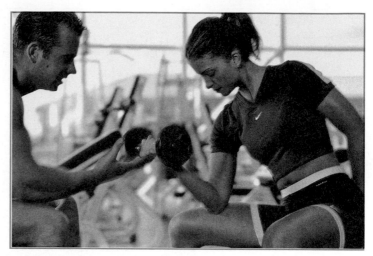

Credentialed trainers provide individualized exercise programs.
Getty Images, Inc.—Allsport Photography

MORE THAN JUST AEROBICS

Aerobic exercise is important because it burns calories. But other types of exercise are also important. Strengthening exercise is important because it increases muscle mass. Additional muscle mass also increases an individual's basal metabolic rate. This is because muscle burns more calories than fat.

TABLE 9–3 • APPROXIMATE ENERGY EXPENDITURE BY A HEALTHY ADULT (ABOUT 150 POUNDS)	
Activity	**Calories Expended per Hour**
Lying quietly	80–100
Sitting quietly	85–105
Standing quietly	100–120
Walking slowly (2.5 mph)	210–230
Walking quickly (4 mph)	315–345
Light work, such as ballroom dancing, cleaning house, office work, shopping	125–310
Moderate work, such as cycling (9 mph), jogging (6 mph), tennis, scrubbing floors, weeding garden	315–480
Hard work, such as aerobic dancing, basketball, chopping wood, cross-country skiing, running (7 mph), shoveling snow, spading the garden, swimming (the "crawl")	480–625

Source: U.S. Department of Agriculture, U.S. Department of Health and Human Services. 1985. *Nutrition and Your Health: Dietary Guidelines for Americans*, 2nd ed. Home and Garden Bulletin No. 232; Rockville, MD.

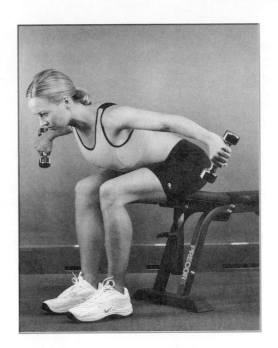

Conditioning exercise leads to
increased muscle mass.
John Davis © Dorling Kindersley

APPETITE SUPPRESSANTS

AMPHETAMINES Drugs used to stimulate the central nervous system. Dependence is a great risk.

In the 1960s, **amphetamines** were used in diet pills. They sped up metabolism, were addictive, and caused mood swings. Amphetamines were replaced by newer appetite suppressants, fenfluramine (Pondimin) and phentermine, that had problems of their own and eventually were pulled off the market.

A new drug, dexfenfluramine (Redux), works like fen-phen increasing serotonin levels in the brain. High serotonin levels decrease appetite in some people. The Food and Drug Administration (FDA) approved Redux in April 1996 and issued guidelines reserving it for people who were at least 30% overweight or at least 20% overweight with weight-related health problems (high blood pressure, high cholesterol, or diabetes).

The FDA announced in September 1997 that about 30% of patients who took Redux and subsequently were evaluated for heart valve function had abnormal echocardiograph readings, even without symptoms (Food and Drug Administration 1997). Redux was also found to cause a rare, but deadly, condition called *primary hypertension*. With this condition, the blood vessels that supply the lungs thicken, making the heart work harder. The manufacturers withdrew Redux and Pondimin from the market upon FDA request. Phentermine was not withdrawn (Food and Drug Administration 1997).

The manufacturer's findings contradict earlier reports of heart valve troubles in Redux users, some of whom took the pill for a longer time than the one recommended.

Other drugs are available on the market that suppress appetite and block fat absorption. Expect to see even more prescription opportunities as drug companies search for more pill solutions to the obesity problem (Welch 1998).

SUMMARY

Getting to the Perfect Weight

Many diets support different people's need for individualized nutrition recommendations. In truth, one diet does not fit everyone. Consequently, there are numerous diet plans from multiple health authorities and organizations. The most important point for individuals is to reduce calorie intake and maintain physical activity.

Health professionals, especially registered dietitians, assess nutritional status to determine weight status. Several formulas and tables are available to assist with this determination. In addition, professionals may employ calipers or bioelectric impedance analysis to measure body fat and lean tissue.

Health professionals use several formulas to calculate calorie need. Some of the most common appear in Box 9–4. Make sure the calculations offer realistic calorie goals, and incorporate reasonable dietary and lifestyle changes for healthy weight loss.

Since no diet is perfect, those who wish to eat more healthfully or lose weight should focus on incorporating manageable dietary substitutions. Finding creative ways to continue enjoying all-time favorite foods—making them with less fat, for example—fosters better eating and better overall health.

A successful weight management plan includes behavior change along with calorie restriction and exercise. Identifying what cues specific behaviors, what the responses to the behavior cues are, and what results from the behavior should be part of any behavior modification program.

CASE RESOLUTION

Franklin is wise to recognize the importance of social interaction for Wheelan's residents. This may play an important role in their mental health and overall well-being. However, the growing dietary problem from the ice-cream service easily negates any positive psychological benefits. The most obvious answer is to serve the correct portion; premium ice cream can be enjoyed, but the amount must be reduced. Also, instead of serving full-fat premium ice cream, Franklin should explore "light" ice cream, sherbets, and sorbets. For toppings, the residents may enjoy cut-up fresh fruit, fresh or frozen berries, and dried breakfast cereals (for example, cornflakes, giving the ice cream a "fried" crunch). That way, the residents can still enjoy the sweets and the social connectivity, as well as receive added vitamins, minerals, and fiber from the toppings.

Wheelan's residents could also increase their exercise to make up for the extra calories in the ice cream. Exercise is an integral component of weight management. Exercise can boost metabolism by building lean tissue and can enhance mood. Individuals should work with a certified personal trainer to design an exercise plan that maximizes health benefit while minimizing risk of injury. Just walking once around the block can be the starting point for improving physical fitness.

REFERENCES

American Heart Association. 2004. *Obesity and Heart Disease*. http://www.americanheart.org (accessed February 27, 2004).

Anderson, G. F., U. E. Reinhardt, P. S. Hussey, and V. Petrosyan. 2003. It's the prices, stupid: Why the United States is so different from other countries. *Health Affairs* 22 (3): 89–105.

Atkins, R. C. 1999. *Dr. Atkins' New Diet Revolution*. New York: Avon.

Baker, R. C., and D. S. Kirschenbaum. 1998. Weight control during the holidays: Highly consistent self-monitoring as a potentially useful coping mechanism. *Health Psychology* 17: 367–70.

Boutelle, K. N., D. S. Kirschenbaum, R. C. Baker, and M. E. Mitchell. 1999. How can obese weight controllers minimize weight gain during the high risk holiday season? By self-monitoring very consistently. *Health Psychology* 18 (4): 364–68.

Centers for Disease Control and Prevention. 2000. *Health Statistics* Atlanta: GA.

Centers for Disease Control and Prevention. 2006. Obesity trends. http://www.cdc.gov (accessed June 25, 2008).

Department of Health and Human Services. 1996. Physical activity and health: A report of the Surgeon General. Superintendent of documents, Washington, DC.

Economic Research Service, U.S. Department of Agriculture. 2008. Food away from home as a percentage of expenditures. http://www.ers.usda.gov/Briefing/CPIFoodAndExpenditures/Data/table1.htm (accessed June 24, 2008).

Flegal, K. M., B. I. Graubard, D. F. Williamson, and M. H. Gail. 2005. Excess deaths associated with underweight, overweight and obesity. *Journal of the American Medical Association* 293: 1861–67.

Food and Drug Administration. 1997. Diet drugs off the market. *FDA Consumer*, 31 (7): 2.

Foran, J. R., M. A. Mont, G. Etienne, L. C. Jones, and D. S. Hungerford. 2004. The outcome of total knee arthroplasty in obese patients. *Journal of Bone and Joint Surgery, American* 85A (8): 1609–15.

International Obesity Task Force. 2003. International Obesity Task Force press statement, August 25. http://www.iotf.org (Media) (accessed June 25, 2008).

Kreb-Smith, S., M. Cook, A. Subar, A. Cleveland, L. Friday, J. L. Kahle. 1996. Fruits and vegetable intakes of children and adolescents in United States. *Archives of Pediatric and Adolescent Medicine* 150: 81–86.

Lin, B., and E. Frazao. 1999. *Away-From-Home Foods Increasingly Important to Quality of American Diet*. Washington, DC: U.S. Department of Agriculture Economic Research Service.

Moskowitz, J. 2004. Obesity to become leading cause of death. *Drug Benefit Trends* 16 (4): 164–65.

National Academy of Science. 2002. Report offers new eating and physical activity targets to reduce chronic disease risk, press release.

Painter, J. E., B. Wansink, and J. B. Hieggelke. 2002. How visibility and convenience influence candy consumption. *Appetite* 38: 237–38

Painter, J. E., and J. North. 2003. Effects of visibility and convenience on snack food consumption. *Journal of the American Dietetic Association* 103 (9): A-81.

Pi-Sunyer, F. 1993. Medical hazards of obesity. *Annals of Internal Medicine* 119: 655–60.

Pritikin, R. 1990. *The New Pritikin Program*. New York: Simon and Schuster.

Putnam, J., L. S. Kantor, and J. Allshouse. 2000. Per capita food supply trend: Progress toward dietary guidelines. *Food Review* 23: 2–13.

Reinehr, T., and W. Andler. 2004. Changes in atherogenic risk factor profile according to degree of weight loss. *Archives of Disabled Children* 89 (5): 419–22.

Rippe, J., and S. Hess. 1998. The role of physical activity in the prevention and management of obesity. *Journal of the American Dietetic Association* 96: S31–S38.

Satcher, D. U.S. Department of Health and Human Services. The Surgeon General's call to action to prevent and decrease overweight and obesity. http://www.surgeongeneral.gov/topics/obesity/ (accessed June 26, 2008).

Schwimer, J. B., T. M. Burwinkle, and J. W. Varni. 2003. Health related quality of life of severely obese children and adolescents. *Journal of the American Medical Association* 289 (14): 1813–19.

Shils, M. E., J. A. Olson, M. Shike, and A. C. Ross (eds). 1999. *Modern Nutrition in Health and Disease*, 9th ed. Media, PA: Williams and Wilkins.

Steinbach, G., S. Heymsfield, N. E. Olansen, A. Tighe, and P. R. Holt. 1994. Effect of calorie restriction on colonic proliferation in obese persons: Implications for colon cancer prevention. *Cancer Research* 54 (5): 1194–97.

Surgeon General. 2004. Overweight and obesity: What you can do. http://www.surgeongeneral. gov (accessed June 26, 2008).

U.S. Department of Agriculture. 2000. Nutrition and your health: Dietary Guidelines for Americans, 5th ed. Home and Garden Bulletin 232. Superintendent of Documents

Vega, G. L. 2004. Obesity and the metabolic syndrome. *Minerva Endocrinology* 29 (2): 47–54.

Wansink, B., J. E. Painter, and J. North. 2005. Bottomless bowls: Why visual cues of portion size may influence intake. *Obesity Research* 13 (1): 93–100.

Welch, C. B. 1998. The miracle that wasn't: Fen/Phen and Redux. *Diabetes Forecast* (April): 40–45.

World Health Organization. 2002. *Reducing Risks, Promoting Healthy Life*. Food and Agriculture Organization, Geneva, Switzerland.

World Health Organization. 2003. Food and Agriculture Organization expert consultation on diet, nutrition and the prevention of chronic diseases. http://www.who.int/hpr/NPH/docs/who_fao_expert_report.pdf (accessed June 26, 2008).

World Health Organization. 2004. Overweight and obesity. http://www.who.int (accessed June 26, 2008).

Young, L. R., and M. Nestle. 2003. Expanding portion sizes in the US marketplace: Implications for nutrition counseling. *Journal of the American Dietetic Association* 103 (2): 231–34.

1. Calculate your ideal body weight using each of the formulas shown in Box 9–1. Which formula gives the answer that is best for you?
2. Keep a 24-hour dietary record. Count your calories for the day.
3. Use one of the formulas shown in Box 9–2 to determine your caloric needs.
4. Compare your answer for question 3 with your answer for question 2. Discuss the reasons for basing a diet on individual needs.
5. Visit www.mypyramid.gov to plan a well-balanced diet using the USDA My Pyramid. How many calories are in the diet you planned?
6. According to the research presented in this chapter, what two environmental factors play a major role in how people eat?
7. Describe two methods used to measure body fat.
8. Explain why you think obesity treatment is difficult.
9. What causes obesity?
10. List five diseases associated with excess body fat.
11. What key factors are used for weight loss?

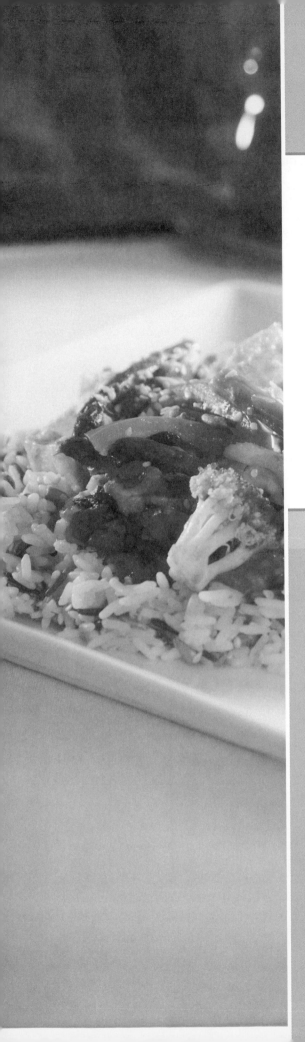

10

Serve Nutritionally Rich Foods through Proper Selection, Handling, and Cooking

KEY CONCEPTS

- The nutritional content for foods reported on food labels assumes ideal conditions for the growth, harvest, and transport of each food ingredient.

- Oxygen, light, heat, pH, water, and cooking reduce the nutrient content in foods as they are packed, shipped, stored, and processed for eating.

- "Fresh" fruits and vegetables are often defined by taste and eye appeal alone; however, "fresh" in this sense does not always equate to "nutritious."

- Ripening fruits and vegetables on the vine or plant and short holding and travel times can help guarantee higher nutrient levels and better retention of important nutrients.

- The more naturally foods are grown, the greater the care given to soils and feed, and the less time it takes to get harvested foods from the field to the table, the higher their nutrient levels are.

- The most dangerous elements affecting the nutritional content of fresh foods in storage are bacteria, mold, and yeast contamination and enzymatic breakdown.
- The nutritional content of seafood species differs significantly, which can directly affect the total nutrition on the plate.
- Important water-soluble nutrients, particularly vitamin C, thiamin, folate, and flavonoids, are washed away by food preparation workers following standard kitchen preparation practices.

Serving foods for the purposes of nutrition and health requires selecting foods with the requisite nutritional makeup, receiving and handling them properly to protect the nutrients they contain, and cooking them according to nutritional cooking guidelines. When chefs apply solid nutritional knowledge to the selecting, handling, and cooking practices they perform every day, they can better predict and protect the nutrient value of the foods they cook and serve. The purchasing, receiving, storage, preparation, cooking, and serving of foods all play a critical role in delivering healthier meals to customers. To protect the nutrients in food, the chef must examine and adjust commonly accepted food selection, handling, and preparation procedures based on scientific evidence describing the availability and stability of nutrients in the general food supply. The presence of food ingredients alone is not enough to guarantee nutrition on the table; careful planning and proper execution are needed to ensure the availability and balance of nutrients in foods served.

Extra time will be needed at first to plan, change, and then execute nutrient protection procedures. Once in place, however, the new procedures could become common practice. The benefits to the customer will be great when nutrition and flavor are both planned for and delivered.

THINK ABOUT IT

Consider all of the TV commercials, newspaper and magazine articles, and books that are written about the health benefits of eating certain foods. You might think that the nearly perfect fruits and vegetables that you get from your supplier or buy at the grocery store are chock-full of vitamins and minerals. But fruits and vegetables begin to lose their vitamins and minerals the minute they are picked from the tree, bush, or field. In light of this fact, just how much nutrition is in the fresh foods that you eat?

CASE STUDY

Local Produce

LaShawnda is a first-year culinary arts student enrolled at the local community college. She studies late at night and is always looking for healthy snacks to eat.

While growing up in the suburban South, LaShawnda had always heard that fresh fruits and vegetables were the healthiest foods to eat. Fresh fruits and vegetables were easy to find in her hometown, as it was surrounded by farms and cattle ranches.

In college, her nutrition classes emphasize the same notion. But now she lives in a major metropolitan area where fresh produce is scarce. Where can LaShawnda find those healthy fresh carrots, celery, and fruits to snack on?

How can LaShawnda obtain local produce for herself and her family in the urban setting in which she now lives? *The resolution for this case study is presented at the end of the chapter.*

NUTRIENT SENSITIVITY IN FOODS

The nutrient content for foods reported in nutritional databases and on nutrition labels assumes ideal conditions for the growth, harvest, and transport of each food ingredient. The data presuppose that foods, especially fruits and vegetables, are grown to full ripeness on the plant; are handled and packed quickly and properly; are used in production very shortly after being harvested; and are prepared and cooked so as to retain nutrients. If any of these conditions is less than ideal, the actual nutrient content of the food, and the meals in which they are served, can no longer be guaranteed.

Many factors affect the nutrient content in foods. Food genetics, farming and herding practices, soil conditions, and the crop maturity at the time of harvest all determine the nutrient levels actually found in the foods as they are harvested and prepared for market. Oxygen, light, heat, pH, water, and cooking continue to reduce the nutrient content in foods as they are packed, shipped, stored, and processed for eating.

The vitamins most affected by oxidation are A, B_{12}, B_6, C, D, K, and riboflavin. The vitamins most affected by acids (pH lower than 7) are A, D, and folate those most affected by alkalinity are C, D, riboflavin, and thiamin.

Food genetics determines the physical structure and appearance of foods as well as their carbohydrate, amino acid, and fat content. The practice of buying foods from around the world and transporting them to distant markets has created a demand for tough-skinned, slow-ripening fruits and vegetables for the purpose of transport and sale. Using genetic engineering, biochemists have created strains of plants that produce crops with all the physical characteristics farmers needs to transport their products to distant markets in salable condition. However, what consideration has been given to their nutritional content?

As early as 1940, biological research determined that the nutritional content of foods was also tied to genetic structure and the heredity of the species. Bioengineers could then use this information to create strains of fruits and vegetables as rich in nutritional content as they were attractive in appearance, color, shape, and size. Unfortunately, genetic study was, and continues to be, extremely expensive, and there have been few incentives to consider nutritional content when engineering new food strains. Consequently, in today's marketplace it is hard to determine which fruits and vegetables were bred for beauty and convenience and which ones also contain high levels of essential nutrients.

Genetics also affects the physical structure of cattle, pork, lamb, and poultry. Specific strains of animals and birds are bred to produce desirable fat-to-lean ratios, fat concentrations, muscle size, egg production, and age to maturity. (Some breeds of animals and poultry mature more quickly and therefore put on weight faster than do other breeds.) While the overall vitamin and mineral content of animal flesh does not vary greatly, the amount of vitamin D found naturally in dairy cows and chicken eggs is determined partly by genetics and partly by herding or breeding practices. The type of feed used and the amount of time the animals were allowed to eat in direct sunlight directly affect their vitamin D content, which is then passed on to humans through the milk and eggs.

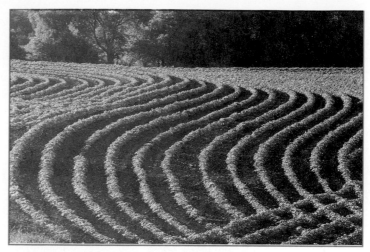

Either the minerals are in the soil, or they are not.
Tom Stack & Associates, Inc.

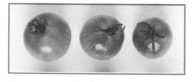

Tomatoes picked green will not develop their full nutritional values.
Steve Shott © Dorling Kindersley

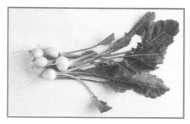

Beets and turnips are often served with their tops, called greens, for added nutritional value.
Steve Gorton © Dorling Kindersley

The condition of the soil in which fruits and vegetables are grown and on which cattle, sheep, pork, and poultry are raised also affects the nutritional content of these foods. The mineral content of plants is directly affected by the composition of the soil in which they were grown and the method and type of fertilization used. The minerals on which these food sources depend for food either are in the soil or are not. The modern farming practice of using nitrogen-rich fertilizers to promote plant growth does not return important minerals like selenium, calcium, and magnesium to the soil; therefore, these minerals never make it to plants or animals raised in those areas.

Scientific studies conducted by L. A. Maynard and K. C. Hammer in the 1940s (U.S. Department of Agriculture, Misc. Publication, 1942) determined that fruits and vegetables reach their full potential of vitamin and mineral content when they are allowed to ripen fully in the ground, or on the vine, plant, or tree from which they came. Particularly high were the ascorbic acid and thiamin content of the foods studied; ascorbic acid content is affected by an increase or decrease in direct sunlight upon the fruit or vegetable; thiamin is created in the plant's leaves as a by-product of photosynthesis and passes to the stem, and then to the fruits or vegetables as they mature.

Therefore, fruits and vegetables that are picked green and allowed to ripen slowly while being shipped never develop their full complement of important nutrients. Nor do root vegetables contain their usual levels of nutrients when they are pulled out of the ground and their nutrient-rich stems and leaves are cut away from them.

The leaves (commonly called greens) of root vegetables like turnips and beets should be kept attached to their roots until the roots are prepared for cooking. Serving the greens separately or in combination with the roots presents the greatest possible amount of nutrients from those particular vegetables.

The nutrients that fruits and vegetables contain when they are harvested can be destroyed or rendered unavailable for human consumption if the foods are handled improperly after they are picked. The nutrients at particular risk are the water-soluble vitamins (C and B), vitamins K and E, beta-carotene, and the minerals magnesium, calcium, and potassium. Carbohydrate content, protein, and fiber do not change significantly as fruits and vegetables mature, rot, and die.

Water-soluble vitamins are at risk when fruits or vegetables become dehydrated. Consequently, the depletion of the moisture content of fruits and vegetables that occurs after harvest decreases their water-soluble vitamin content. Other vitamins also deteriorate with the passing of time, so the older a fruit or vegetable becomes, the less its nutritional worth.

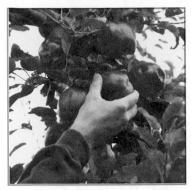

Fruits, like apples, are at their peak of nutritional value when first picked; immediately afterward that nutritional value begins to go down.

Peter Anderson © Dorling Kindersley

THE RIPENING OF PICKED FRUITS AND VEGETABLES

Not all fruits or vegetables mature and ripen after they are picked; some simply begin rotting immediately. Generally, fruits and vegetables grown on vines, particularly melons, yellow squash, zucchini, cucumbers, and all forms of winter squash, do not ripen after they are separated from their host plant. Without the flow of needed nutrients, these fruits and vegetables begin to deteriorate right after picking. Tree fruits like apples, pears, peaches, nectarines, and plums do continue to ripen after harvest. These ripen very quickly (within a few days) if not refrigerated. Citrus fruits and berries do not ripen after they are picked.

Some vegetables continue to mature after harvesting. Broccoli, cauliflower, eggplant, tomatoes, and peppers (all forms of capsicum peppers) all ripen after they are picked, eventually becoming inedible if stored too long after harvest. Other vegetables do not mature after harvest; they start to rot as soon as they are picked. Lettuces, cabbages, and all root vegetables are harvested fully mature and do not continue to mature once removed from their host plant or pulled from the ground.

Fruits and vegetables continue to feed, drink, breathe (expel gases), and conduct photosynthesis (where appropriate) for several days after they are separated from their host plant. These living processes use nutrients from the cells for these changes rather than those from the tree or roots from which they had been taken, thus using up these important resources from the food's own structure and juices. Most fruits and vegetables actually "cannibalize" themselves to sustain life as long as possible after harvest. When the fruits and vegetables exhaust their own natural resources to sustain their own life processes, they begin to wither, rot, and die. So, too, do the nutrients they contain change, becoming denatured and eventually unavailable for human health.

Chilling fruits and vegetables immediately after they are harvested as well as maintaining cool temperatures throughout packing, shipping, and storing is the best way to preserve the nutrients they contain. Iceberg lettuce, for example, can lose as much as 50% of its vitamin C content after only one day at room temperature storage, yet it may retain nearly all of its vitamin C for up to three days when refrigerated properly. Refrigeration, however, often does not occur quickly enough in the field, and storage units and transportation vehicles are subject to temperature fluctuations. The time needed to get produce from the field to the table dramatically affects nutrient retention.

Freezing fruits and vegetables after they are harvested preserves their nutritional content even longer than does normal refrigeration. This occurs for two reasons. First, the fruits and vegetables ripen fully on the vine or plant since they do not have to be shipped over long distances; at the same time their vitamin and mineral content rises to its full potential. Second, the speed at which these fruits and vegetables are harvested, prepared, and frozen decreases their exposure to the sunlight and high temperatures that cause produce to deteriorate and lose their nutritional content.

The valuable vitamins and minerals, allowed to mature in the fruits and vegetables, are sealed tightly in the frozen cell walls before deterioration can begin. Frozen foods that are thawed properly and cooked quickly often contain more vitamins and minerals than do fresh (nonfrozen) or canned varieties of the same foods.

Oxygen, light, and heat are known destroyers of vitamins. They accelerate the decomposition of harvested fruits and vegetables, meat, poultry, and fish, and they have a similar effect on vitamins. Long exposures to these elements can significantly reduce nutrient retention as outlined in Table 10–1.

TABLE 10–1 • CAUSES OF VITAMIN LOSS IN FOOD

Vitamin	% Loss	Cause of Loss
Vitamin A	0 to 60	oxygen, heat, light
Vitamin B_1	30 to 80	water, alkaline pH, heat
Vitamin B_2	9 to 39	water, alkaline pH
Niacin	3 to 27	water
Vitamin B_6	30 to 82	water
Biotin	0 to 50	oxygen, alkaline pH
Vitamin C	0 to 100	oxygen, heat, alkaline pH, water
Vitamin D	0 to 40	oxygen, light
Vitamin E	0 to 60	oxygen

Source: Adapted from Vitamin and Information Service (Hoffman LaRoche).

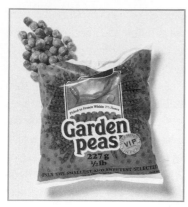

Vegetables retain their nutrients when properly frozen.
© *Dorling Kindersley*

Chilling foods as soon as possible after harvest or slaughter, keeping them out of the light, and leaving whole until ready for cooking or serving helps to preserve nutrient content. Even whole fruits and vegetables may have their nutritional content reduced in their exterior layers, although good levels of vitamins remain below the surface. Cutting, chopping, slicing, and otherwise mechanically breaking down animal and plant tissues expose more of the food's cells and therefore more of its vitamins to oxygen and light; the longer this exposure exists, the greater the vitamin loss.

BUYING NUTRIENT-RICH FOODS

Nutritional knowledge imposes a new set of guidelines for purchasing foods for healthy meals. The common purchasing specifications of variety, size, color, and shape do not guarantee the nutritional content of foods. How truly fresh are "fresh" foods given the instability of nutrients in the host fruits and vegetables from the moment they are picked from the fields? When you buy peeled carrots, diced onions, or chopped tomatoes, what is the cost in nutritional loss for the convenience? Furthermore, what nutrients remain after processing, shipping, and storage? Fortunately, a knowledge of nutrient availability and vulnerability enables chefs to purchase foods rich in nutritional value and pass these nutrients to their customers through the dishes they prepare.

Freshness is the most significant factor in determining the potential nutrient content of food ingredients. However, the term "fresh" as commonly used does not take into account the full nature of the product. Foods may have a fresh appearance, texture, and even taste, yet their vitamin and mineral content could be low or missing altogether. The demand for fresh-looking fruits and vegetables throughout the year and a new demand for convenience fresh-food products have created whole product lines that offer the appearance of good nutrition without providing any substantive nutrition. When used to describe quality foods for nutritional cooking, the word "fresh" must also refer to the quality and availability of the nutrients they contain. Accordingly, "fresh foods" refer to foods that are grown properly; harvested at their peak of readiness (ripeness in fruits and vegetables); protected from outside elements of air, light, and heat; and prepared as soon as possible after harvest.

Buying locally raised fruits and vegetables ensures the greatest amount of nutrition in the foods you cook and serve. These products often are allowed to ripen more fully in the fields than produce shipped across the country. This allows for their nutrients to develop completely. In addition, locally grown produce is sold and prepared within days of harvest rather than weeks. This helps local produce retain the vitamins it does contain. The combination of being fully ripened on the vine or plant and short holding and travel times can help guarantee higher levels of important nutrients and better retention.

Purchase root vegetables, cauliflower, broccoli, and other vegetables produced by leafy plants that have been trimmed as little as possible to allow as many important nutrients as possible to transfer from the host plants to the vegetables themselves. This transfer of nutrients continues well past the harvest if the nutrient-rich leaves and branches are left intact. These outer leaves and branches can then be eliminated during final preparation and cooking, leaving behind the valuable nutrients.

Cabbage, iceberg lettuce, and other headed vegetables should not have their exterior leaves trimmed until ready for use. These leaves are the first to deteriorate during storage

BIOAVAILABILITY OF NUTRIENTS

The nutrient content of foods is not enough to ensure that those nutrients are passed on to the persons consuming them. Not all nutrients are available for human digestion. Although consumed, the form in which they exist may prevent the body from digesting or otherwise utilizing them for normal bodily functions. Bioavailability of nutrients describes the fraction of an ingested nutrient that is available to the human body for utilization in normal physiological processes or for storage.

Some factors that affect the bioavailability of nutrients for human consumption are:

- Specific form of the nutrient
- Molecular linkage of nutrients to other food components
- Amount consumed in a single meal
- Nutritional health of the consumer
- Individual person's genetics
- Human health factors, particularly digestive and absorption problems

While some nutrients are lost or destroyed through food processing and cooking, the nutrients that remain have been shown to be more bioavailable to the consumer. Arguments to at least partially cook all foods for better health can be easily defended.

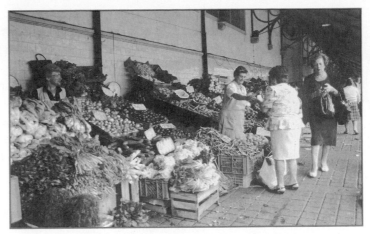

Fresh local produce can be bought at farmer's markets and roadside stands.
Linda Whitwam © Dorling Kindersley

and can be removed easily before prepping the vegetable for cooking. Allowing these leaves to remain on the head until the vegetable is ready for use protects the inner leaves from dehydration and exposure to air and light.

Pretrimmed vegetables, cut lettuce, peeled carrots, and other convenience fresh-food products can save an operator a lot of preparation time and require fewer skilled workers to cook and serve them; their nutritional content, however, drops with each process or technique performed on them before they reach the table. Valuable nutrients are either torn away by mechanical peeling machines and scrapers, or they deteriorate quickly under the added exposure of light and oxygen. In either case, preprocessed vegetables and fruits do not provide the high levels of nutrition they otherwise would contain.

Frozen vegetables and fruits can be good nutritional sources if fresh local fruits and vegetables are not available. Most frozen produce is harvested at the peak of ripeness and frozen within hours of being picked, which preserves and protects its nutritional content. For quality

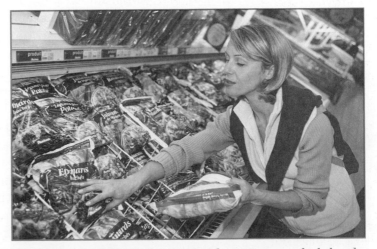

Preprocessed vegetables may not contain the nutrients you think they do.
Photo Researchers, Inc.

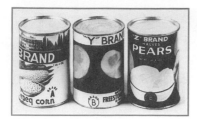

Canned fruits have their nutrients locked inside.

U.S. Department of Agriculture

food production, frozen vegetables may not be appropriate as the main menu choices; but frozen corn, peas, beans, cut greens, and other vegetables do retain their quality and can be used in a variety of cooking applications with practically no loss in the final dish's presentation or taste.

Some canned fruits and vegetables are also good sources of vitamins and minerals. Even though the canning process causes significant losses of vitamin C, niacin, riboflavin, thiamin, vitamin A, and beta-carotene, these same vitamins are lost during standard cooking practices. To recapture as many of these nutrients as possible, the chef should use the liquid or broth, which contains the leached-out vitamins, in the final meal preparation.

Like frozen produce, fruits and vegetables used for canning often are allowed to ripen on the plant or vine and are processed very soon after harvest.

Canned tomato products like whole tomatoes, diced tomatoes, tomato sauce, and tomato paste are excellent examples of quality canned food products. Tomatoes targeted for canning are ripened fully on the vine and in direct sunlight, developing maximum nutrition as well as flavor. Then they are canned quickly, which locks in their nutritional vitamins and minerals until needed. Fresh tomatoes from the typical vendor (not local vine-ripened tomatoes) cannot match the nutritional content of canned ripe tomatoes.

Fruits canned in water can often be used in place of fresh fruits in production cooking and baking, particularly in pies, tarts, and fruit sauces, without sacrificing the quality of the finished product. Fruits canned in syrup, however, should be avoided in nutritional cooking; the syrup supplies a lot of calorie content with little nutritional value.

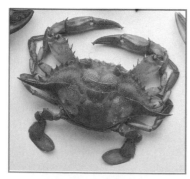

Canned sardines are an excellent source for omega-3 fatty acids and calcium.

Andy Crawford © Dorling Kindersley

Nutritional food choices can also be made based on the food itself. This is particularly true when ordering seafood for the menu. Seafood includes many different species of fish and shellfish, and each contains different nutrients depending on their environment (salt water or fresh; cold water or warm) and what they eat. In particular, the omega-3 fatty acid content of seafood varies depending on the species. (See the benefits of eating seafood with omega-3 fatty acids in Chapter 5.)

Many nutritionists and chefs consider seafood to be an inherently healthy food. In general, seafood contains a fraction of the fat found in beef and poultry and is a good source of vitamins and minerals. The nutritional value of seafood combined with its versatility in cooking makes serving seafood both healthy and fun. But significant nutritional differences exist between seafood species, which can directly affect the total nutrition of the dish to be served. For the chef who wants to provide the highest nutrition possible, the omega-3 fatty acid, cholesterol, sodium, and calcium content of different species of seafood can help deliver healthier dishes to the table.

The best seafood sources of omega-3 fatty acids are cold-water fatty fish like salmon, halibut, trout, herring, tuna, and sardines. Because these fish live in cold water, their bodies naturally contain higher levels of fat for warmth. These fats contain high levels of omega-3 fatty acids, which can be passed on to consumers at the time of consumption. The small bones of sardines and salmon (canned) are a good source of calcium when consumed as part of the final dish.

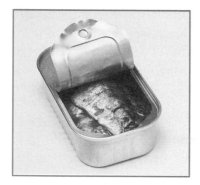

Blue crabs are a good source of calcium.

Philip Dowell © Dorling Kindersley

Crab, shrimp, lobster, and clam are also good sources of calcium; so are some bottom-feeding fish, such as grouper and orange roughy, that eat them. Crustaceans in general, however, contain more cholesterol than do other species of seafood. To prepare crustaceans nutritiously, use no-fat cooking procedures and serve them with low- or nonfat sauces made from reduced or vegetable purées.

TABLE 10–2 • NUTRITIONAL VALUES OF COMMON SEAFOOD

Species	Calories	Total Fat g	Sat. Fat g	Cholesterol mg	Sodium mg	Protein g	Calcium mg	Phosphorus mg	Iron mg	Potassium mg
				Approximate Values for 3 Ounces of Edible Portions						
Bluefish	130	3	1	59	60	20	7	227	0.48	372
Catfish	95	2.8	0.5	58	43	16.4	14	209	0.3	358
Clams	74	1	0.09	34	56	12.7	46	169	14	314
Crab, blue	87	1	0.22	78	293	18	89	229	0.74	329
Flounder	91	1.1	0.28	48	81	18.8	18	184	0.36	361
Grouper	92	1	0.23	37	53	19.4	27	162	0.89	483
Halibut	110	2.3	0.32	32	54	21	47	222	0.84	450
Lobster	90	0.90	0.18	95	296	18.8	48	144	0.30	275
Mackerel, king	120	2	0.5	55	65	23	4	248	10	435
Orange roughy	69	0.7	0.02	20	63	14.7	30	200	0.18	300
Oyster	81	2.3	0.51	50	106	9.45	8	162	5.1	168
Salmon, Atlantic	142	6.34	0.98	55	44	20	12	200	0.80	490
Shrimp	106	1.7	0.32	152	148	20.3	52	205	2.4	185
Swordfish	121	4	1.1	39	90	19.8	4	263	0.81	288
Trout	148	6.6	1.1	58	52	21	43	245	1.5	361
Tuna, bluefin	144	4.9	1.3	38	39	23.3	8	254	1.02	252

Source: U.S. Department of Agriculture. 2003. *USDA National Nutreint Database for Standard Reference.* http://www.nal.usda.gov/fnic/cgi-bin/list_nut.pl.

Shrimp with 148 milligrams, crab with 293 milligrams, oysters with 106 milligrams, and lobsters with 296 milligrams of sodium per 3-ounce edible portion (Table 10–2) provide a lot of sodium in a single dish. Cooks and chefs should avoid using excessive salt when preparing these shellfish, and should not put them on the menu for patrons on sodium-restricted diets without knowing and communicating their true sodium content.

Clams, oysters, shrimp, and king mackerel contain large amounts of iron compared to other seafood choices. Most seafood choices are good sources of protein, potassium, and phosphorus.

Free-range chickens and the eggs they produce contain higher levels of minerals and vitamin C than do chickens grown by modern high-production methods and the eggs of caged, grain-fed production hens. Nutrients are naturally passed on to free-range chickens from their food source. Although free-range chickens are primarily fed on grain, as other

Jean-Anthelme Brillat-Savarin
(1755–1826), who wrote a
treatise on gastronomy and the
development of culinary arts,
La Physiologie du Goût (*The
Philosopher in the Kitchen*),
was living and writing at a time
when culinary innovations like
coffee and chocolate first became popular in European communities. Brillat-Savarin was a
gourmet of great importance.
As the mayor of Belley, France,
during the French Revolution,
he enjoyed many fine meals in
restaurants (another innovation
of the late eighteenth century),
hotels, and palaces; courted
royalty and political leaders at
his own home; and shared the
finest meals available with
friends and associates throughout Europe and America.

One of the food industry's
innovations at the time, with
which Brillat-Savarin was not
pleased, was the mass raising
of chickens in cages, fed solely
on processed grains. To Brillat-
Savarin, free range was the normal process by which chickens
were raised, the complete opposite of what it is like today. This
is what Brillat-Savarin had to
say about the new chickens in
1825.

> We have not been content, how-
> ever, with the natural qualities
> of the gallinaceous species
> (poultry); art has laid hands on
> them, and under the pretext of
> improving them, has con-
> demned them to martyrdom.
> Not only do we take away their
> means of reproduction, but we
> keep them in solitary confine-
> ment, cast them into darkness,
> force them to eat willy-nilly, and
> so blow them up to a size for
> which they were never in-
> tended. (Brillat-Savarin 1984)

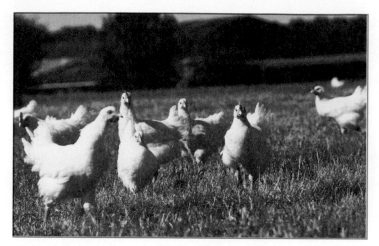

Free-range chickens contain higher amounts of nutrients than cage-
raised chickens.
Andres Holligan © Dorling Kindersley

chickens, they also forage in open fields and pastures for natural foods like insects, grasses, and wild seeds.

These natural foods are loaded with rich nutrients, especially minerals taken from the ground, which are not available in processed foods. These nutrients are then passed on to the chickens and end up in their eggs. The vitamin C content of free-range chickens and eggs also increases naturally with the extra sunlight exposure the chickens get as they forage in the open air.

Chickens that are raised for rapid maturing and for size are kept in cages, are given diets of 100% processed grains, and live their whole lives in artificially lit enclosed buildings. These chickens are safe to eat and have a low-fat content, but they do not contain the levels of vitamins and minerals that more naturally raised chickens have.

In most cases, growing foods more naturally, taking better care of soils and feed, and reducing the amount of time transporting harvested foods from the field to the table increase the levels of nutrients the foods contain. Buying locally raised produce and poultry and meat from free-range breeders and purchasing seafood selectively for nutrition can also dramatically increase the vitamin and mineral content of foods served.

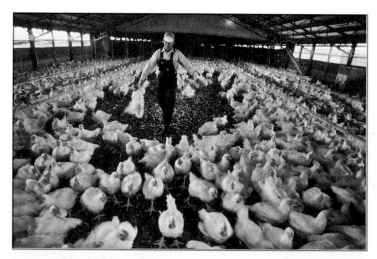

Mass-produced poultry.
Aurora Photos, Inc.

STORING FOODS TO PRESERVE NUTRIENTS

Once you have specified and ordered healthier foods, you must store them properly in order to maintain the nutrients all the way to the table. The nutrients in foods continue to deteriorate when they are received into the food service establishment. Speedy receipt and proper storage of foods in refrigerators, freezers, or dry store rooms help reduce the speed at which these nutrients deteriorate.

The most dangerous elements affecting the nutritional content of fresh foods in storage are contamination by bacteria, molds, and yeasts and the enzymatic breakdown of plant cells that begins when the product is harvested. Cleaning refrigerators properly, providing ample air flow around each product, storing raw protein foods below all other foods, and rotating stock (first in, first out; or FIFO) must be part of the normal kitchen routine. Dirty or damp refrigerators where ice or spills are allowed to stay on the floor are great environments for bacteria, molds, and yeasts to thrive and contaminate foods. The same factors that make foods unsafe to eat also compromise their nutrient content.

The best refrigerator temperatures for retaining vitamins and minerals in most fresh foods are between 32°F and 35°F (0–2°C). Produce should be stored in dark closed containers to protect it from unnecessary exposure to light or heat and from dehydration.

Humidity is also important for protecting nutrients in foods. Fresh foods should be stored between 90% and 95% humidity. Commercial refrigerators are designed to maintain proper humidity and temperatures, yet excessive water pooled on the floor or in open boxes, overcrowding of shelves, and opening the door too frequently drastically alter these delicate storage environments.

A good way to protect the moisture of foods in cold storage is to sprinkle them lightly with freshwater and store them in plastic or polyethylene food storage bags. (Berries, grapes, or cherries, however, should not be sprinkled with water, as they are more susceptible to mold and yeast contamination.)

Some fruits and vegetables are better preserved in slightly warmer temperatures. Bell peppers, ripe tomatoes, summer squash, watermelons, and okra, for example, keep better in temperatures between 45°F and 50°F (7–10°C). Place these foods in the front part of

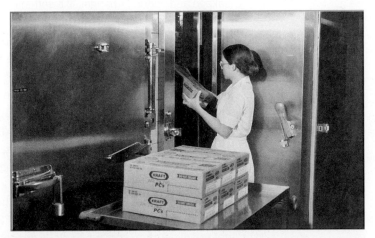

Refrigerators should be set between 32°F and 35°F to help retain the nutrients in fresh foods.
Pearson Education/PH College

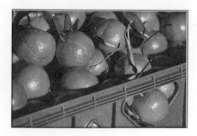

Oranges are often stored at or near room temperature to help preserve their freshness and, therefore, their nutrient levels.

Getty Images, Inc.—PhotoDisc

the refrigerator; this area is usually warmer than the others because it is exposed to outside air every time the door is opened. The coldest section of a refrigerator is in the rear or back wall area (usually below the fans). Brown paper food service bags are ideal containers for foods stored in this temperature range; these bags insulate the foods from the colder outside air temperature of the refrigerator.

Other produce keeps better in even higher temperatures, often temperatures too high for refrigerated storage. Cucumbers, eggplants, pumpkins, sweet potatoes, winter squash, oranges, limes, lemons, mangoes, bananas, papayas, grapefruits, and avocados should be stored at temperatures between 50°F and 65°F (10–18°C).

Usually, food preparation areas in kitchens offer the coolest room temperatures. They are often located near the front of walk-in refrigerators and freezers, or close to the dry storage areas far away from the cooking line where all the kitchen heat is generated. Temperatures of 50°F, to 65°F (10–18°C) are often possible in these cool areas without any extra air-conditioning. The closer the storage areas are to the cooking line, however, the higher the overall temperature and the greater the nutrient loss even in cold-sensitive foods. Large production facilities and food suppliers have rooms for each type of produce that are set at the appropriate temperatures and humidity levels.

In warm climates, the entire kitchen's air temperature, including the preparation area, may be consistently higher than 65°F (18°C). All produce will deteriorate if left at these temperatures for extended periods of time. In these cases, use insulated containers to store cold-sensitive foods inside refrigerators. This will allow them to stay near their ideal storage temperature without being exposed to either the colder air in the refrigerator itself or the warmer air in the kitchen.

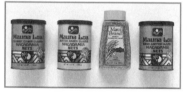

Keep roasted nuts in tightly sealed containers to prevent them from turning moldy or rancid.

Steve Gorton © Dorling Kindersley

Nuts stay fresh longer under the cooler temperatures of 32°F to 35°F (0–2°C), but can become moldy and rancid if stored at the high humidity needed for other cold storage foods. To keep humidity low for foods like nuts in refrigerated environments, store them in sealed, vacuum-packed, or moisture-proof containers.

As previously mentioned, freezing is a very efficient way of preserving the nutrients in foods. Most vitamins (for example, beta-carotene) keep well within frozen foods. To preserve frozen foods properly, as well as their nutrients, keep freezers between 0°F and −18°F (−18 to −28°C). Temperatures higher than 0°F (−18°C) can increase the rate of deterioration of fatty foods, cause colors in foods to fade, and interfere with vitamin retention. Although proteins and carbohydrates appear to be stable in the frozen state, freezing, thawing, and refreezing foods can break down proteins and carbohydrates, causing cell leakage and textural changes like softening.

The best way to retain vitamins and minerals when cooking frozen vegetables is to place them in a steamer or directly into boiling water while they are still frozen. Thawing them out first in a refrigerator allows some of their natural juices to escape, which carry valuable vitamins and minerals with them.

Dry storage areas should be maintained in cool, dry condition. Temperature ranges should be kept between 50°F and 70°F (10–21°C) with humidity no higher than 50% to 60%. Higher temperatures can cause vitamin loss. Higher humidity can cause slight hydration of dried grains, cereals, and pastas, which can leading to bacteria or mold growth and rapid deterioration. (Dry foods must maintain a low moisture content of 10% or lower if stored for a long time.) Consistently high levels of humidity in dry storage can also cause food cans to corrode, contaminating food through oxidation and leakage.

High storeroom temperatures of 100°F or more significantly affect vitamin and mineral retention of dry storage foods. Extended storage times also have a negative effect on nutrient retention. Dry foods should be used within six months of receipt to ensure good food quality, sanitation, and nutrition.

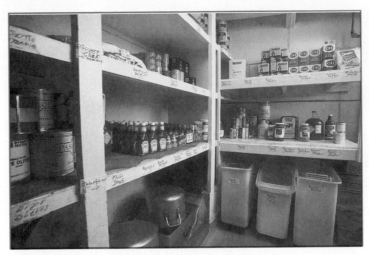

Dry storage areas should be kept dry and cool.
PhotoEdit Inc.

Light can also affect nutrient retention in dry foods, particularly enriched pastas, cereals, and grains. The fluorescent lighting used in many dry storage areas has the same negative effect on vitamin retention as does natural sunlight. Vitamins that are particularly unstable in light are C, B_6, and riboflavin. Significant losses of riboflavin can occur in as few as 12 weeks of dry storage under fluorescent lighting. Enriched cereal in dry storage shows a significant loss of vitamin A when stored longer than six months. Even perfectly preserved foods after one year of dry storage show a reduction of major vitamins: 50% reduction in vitamin A, 41% in vitamin C, 23% in riboflavin, 19% in folate, and 17% in vitamin B_{12}.

Proper environmental factors in dry storage can extend the shelf life of foods. The best practice to implement, however, is still proper stock rotation of first in, first out (FIFO). When new dry storage food items are received, place them in back or below similar foods already in storage. Marking containers with the date of receipt can help ensure that the oldest product is always used first. Dry storage areas should not have windows that allow natural light to come in. If there are exterior windows in your dry storage area, keep them closed and covered all the time. Dry storage areas should be fitted with incandescent lighting whenever possible to reduce exposure to harmful synthetic light rays. If fluorescent lighting is already in place, turn them on only when you need to work in the storeroom. Turn fluorescent lights off every time you leave the room or the room is left empty.

Proper storage helps extend the shelf life of nutrient-rich foods and keeps their nutritional value high. Improper storage of nutrient-deficient foods will cause them to lose even more nutrients at accelerating rates.

PROCESSING FOODS TO PRESERVE NUTRIENTS

The conscientious chef forgoes the benefits of speed production in order to provide higher levels of nutrition to their guests. A lot of "tricks of the trade," or shortcuts, to proper food preparation can cause significant losses of vitamins and minerals. Cooks and chefs inadvertently destroy or remove nutrients from food every day.

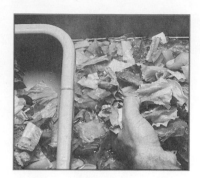

Soaking vegetables in water can rob them of valuable vitamins and minerals.
Pearson Education/PH College

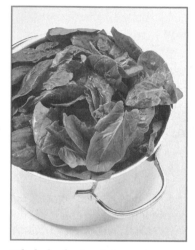

Whole-leaf spinach has more nutrition when cooked quickly without chopping the leaves.
Dave King © Dorling Kindersley

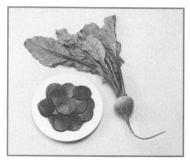

Cook root vegetables and tubers in their skins to help retain nutrients.
Pearson Education Corporate Digital Archive

The sensitivity of nutrients to light, oxygen, pH, heat, and water dictates that chefs process and cook food cautiously in their kitchen operations. Even commonly accepted food preparation techniques significantly diminish the nutritional value of fresh foods and must be reexamined, altered, or dropped altogether for the sake of nutrient retention.

Food preparation workers wash away important water-soluble nutrients, particularly vitamin C, thiamin, folate, and flavonoids, when following standard kitchen preparation practices. These techniques are designed for efficiency of operation and for the speed and accuracy of the employee. Produce is cleaned and washed to remove contaminants. But if it is also left to soak in water or is chopped prematurely, a significant loss of valuable nutrients results.

Foods should not be washed, cut, chopped or otherwise broken down into smaller pieces until just before they are needed for service. Exposing food cells to air (oxygen), light, and heat causes their nutrients and antioxidants to deteriorate. Nutrients in foods deteriorate in direct proportion to the amount of cell exposure to outside elements. Purchasing chopped, sliced, and otherwise previously prepared vegetables eases in-house preparation demands, but these products provide significantly less nutritional value than those that are pealed and prepped just before cooking and serving.

Severe chopping and puréeing of plant foods accelerates the loss of nutrients even faster. Plant cells are broken by these processes, releasing enzymes that can destroy antioxidants, thiamin, and flavonoids. Even the carotenoid content of foods like carrots and sweet potatoes suffers when these vegetables are chopped or puréed. The faster the cooked and puréed vegetables get to the customer, the more nutrients they will contain.

Whole carrots, leaf spinach and other leafy vegetables, whole or large diced sweet potatoes, and whole cooked mushrooms provide more nutrition than they would in any processed form. For example, while a spinach timbale may sound appealing nutritionally, steamed whole-leaf spinach contains much more nutrients for the same portion weight.

Washing produce and cut fruit also washes away water-soluble vitamins. Although it is necessary to wash produce before preparing it to remove contaminants like dirt and pesticides, do not soak produce or cut fruit in water any longer than is absolutely necessary. Washing uncut produce quickly in large amounts of water is the best method for washing and preserving nutrients at the same time.

Peeled potatoes, cut celery, and produce for salad preparations and salad bars are often left soaking in water to keep them hydrated, crispy, and fresh looking. The appearance may be preserved, but major amounts of water-soluble vitamins and minerals are leached into the water. And the water does not have to be heated to absorb valuable nutrients. The mere contact of water with produce and meats containing water-soluble nutrients is enough to leach away those nutrients.

Another food preparation technique that speeds up production yet removes valuable nutrients is the peeling of root vegetables and tubers (potatoes) before cooking them. Cooking them whole and then peeling them later may take longer, but their nutritional value will be protected.

Most nutrients in root vegetables and tubers are found in or directly under their thin skins. A handheld vegetable peeler or paring knife can cut deep into the flesh of potatoes, carrots, beets, and other root vegetables, stripping away valuable nutrients with every scrape or cut. And machine-operated vegetable peelers can do even more damage to the nutrient content of these foods.

Cooking root vegetables in their skins allows the flesh of the vegetables to absorb some of their valuable nutrients as they are drawn out of the skins during cooking. After the vegetables are cooked, the nutrient-depleted skins can be removed and the final dish prepared. This leaves valuable nutrients in the vegetables themselves, which can then be passed on to the dining guest.

You go through a lot of work in specifying, ordering, and receiving nutritious foods. Do not process those nutrients away for the sake of speed and efficiency.

COOKING FOODS TO PRESERVE NUTRIENTS

Cooks and chefs have many options when deciding on a healthier way of cooking and serving foods. A good understanding of the effects of heat, pH, oxygen, light, and exposure to water on nutrients enables cooks to select cooking methods and procedures that preserve nutrients or capture them for later use.

Many nutrients simply leach into the liquid they are cooked in. Even greater amounts disappear if that liquid is alkaline (pH greater than 7). Water-soluble vitamins like vitamins B_1 and B_2, biotin, and vitamin C; minerals; and flavonoids are reduced significantly when foods are simmered or boiled in water. That water is all too often thrown away, sending valuable nutrients down the kitchen drain.

Do not add baking soda or any other alkaline substance to your cooking water. A slightly alkaline cooking liquid may help retain the color in green vegetables like green beans, asparagus, and broccoli, but it is at the sacrifice of valuable nutrients.

The best method of cooking vegetables in water is to cut them into small pieces (to speed the cooking process) and cook them in small batches in plenty of plain boiling water so the cooking liquid never drops below the boiling point. You can use the cooking liquid in the final preparation of the dish or in another dish to return leached nutrients back into the foods you serve. A sauce, stock, or soup is a great way to use cooking liquids rich in water-soluble nutrients.

Keep lids on pans and pots during cooking as much as possible. This will prevent exposure to air and light, which would cause additional nutrient loss. Protect water-soluble nutrients even more by steaming foods instead of poaching or boiling them.

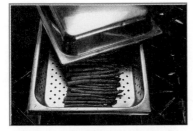

Steam cooking offers the benefit of fast cooking while retaining nutrients.
Pearson Education/PH College

Steam cooking offers the benefit of extremely fast, no-fat cooking with little loss of vitamins or flavor. Although the steam is created by boiling water, there is no liquid cooking medium to trap the flavors or leach out nutrients. Most foods can be cooked by steam. The temperature of steam is only slightly higher than boiling water (212°F [100°C]), and browning will not occur. (Browning requires temperatures of 310°F [154°C] or higher.)

To preserve the greatest amount of nutrients in boiling, poaching, or steam cooking of vegetables, cook only the amount needed for immediate service. Production facilities usually blanch (partially cook) vegetables first to speed the final cooking for service to a larger number of customers. Typically, blanched vegetables are placed immediately in ice cold water to stop the cooking process and preserve the natural vegetable colors. It is important when blanching to cool off the vegetables as fast as possible and then drain off all excess water. Allowing raw or blanched vegetables to soak in water will accelerate nutrient losses.

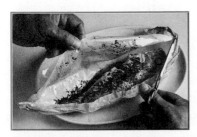

En papillote cookery creates steam to cook its contents using natural juices and flavorings.
Jerry Young © Dorling Kindersley

The *en papillote* technique uses steam to cook seafood, meats, poultry, and vegetables. Foods are placed onto cut heart-shaped pieces of baker's parchment paper or aluminum foil; doused with some liquid like wine, juice, or sauce; and sealed by folding the paper over the product and crimping the edges. The tight package is placed into a hot oven, which quickly turns the trapped liquid into steam. The trapped steam then puffs the package, creating a miniature steam oven. When the cooking is finished, the steam condenses back into a liquid that contains all the flavors originally wrapped inside.

Poaching is an excellent no-fat cooking technique, although vitamins and flavor are leached into the cooking liquid. Poaching occurs at lower temperatures than boiling or steaming, so foods take longer to cook with this cooking technique. And the longer a food takes to cook in water, the greater the nutrient loss; however, flavor and nutrients can be returned in the final dish.

The recipe used for the cooking liquid in poaching preparations can add some flavor back to the dish by utilizing aromatic and vitamin-rich vegetables (e.g., carrots, celery, and onions) and herbs for a full-flavored cooking liquid. In these cases flavor exchanges between those leached into the cooking liquid and those absorbed from the cooking liquid itself can create a finished product bursting with flavor and full of nutrients. Return water-soluble vitamins and extra flavor to the dish by utilizing the cooking liquid in an accompanying sauce or soup.

Water-soluble vitamins (particularly thiamin, vitamin C, and folate) and flavonoids are sensitive to heat and are destroyed if exposed to high temperatures (100°F [38°C]) for extended periods of time. Minerals are not heat sensitive.

Baked vegetables, like baked potatoes, acorn squash, tomatoes, grilled vegetables, baked breads, roasted and grilled meats, poultry, and seafood retain most water-soluble nutrients because of the dry cooking methods used, but lose other nutrients because of the high cooking temperatures. Bake only the number of items required for immediate service; this ensures that the product can go directly from the oven to the customer's plate as fast as possible. The practice of baking full sheet pans of baked potatoes or multiple pieces of prime rib at the beginning of service and holding them in a hot oven for an extended service time (two or more hours) should be avoided for the sake of better nutrition.

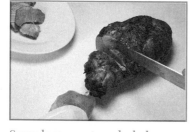

Serve large roasts and whole roasted birds as soon as possible after cooking to retain as many nutrients as possible.
Pearson Education/PH College

If it takes one hour to bake a potato, bake only what is needed for approximately one hour of service and place more in the oven at one-hour intervals. This allows the cook or chef to supply the service line with fresh baked potatoes every hour while their nutrient levels are still high. Baked potatoes held in warm ovens for two or more hours suffer significant losses of nutrients. Prime rib, roasted whole turkeys, and other large roasted foods also require long cooking times. This in itself has a negative effect on nutrient retention. Large roasts are often stored in heated cabinets for the entire service period. The longer they are held in heated cabinets or ovens over 140°F (60°C), the lower their nutrient content becomes.

Preparation and cooking techniques for rice and dried beans can also be improved to retain more nutrients in the final dish. Always cook rice and dried beans in the liquid that will be served with the dish, and use only the quantity of liquid required to complete the job. For rice, an exact measure of liquid to rice (usually two parts flavored liquid or stock to one part rice) allows the rice to fully absorb all of the liquid. Washing enriched white rice before cooking or rinsing it after it is cooked robs the rice of the valuable vitamins added back to the processed grains in the enrichment process.

Dried beans require much more than two parts liquid to one part dried beans to cook, but not as much as cooks and chefs commonly use. Often, dried beans are cooked in much more liquid than the beans can absorb, so a lot of residual liquid remains after the beans are served. A better practice is to use only the amount of liquid required to cover the dried beans and to add additional liquid as the beans cook. The beans absorb the liquid as they cook, and more liquid can then be added to finish the process. Adding a measurable amount of liquid at various times during the entire cooking process ensures that only the needed amount of liquid is used; all the liquid is either absorbed or served along with the cooked beans as an accompanying sauce.

If low-fat cooking is the goal as well as nutrient retention, pan frying and deep-fat frying should be avoided. Use of fats at high temperatures to cook foods reduces nutrient

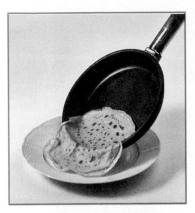

Nonstick pans are a good tool to use in low- and no-fat cooking.
Dave King © Dorling Kindersley

content dramatically and exponentially increases fat calories in a person's diet. There are many alternative cooking techniques that provide nutritionally balanced foods.

Sautéing, if done properly, can be considered a low-fat cooking process. Using nonstick coated cooking pans will help reduce the amount of fat needed in cooking. Measure the amount of fat used carefully. In a nonstick pan, you can reduce the amount of fat needed as a cooking medium to one-half teaspoon, or approximately 4 grams of fat, per serving. In contrast, as much as 1 tablespoon of fat may be needed if noncoated pans are used.

Sautéing foods in even a small amount of fat will cause fat-soluble nutrients to leach from the foods into the cooking fat. Always use as little fat as possible and incorporate the pan drippings, which include any residual fat and the fat-soluble nutrients it contains, in the final sauce. Cooks and chefs, unfortunately, tend to use too much fat even when sautéing foods, then pour off all the excess fat just before finishing the sauce, throwing away valuable nutrients. Nonstick pans allow cooks and chefs to sauté using very little fat, thus reducing the fat in the final preparation and preventing fat-soluble vitamins from leaching out. The high temperatures of the sautéing technique, however, also have a negative impact on nutrient retention. All foods should be cut into small pieces or portions before sautéing them quickly over high heat in order to preserve as many nutrients as possible.

Stir-frying is another technique that cooks foods rapidly with only a fraction of the amount of fat needed for pan frying. The large, round shape of the wok; the high cooking temperatures required; and the fine chopping, slicing, or dicing of foods all add up to fast cooking with little need for fat. (Just remember to chop the foods immediately prior to cooking.) If the wok is properly seasoned (that is, prepared in a way that prevents foods from sticking) or coated with a nonstick material, the amount of fat needed is minimal.

Wok cooking typically incorporates drippings or residual cooking fats or liquids in the accompanying sauces (except when the woks are used for deep-fat frying or poaching); this is a good way to return nutrients leached out by water or fat to the dish being served.

One criticism of stir-frying is that the amount of fat it uses is still more than the 30% of daily caloric intake recommended by the American Dietary Association. Pouring oil into the wok without proper measuring is the biggest culprit. Because fat contains 9 calories per gram, every tablespoon of fat that is used—about 1/2 ounce or approximately 14 grams of fat—contains 126 calories. When oil is poured freely into the wok, two or more ounces (4 tablespoons or more) can easily end up in the pan. If the wok is prepared properly or is coated with a nonstick material, only a small amount of fat (as little as one teaspoon) is needed to help keep the food moving quickly in the pan.

Using vegetable oil sprays or a pastry brush to dispense oils and melted fats reduces the amount of fat by controlling the amount used. Whereas 1 tablespoon of butter contains approximately 104 calories and 1 tablespoon of oil contains 122 calories, one spray from a commercially prepared vegetable oil cooking spray may contain as few as 2 calories and work just as well in a properly prepared pan or nonstick pan. A single brush stroke from a pastry brush dipped into liquid fat will distribute slightly more fat but still in a controlled amount. Pouring oil or other fats into cooking pans adds more fat than is required and can easily turn a nutritious meal into a high-fat one.

A chef who wants to add the traditional flavor of sesame seed into a stir-fry preparation can add two or three drops of sesame oil (less than 1 gram of fat) for flavor at the end of the cooking process. That way, the chef reaps the benefits of low-fat cooking and the rich flavor of the oriental oil.

Braising and stewing are great ways to prepare nutritional dishes because they use leaner and tougher cuts of meat and incorporate the cooking liquids in the final dish.

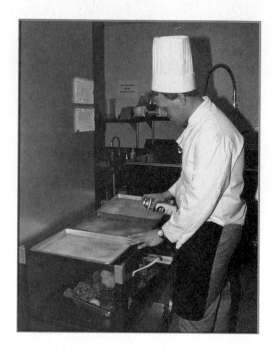

Cooking oil sprays provide less than 1/2 teaspoon per use, an ideal way of controlling the fat used in cooking.
PhotoEdit Inc.

Trimmed chuck roasts, first-cut brisket, and flank steak are ideal for braising and stewing. These cuts are naturally low in fat (compared to other cuts) and therefore make excellent nutritional choices. In braising and stewing, meats are served along with the cooking sauces, so nutrients that leach out during the cooking process remain with the dish.

Roasting is a low-fat cooking process, but the extended cooking times required for roasting can affect nutrient retention. When roasting meats, cut the meat into smaller pieces to speed the cooking process and decrease exposure to high cooking temperatures. For example, cutting a 20-pound top round roast into four equal pieces of 5 pounds each will accelerate the cooking time, as if each piece were cooked separately. Roast all meats and poultry on a rack, which allows melted fats to settle on the bottom of the pan, away from the meat.

Grilling and broiling are fast becoming the two most popular cooking techniques for nutritional cooking. Direct heat cooks items rapidly and requires no additional fat. The high temperatures do destroy some nutrients, but the quick cooking speed reduces the overall risk of nutrient destruction.

All exterior fat can be trimmed from meats and poultry before they are broiled or grilled to reduce the overall fat content of the finished dish: the fatty edge can be trimmed from steaks and chops and the skin from poultry. The items are cooked so rapidly that vitamin retention is high and excess interior fat melts and falls away from the food. Although some fat-soluble vitamins are discarded along with the melted fat, the rapidity of the cooking process minimizes the amount of exposure.

Brushing extremely lean cuts of poultry or fish with a seasoned oil mixture helps prevent them from sticking to the grill and adds some flavors to the final dish. Most of the oil is cooked off the product, whereas the flavors from the seasonings remain. Use well-trimmed meats and poultry parts and cook quickly, without charring the outsides.

The blackening technique, attributed to chef Paul Prudhomme of Louisiana, is also a no-fat cooking procedure, but the extremely high temperatures required can have a significant negative effect on some nutrient retention. The blackening technique requires a cast-iron skillet and a relatively thin cut of chicken, fish, or steak. The pan is put onto a very hot fire with no oil or fat added. Once the pan is smoking hot, the seasoned meat item is added to the pan. The extreme heat from the pan actually lifts the item off the pan (the meat's natural juices vaporize in contact with the extreme heat). In this way, meats can be cooked rapidly without sticking to the pan and without oil, fat, or any other liquid cooking medium. Water- and fat-soluble nutrients are not affected, except those destroyed or reduced by the high heat required in this style of cooking.

The American Cancer Society warns that charred meats produced by broiling, grilling, and blackening techniques may contain carcinogens (cancer-causing compounds), but the studies are not conclusive. The amount of charred meats a person would have to consume every day to cause a health risk is greater than the average person would ever consume. Broiling, grilling, and blackening of foods give consumers no-fat and low-fat cooking choices that retain natural nutrients due to minimal exposure to fats and liquids. Warnings on health risks should be considered, but the lack of evidence suggests that these foods are safe and healthy to eat when part of a nutritionally balanced diet. Complete diets should not be based on any one of these cooking methods alone.

Much more remains to be studied and learned about the nutrient content of natural and processed foods and how to retain those nutrients through handling and cooking. Buying, handling, storing, and cooking foods intelligently, based on validated nutritional knowledge, can help ensure that healthier foods are cooked and served to the guests.

SUMMARY

Buying Nutritious Foods to Cook Nutritiously

Serving foods for the benefits of nutrition and health is predicated upon selecting foods with the requisite nutritional makeup, receiving and handling them properly to protect the nutrients they contain, and cooking them while utilizing nutritional cooking guidelines. When chefs apply solid nutritional knowledge to the selection, handling, and cooking practices they perform every day, they can better predict and protect the nutrient value of the foods they cook and serve. The purchasing, receiving, storing, preparing, cooking, and serving of foods all play a critical role in delivering a healthier meal to the customer.

The nutrition content for foods reported in nutritional databases and on nutrition labels is based on ideal conditions for the growth, harvest, and transport of each food ingredient. The data presuppose that foods, especially fruits and vegetables, are grown to full ripeness on the plant; are handled and packed quickly and properly; are used in production very shortly after being harvested; and are prepared and cooked with the retention of nutrients as key deciding factors. When any of these conditions are less than ideal, the actual nutrient content of the food and the food products they produce can no longer be guaranteed.

Many factors affect the nutrient content of foods. Genetics, farming and herding practices, soil conditions, and the degree of crop maturity at time of harvest all determine the levels of nutrients actually found in the foods as they are harvested and prepared for market. Oxygen, light, heat, pH, water, and cooking continue to reduce the nutrient content in foods as they are packed, shipped, stored, and processed for eating.

CASE RESOLUTION

For the best nutritional values, LaShawnda can obtain locally grown fruits and vegetables from a farmer's market, a place in the city where local farmers sell their goods. Cities often announce the schedules for these markets and locate them in areas that are convenient to visit. Check city and state Web sites for more information, or refer to the U.S. Department of Agriculture's Marketing Service Branch at http://www.ams.usda.gov/farmersmarkets/map.htm for a listing of farmer's markets by state. Some markets offer natural items like juices, honey, baked goods, seafood, and nuts in addition to produce.

REFERENCES

Brillat-Savarin, Jean-Anthelme. 1984. *The Philosopher in the Kitchen*. New York: Penguin.

Maynard, L. A. and K. C. Hammer, *Journal of Farm Economic*. 29 (1): 120–24.

REVIEW QUESTIONS

1. Describe the *en papillote* technique.
2. True or False: You should submerge produce in water and wash it at least three days in advance of using it.
3. Where is the warmest part of the refrigerator, and why?
4. List four environmental elements that cause nutrients to deteriorate.
5. When should vegetables be peeled and trimmed?
6. Is it best to purchase fully ripe produce from a local vendor or from a well-known food provider who ships cross-country?
7. Decide the debate: canned, fresh, or frozen, which is best?
8. Define FIFO.
9. What is the warmest area of the kitchen?
10. Would you favor broiled, grilled, or fried meat for taste? What about nutrition profile?

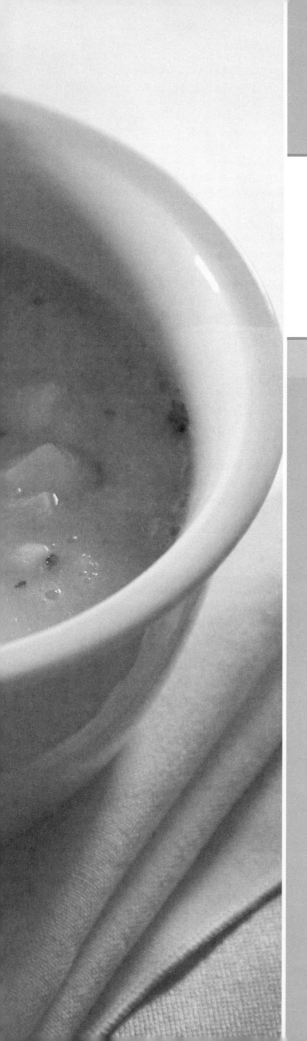

11

The Mechanics of Taste

KEY CONCEPTS

- The perception of flavor in food is influenced by the sense of smell; the five basic tastes of sour, sweet, bitter, salty, and savory (umami); texture; heredity; and even cultural traditions.

- The sensation of a peppery taste is not a true taste sensation; this sensation is a physical response to acid-like irritants burning the tissues in the mouth and tongue.

- At least seven primary odors can be detected by the olfactory neurons in the human nose: camphoraceous, musky, floral, pepperminty, ethereal, pungent, and putrid.

- Flavors can be divided into ten different categories: sweet, sour, bitter, salty, savory, peppery, floral, peppermint, pungent, and putrid.

The art of nutritional cooking is more than following dietary guidelines when designing recipes. Reducing the fat and salt and increasing the fiber and nutrients in a finished dish are important, but not if the execution and presentation of the foods are not also of a very high culinary standard. Preparing healthier foods that look good, taste great, and satisfy a discriminating consumer's appetite is the modern chef's job.

While food presentation depends solely on the physical properties of the food, such as shapes, colors, and sizes, flavors are a combination of sensory and physical influences. The perception of flavor in foods is influenced by the sense of smell; the five basic tastes of sour, sweet, bitter, salty, and savory; texture; heredity; and even cultural traditions. Building flavors in foods is achieved by examining each of these components and applying the knowledge gained to the thousands of potential flavors that are either found naturally in foods or can be created by cooking or otherwise altering the ingredients.

THINK ABOUT IT

Warm apple pie, freshly brewed coffee, and curry dishes often have special places in our memories. Smells remind us of past experiences, perhaps a holiday celebration, a first date, or a new leather bag. In addition to the pleasant, welcoming smells and their corresponding memories are those we could do without, maybe cigarette smoke, a bar after a busy Friday night, or an aged cheese.

Take a moment to collect your thoughts about the smells you associate with positive memories and a few you associate with not-so-positive ones. Share these with your classmates.

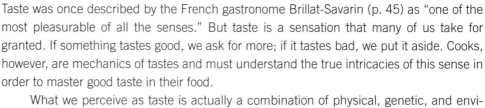

CASE STUDY

An Apple Pie Overload

Albert, the new stockroom clerk at Boyd County Hospital, received a larger-than-usual delivery of frozen apple pies. By the time he discovered the mistake, the delivery truck driver was gone. Albert is concerned because he thinks the pies will take up too much space in the freezers. He also doubts the cooks will even need these pies because apple pie is not served to the patients. Albert plans to meet with the food service operations manager to discuss his concerns and to have the pies returned later in the week.

If you were the operations manager, how would you respond to Albert's predicament? Collect your thoughts before reading this chapter, and then share them with your classmates once you have studied the chapter. *The resolution for this case study is presented at the end of the chapter.*

THE COMPONENTS OF TASTE

Taste was once described by the French gastronome Brillat-Savarin (p. 45) as "one of the most pleasurable of all the senses." But taste is a sensation that many of us take for granted. If something tastes good, we ask for more; if it tastes bad, we put it aside. Cooks, however, are mechanics of tastes and must understand the true intricacies of this sense in order to master good taste in their food.

What we perceive as taste is actually a combination of physical, genetic, and environmental stimuli that come together in the brain to form flavor impressions. Impressions are what we remember regarding the particular food or drink consumed; the look, the feel, the odor, and the taste combined with every past experience we ever had regarding that same item. What we perceive as a flavor, therefore, is a combination of stimuli of which smell and taste are primarily, yet not solely, important.

The physical properties of taste are a combination of smell (the olfactory process) and taste sensations that come by way of more than a thousand taste buds implanted in the tongue and the roof and back of the mouth (Figure 11–1). Sometimes our sense of taste tells us instinctively what is safe to eat and what is better left alone. Poisonous mushrooms and toxic chemicals, for example, often have a bitter taste, which naturally repels humans.

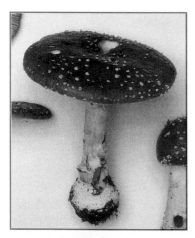

Poisonous mushrooms have a bitter flavor, perhaps as a warning that they are not safe to eat.
Neil Fletcher © Dorling Kindersley

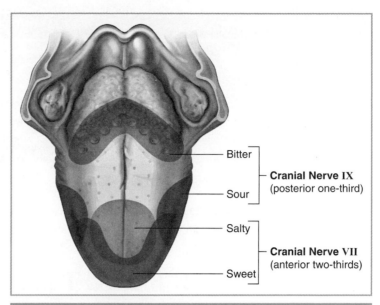

Bitter — ⎤
            ⎱ **Cranial Nerve IX**
Sour — ⎦   (posterior one-third)

Salty — ⎤
            ⎱ **Cranial Nerve VII**
Sweet — ⎦   (anterior two-thirds)

FIGURE 11–1 • THERE ARE THOUSANDS OF TASTE BUDS IN THE HUMAN TONGUE AND MOUTH
Source: Pearson Education/PH College

Environmental stimuli come from family traditions and customs. Family practices that shape our lives influence our desire to eat certain foods and drink certain beverages. Although they do not affect the physical sensation of taste, they do affect our willingness to try various foods as well as the enjoyment we may derive from them. What we learn to eat as children, for example, may influence our own food choices for the rest of our lives.

Traditional food choices are partly influenced by the indigenous foods available to a certain population, their cultural heritage, and their religious and philosophical beliefs. The decision to eat ham or not, for example, may be based on religious or ethical influences; the person may be an orthodox Jew or a vegetarian. Both groups choose not to eat ham yet for totally different reasons.

It is generally assumed that our entire sense of taste arises in the mouth, because this is where food generally enters the body. In fact, only five basic taste sensations are detected there; the rest occur in the olfactory passages above our nasal cavity.

In the mouth the tongue has a dual purpose: (1) to hold food in place for chewing and then carry it to the back of the mouth for swallowing; and (2) as a harbor for tiny organs known as taste buds. Similar taste buds are also found on the roof of the mouth and in the air passageway at the rear of the mouth known as the pharynx.

Taste buds are classified as organs because they have a very specific function in the human body: taste discrimination. They are among the few human organs that completely regenerate themselves almost weekly.

Each taste bud is a collection of modified epithelial cells, or taste cells, which act as receptors for the stimuli created by the ingestion of food. Taste buds themselves are somewhat spherical, with small openings on their surfaces known as taste pores. The flavors of foods dissolved in the saliva pass through these pores and then onto tiny hairs (microvilli) called *taste hairs*. The taste hairs are believed to be a part of the receptor cells. The receptor cells convey the taste impulses to connecting links that lead into the front of the brain where memories and emotions are stored.

The brain then identifies the taste by linking the impulse sensation with similar sensations already learned and stored in its specific memory. Thus we remember what an

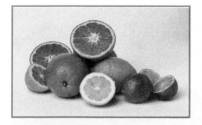

Our brain remembers what an orange tastes like before we even put it into our mouths.
Andy Crawford © Dorling Kindersley

orange tastes like so that when we eat another orange, we know it is an orange and not an apple that we are eating.

FIVE BASIC TASTES

Microscopically, taste cells in all taste buds appear quite similar, yet evidence indicates that at least five types of taste cells exist. Each type of cell identifies one or more of the basic five tastes (sweet, sour, salt, bitter, and umami).

Umami comes from a Japanese word that means "wonderful taste," and refers to the newest taste to be identified and studied by sensory and food scientists. The English word "savory" best describes the umami taste. Researchers at the Monell Chemical Senses Center in Philadelphia are trying to understand the biological basis of this "new" taste and to identify some of its natural sources. One primary source is monosodium glutamate, or MSG, the sodium salt of the common amino acid glutamate that is commonly used as a flavor enhancer.

Although all taste cells can detect a variety of tastes, some collections of cells on the surface of the tongue appear to be more sensitive than others to a specific taste sensation. The taste cells that are predominantly sweet sensitive are near the tip of the tongue. The sensation of sweetness can be created through the ingestion of either organic or inorganic sources. Organic sources are from the family of sugars (cane and beet sugars, honey, and fructose). Other sources are organic chemicals such as saccharine and aspartame. Inorganic sources include lead and beryllium salts.

Using any one or a combination of the vegetables listed in Box 11–1 will contribute sweetness to the final dish.

The sour taste is detected primarily along the right and left margins of the tongue. This sensation is generated by many of the acids present in foods: citric (in oranges, lemons, and limes), malic (in apples), tartaric (in grapes; tartaric acid is a by-product of the wine industry), and oxalic (in rhubarb, spinach, and other green leafy vegetables). In fact, all plant tissues are acidic to some degree, with pH levels at or below 7. Sour is the easiest flavor to produce in cooking because of the pronounced flavors of its host sources (Box 11–2).

BOX 11–3 • COMMON BITTER-TASTING FOODS

Endive (escarole)	Collard greens	Turnip greens
Belgium endive	Watercress	Kale
Radicchio	Dandelion greens	
Mustard greens	Turnips	

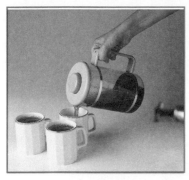

Coffee contains an alkaloid that is slightly bitter in taste, reminiscent of the poisonous alkaloids found in nature.
© *Dorling Kindersley*

Saltiness in food is detected at the tip and upper front portion of the tongue. This sensation is generated by a number of ionic compounds regardless of the positive or negative nature of the present ions. Sodium chloride (table salt) is the most common source, but other chlorides, fluorides, and nitrates also create a salty taste.

The fourth basic taste, bitter, has the majority of its taste receptors at the back of the tongue. Most bitter flavors are caused by organic materials, although some inorganic salts, like magnesium and calcium, also generate a bitter sensation from the taste buds. The bitter taste, almost like a primal reflex, indicates the presence of poisonous alkaloids in some plant and animal species, thus sparing unsuspecting animals from ingesting poisonous foods. The common rejection of bitter foods may be related to this protective mechanism, which is at work in even the most primitive of life-forms. Examples of poisonous alkaloids are strychnine, nicotine, and morphine; similar alkaloids are present in minute amounts in coffee, tea, and chocolate.

There are many bitter-tasting foods and ingredients to choose from, ranging in flavor from mild to strong. Whether a bitter taste is needed to balance other flavors (as in adding turnips to creamed potatoes) or on its own (as in braised Belgian endive), bitter foods play an important part in world cuisine (Box 11–3).

The savory taste, or umami, has not yet been well defined. Scientists worldwide are trying to isolate flavors that trigger this sense. Thus mushrooms, truffles, sage, and many wildflowers that share a similar earthy taste may one day be reclassified as umami foods.

The flavor of pepper is not a true taste sensation. The taste buds do not generate a sensation of pepper as a specific taste; this sensation is a physical response to irritants burning the tissues in the mouth and tongue. Chili peppers, peppercorns, and ginger contain alkaloids that stimulate pain receptors in the mouth, which causes the burning sensation we associate with spicy food (Box 11–4). Capsaicin in chili peppers and jalapeños and piperine in black and white peppercorns are the alkaloids that cause the peppery sensation.

You can use any of several hot capsicum peppers to create a peppery taste easily. But remember that hot pepper seeds can be as much as four hundred times hotter than the pod itself. Therefore, to create a slight peppery taste, use the pod or part of the pod only; to create more heat, use some or all of the seeds and seed membranes as well as the pods.

The basic tastes just described and the taste of pepper only begin to define flavors in food. The sense of smell gives flavors greater dimension and complexity as well. As Brillat-Savarin (p. 41) put it so elegantly, "Smell and taste form a single sense, of which the mouth is the laboratory and the nose is the chimney."

BOX 11–4 • COMMON PEPPERY-TASTING FOODS

Jalapeño	Jamaica Gold	Habanero
Cayenne	Ancho	Serrano

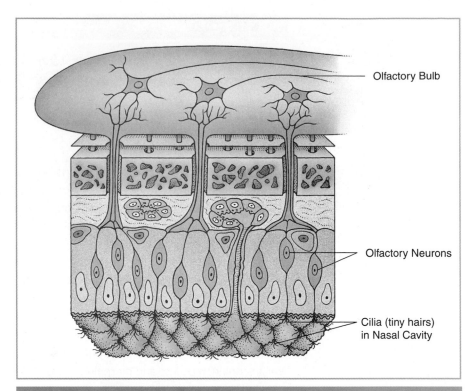

FIGURE 11–2 • THE OLFACTORY LOBES, NEURONS, AND HAIRLIKE CILIA THAT PROTRUDE INTO THE NASAL CAVITY.
Source: © Dorling Kindersley

PRIMARY ODORS

As air is breathed into the nose, thousands of microscopic organic and inorganic particles are carried in with it. These particles then come in contact with olfactory neurons (from the Latin *olfacere*, which means "to smell"), which act as smell receptors and protrude into the nasal cavity as seen in Figure 11–2. The olfactory lobes in the brain translate the many different scents into recognizable smell sensations. The olfactory bulbs in the front of the brain in turn connect to the centers of the brain in which, according to Monell scientists, association and other higher mental processes, including pleasure, take place.

This theory is partially proved by our many experiences in which smells, and therefore tastes, are triggered by memory. Memory can affect olfaction more than any other human sense.

At least seven primary odors can be detected by the olfactory neurons in the human nose:

1. *Camphoraceous:* the scent of camphor, a chemical present in some insect repellents and lacquers as well as in sage and used as a stimulant, expectorant, and diaphoretic
2. *Musky:* the scent of sexual attraction between the sexes in both animals and humans
3. *Floral:* the scent associated with flowering vegetables, herbs, and plants
4. *Pepperminty:* the scent found in various strengths in all members of the mint family (peppermint, basil, marjoram, and oregano)
5. *Ethereal:* the scent of ether, any of a class of organic compounds derived from the distillation of ethyl alcohol and sulfuric acid and used widely as an anesthetic

6. *Pungent:* the scent of spices
7. *Putrid:* the scent of decay, of aged meat, and of some cheese molds

Any odor may be described as one or a combination of these primary odors.

Scientists at Monell are also studying the effects of time on the perception of smell. When we are first exposed to an odor, it is very distinct; but after continued exposure, the smells often seem to fade or disappear altogether. Examples include cigarette smoke (smokers often cannot smell their own smoke) and perfumes or colognes, which often smell very strong when first applied and then seem to fade away a few seconds later. The source of the odor may remain, so others who approach us can still detect the scents, but our own ability to detect the same odor fatigues quickly and soon vanishes.

Because taste is linked to the sense of smell, it, too, is affected by this fatigue phenomenon. As the odors of foods and seasonings used in a particular dish become faint, so, too, does their taste and appeal fade away.

To keep every bite of the meal exciting, the chef must take great care not to repeat dominant flavors or textures in the foods being presented lest the benefit of these flavors be altogether lost. For example, a chef should never use the same seasonings for the appetizers as those used for the day's soups, entrees, or sauces. This is especially critical in a table d'hôte, banquet, or other full-menu service in which the customer does not choose the components of the meal. Using multiple flavorings in every dish and throughout the meal will keep your customer's olfactory neurons stimulated, heightening their sense of taste and keeping their satisfaction intact.

A cold or any other nasal infection or obstruction can cause the olfactory neurons to temporarily lose their ability to send accurate messages to the brain. (This is why the sense of taste is diminished in such circumstances.) Unfortunately, the direct exposure of the olfactory neurons to external elements makes them susceptible to long-term damage and destruction as well. Olfactory neurons are not easily regenerated, so the damage caused by heavy smoking, chemical abuse, and aging can be permanent.

A complete loss of the sense of smell is known as *anosmia.* Partial anosmia usually afflicts people whose olfactory center is damaged or who have some temporary malady that interferes with the reception and transmission of smell impulses. People with partial or total anosmia, including the elderly, need special encouragement to eat balanced meals. They may eat primarily fatty and high-sodium foods in an attempt to experience the sensations of taste. (As noted previously, consuming too much of these foods can cause serious health problems.)

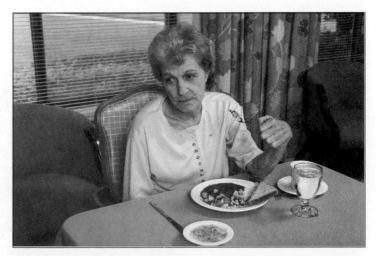

The elderly often suffer from taste depravation, known as anosmia.
Pearson Education/PH College

Continued disinterest in eating will lead to malnutrition, sickness, and possibly death. So people with partial anosmia should eat foods that stimulate the basic taste sensations assimilated in the mouth rather than in the nose; for example, foods flavored with sour, salty, bitter, sweet, or savory ingredients. In this way, they can still sense the flavors in their food while bypassing the need for olfactory stimuli.

People with a normal sense of smell can usually judge whether they would like to eat a food by smelling it, even before they put it into their mouths. Hot foods give off more odors than warm or cold foods. The smells of hot foods travel to the nose even as the fork or spoon approaches the mouth. Cold foods, however, must first be placed in the mouth for taste to occur. As the foods are warmed by our body, their smells are released and carried to the nasal cavity through the pharynx at the back of the throat.

FLAVOR CONSTRUCTION

Flavors are a combination of tastes, textures, and smells. A good analogy can be drawn between the building of flavors and the creation of music. Musical notes, by themselves, do not generally invoke great emotion; when they are combined together to form musical chords, however, they begin to sound wonderful and pleasing. The chef creates similar flavor chords by combining various tastes that are either harmonious or purposefully discordant, either naturally or through the application of cooking and other food preparation strategies and techniques.

Paul Prudhomme, the famous Louisiana chef and inventor of blackened redfish (well-seasoned redfish fillets seared in a hot iron skillet to intensify flavor while creating a blackened crust), has a particular liking for certain flavors. So he adds a simple procedure to many of his recipes to ensure the continuation of these flavors throughout the cooking process. He often begins cooking a dish with the tastes of certain herbs, flavoring vegetables, wines, or brandies. Then, about halfway through the cooking process, he adds more of these same ingredients. At the end, just before plating, he may add the same key flavoring elements a third time.

The flavors of the dominating ingredients thus evolve along with the dish itself. The original flavor ingredients cook, mellow, and blend with the other ingredients; the second addition of ingredients does the same thing but at a different pace. The third addition returns the original taste of the ingredients to the dish at the very end, just before plating, and ties together the beginning, middle, and end of the cooking process.

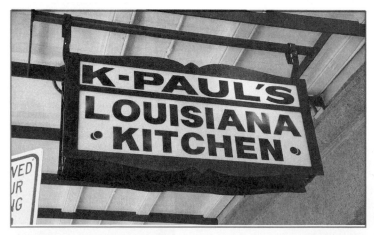

K-Paul's Louisiana Kitchen, New Orleans, LA, where chef Paul Prudhomme masterfully crafts great-tasting natural foods.
Greg Ward © Rough Guides

Flavor building, or *flavor profiling* as it is sometimes called, is the construction of flavors through a combination of tastes, textures, and other sensory and memory indicators. The diner's perception of flavor is the blending of all these factors; it arises from the strengths of the flavors used, the variations in taste caused by different cooking processes (sweating versus browning or caramelizing), the physical structure of the food (firm and crisp versus soft and smooth), and the smell, appearance (presented appealingly), and temperature (hot versus cold) of the foods and beverages being served.

Flavors can be categorized into ten distinct major groups (Box 11–5). The variations are too numerous to mention. Sweet, sour, bitter, salty, savory, peppery, floral, peppermint, pungent, and putrid are the major categories of flavors under which most foods can be grouped. To give depth to flavors in foods and beverages, the cook can use various items from a single category instead of a single dominant flavor; to expand flavor laterally, the cook would choose items from various categories. Foods from a single category emphasize a certain taste, while items from multiple categories create interesting contrasts and pleasant discord.

SWEATING VERSUS BROWNING TO CREATE FLAVORS

The taste of cooked flavoring vegetables can easily be varied by changing the cooking process. These are what chefs refer to as browned versus sweated vegetables.

Cooking vegetables uncovered in hot oil (310°F) allows cooked moisture to escape through evaporation, caramelizing their natural sugars and turning them brown. These vegetables will add color and a slightly sweet taste to the final product.

Cooking vegetables in a covered pan traps the evaporated liquids in the pan during the cooking process. This moisture condenses on the lid of the pan and falls back down onto the vegetables and the cooking medium (thus the descriptive term sweating). This prevents browning because the moisture keeps the fat from reaching the high temperature needed for browning. Sweated vegetables have the most natural taste.

Both browned and sweated vegetables have a place in culinary preparations depending on the desired taste of the end product. Some recipes may even use both to deepen the taste sensation. A recipe for French onion soup, for example, may start with browning a portion of the onions in hot fat for color and flavor. Another portion of onions is then added, which are sweated just before adding the flavored stock. Combining browned and sweated vegetables this way in a recipe gives a unique depth of flavor not possible using only one of the vegetable preparations.

CARAMELIZATION OF SUGAR

Caramelization of sugar is a nonenzymatic browning in which the sugar begins to decompose at about 338°F (170°C). Caramelized sugar is noncrystalline and water-soluble with a slightly pungent and sometimes bitter taste.

The caramelization of sugar is key in the making of peanut brittle. The organic acids formed during the caramelization process react with the baking soda to produce carbon dioxide bubbles. These bubbles produce the characteristic holes and opaqueness of the brittle.

Different sugars caramelize at different temperatures. Maltose, for example, caramelizes at 356°F (180°C), while fructose caramelizes at the lower temperature of 230°F (110°C).

SEARING MEATS
FOR BETTER FLAVOR

Searing meat in hot fat or on top of a red-hot grill dramatically alters the flavors and color of the meat. When protein-based foods like meat are cooked at high temperatures (over 310°F), the food molecules themselves begin to change, browning the food and developing roasted aromas. This process is known as the Maillard reaction.

Meats are fried or grilled at high temperatures to quickly alter their color and flavor. This is usually the first step in another process known as braising, which continues the cooking of the meat in a flavored liquid over a long period of time. Simply cooking the meat in the flavored liquid would not give the final dish the color and flavor that usually develop in a properly braised item. The temperatures of cooking something in water (not more than 212°F, the boiling point of water) are too low to brown the meat; rather, the meat turns gray as the fresh color is drawn out, creating a pallid (and tasteless) product. Searing the meat at high temperatures in fat or over a grill, however, gives it a brown color and flavorful texture.

The Maillard reaction also gives toast its distinctive flavor, beer its distinctive color, and self-tanning products the power to turn skin brown. It is responsible for literally hundreds of flavor compounds and is also used to make artificial maple syrup.

SUMMARY

Foods Are Rich in Flavors to Be Explored

What we perceive as taste is actually a combination of physical, genetic, and environmental stimuli that come together in the brain to form flavor impressions. Impressions are what we remember regarding the particular food or drink consumed: the look, the feel, the odor, and the taste combined with every past experience we ever had regarding that same item. What we perceive as a flavor is a combination of stimuli of which smell and taste are primarily, yet not solely, important.

The physical properties of taste are a combination of smell (the olfactory process) and the sense of taste that arises from more than a thousand taste buds implanted in the tongue and the roof and back of the mouth.

The cultural factors that shape our lives also influence our desire to eat certain foods and drink certain beverages. Although they do not affect the physical sensation of taste, they do affect our willingness to try various foods and the enjoyment we may derive from them. What we learn to eat as children, for example, may influence our own food choices for the rest of our lives.

Flavors, as opposed to tastes, are a combination of tastes, textures, and smells. Flavor building, or *flavor profiling* as it is sometimes called, is the construction of flavors through a combination of tastes, textures, and other sensory and memory indicators. For the diner, the perception of flavor is the blending of all these factors.

CASE RESOLUTION

In an ideal food service operation, Albert would have checked and double-checked his delivery to ensure receipt of the proper items. Sometimes, however, circumstances are beyond one's control. In this case, the delivery truck driver departed while Albert was checking his delivery.

From the information presented in this chapter, you should now have a better understanding of the impact of the sense of smell and the olfactory system on nutritional intake. This understanding is especially important for helping individuals who have a diminished sense of smell, such as the elderly.

Boyd County Hospital has one floor devoted to geriatric patient care. Many of the patients on this floor stay there for several weeks at a time, and they grow tired with the hospital's same weekly menu. Albert and the operations manager could keep the apple pies and serve them in the geriatric unit as a monotony breaker. The pies should be delivered piping hot so that their pungent and floral scents will permeate the air. These strong odors can help enhance appetite and intake. Although apple pie is not considered to be a nutritious food, one slice is a nice treat for someone who normally has a low appetite.

REFERENCES

Brillat-Savarin, Jean-Anthelme. 1984. *The Philosopher in the Kitchen*. New York: Penguin.

Cook, J. 1983. Nutritional anemia. *Contemporary Nutrition* 8 (4): 112–14.

REVIEW QUESTIONS

1. List the five basic tastes.
2. Explain why peppery is often described as a taste when in fact it is not.
3. Describe the tongue's dual purpose.
4. Name five vegetables that contribute to a dish's sweetness.
5. Where is the bitter taste detected on the tongue? Explain the significance of this location.
6. Define anosmia. What impact does anosmia have on human health?
7. List the 10 flavor categories; then create three recipes or meals that each combine two or more flavors.
8. Compare and contrast sweating to browning.

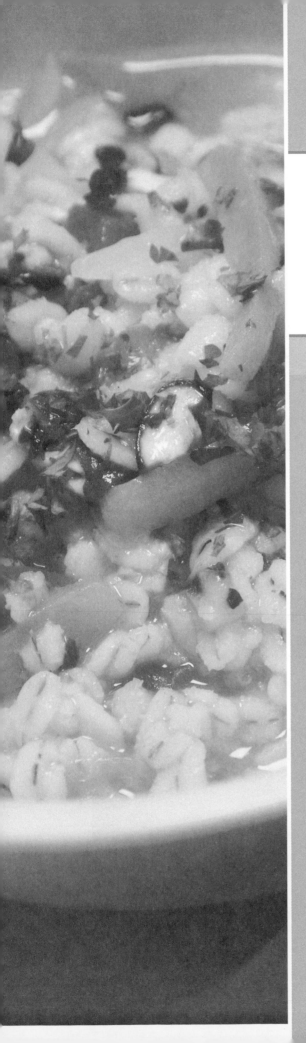

12

The Natural Flavor of Foods

KEY CONCEPTS

- Herbs and spices play critical roles in flavoring healthy foods. Their price, quality, and availability are more consistent today than ever before.
- For the freshest flavor, use fresh herbs whenever possible, dry leaf forms next, and ground forms last.
- Vegetables and other natural flavoring foods, often overlooked, are as much tools of the trade as they are food for the table.
- Some fats add flavor to foods but require strict control due to their caloric density.
- Alcoholic beverages represent part of a spectrum of flavors that can blend with or dominate flavors of any particular dish, adding character.

Herbs and spices have long been used to season cuisines around the world. Used since ancient times, they have a long history of intrigue, suspense, and adventure. Once worth their weight in gold, they are now readily available year-round for the average consumer and cook. Despite their ubiquity, herbs and spices can still transform an ordinary dish into something quite delicious, even spectacular.

In addition to herbs and spices, cooks use an array of highly flavorful foods to heighten tastes. These include flavoring vegetables, oils, and vinegars. Accomplished cooks apply these ingredients as freely as they do spices and herbs to create great taste.

Wines, beers, and spirits also are versatile flavoring ingredients used extensively in cooking and baking around the world. Their unique set of flavors can be paired or contrasted with other natural food flavors to build dynamic flavoring profiles.

THINK ABOUT IT

Traditions are the fabric of our daily lives. Never is this more apparent than during holiday celebrations and festivities. Families and friends gather to commemorate special occasions where certain food and drink are paramount. Holiday menus, planned days and weeks in advance, are serious matters.

Consider your holiday gatherings. Do you assemble with friends and family members and consistently enjoy the same traditional foods? For example, suppose that your family partakes of a specialty dessert and coffee containing Sambuca during the winter holidays. Some may find this dessert unpalatable, while others may thrive on it. Share a few of your enjoyable holiday traditions.

CASE STUDY

To Use Alcohol in Cooking, or Not

Chef Adam Christopher, the new executive chef at Southeast County Hospital, insists on cooking with alcohol. He has always cooked with alcohol, especially for one recipe. In fact, this recipe received numerous rave reviews at a ski resort in Colorado. There are just no exceptions to this recipe.

But there are objections. The social worker who leads Alcoholics Anonymous meetings with staff members at Southeast County Hospital feels that serving alcohol, even when cooked in food, is an unacceptable temptation. If you had to determine alcohol's rightful place at this hospital cafeteria, what would you decide? *The resolution for this case study is presented at the end of the chapter.*

HISTORICAL USE OF SPICES

Over the centuries, some spices have been of great value and importance. Their worth was a type of currency used to obtain other goods. Cassia and cinnamon, for example, were once bartered for fine silks and jewelry. Sesame seeds were used to pay ransoms and taxes for ancient kingdoms. The ancient Egyptians used anise, cumin, and marjoram in their embalming processes.

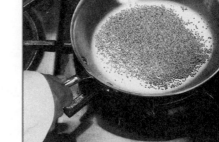

Sesame seeds are an ancient spice and have been used for thousands of years.
Pearson Education/PH College

The history of the spice trade is associated with the development of world cuisine, cultures, and civilizations. For centuries, the city or nation that controlled the flow of spices from the Orient to the Mediterranean settled the issue of sovereign power in Europe and the Middle East.

Entire civilizations and cities depended on the spice route. From India and the Orient through the Middle East and into Europe, traders along the spice route determined which ancient cities would last through the centuries and which would perish. Constantinople and Alexandria, for example, evolved into great market centers for the collection of precious spices and for their further sale and transport into Europe. Venice, with its beautiful Italian canals, owed much of its development as a major European city and political power to the spice trade. Situated at the head of the Adriatic, Venice's maritime position enabled it to control all shipping in the Mediterranean Sea, including the shipment of spices from the East to the West. Spices became Venice's most valuable commodity.

The Portuguese Quest

The search for a direct sea route to India and China, the land of spices, led the Portuguese south along the western coast of Africa. Their quest for valuable spices hinged on a plan to sail south around the great continent of Africa and then back north to China and India, completely circumventing the land route. In doing so, they could navigate around the Arabs and Venetians to obtain their spices.

Prince Henry of Portugal was a well-learned fifteenth-century man with a keen interest in maritime adventures, astrology, and cartography (the science of map or chart making). He was also a shrewd ruler who knew that finding a sea route to the land of the spices would secure a dominating position in world trade. Because of their exotic appeal and the difficulty in obtaining them, aromatics were beginning to cost as much as precious metals and jewels.

Prince Henry died in 1460, 27 years before Bartholomew Diaz rounded the Cape of Good Hope and 38 years before Vasco da Gama completed the journey to India with three small ships on May 20, 1498. Prince Henry's dream was finally realized, albeit posthumously, and Portugal became a major player in the trading of priceless aromatics.

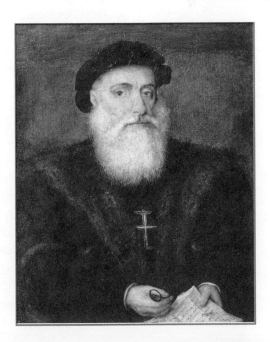

Vasco da Gama.
Picture Desk, Inc./Kobal Collection

The Natural Flavor of Foods **231**

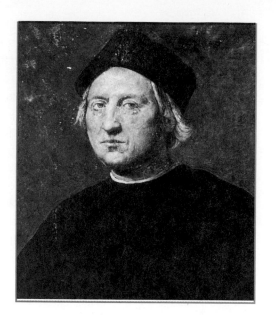

Christopher Columbus.
Ridolfo Ghirlandaio (1483–1561)
Christopher Columbus. Museo Navale
di Pegli, Genoa, Italy. Scala/Art
Resource, NY.

Christopher Columbus

The adventures of the famous Italian captain Christopher Columbus were merely an attempt to outdo the Portuguese in discovering a sea route to the spice lands. Whereas the Portuguese were headed south, Columbus was able to convince King Ferdinand and Queen Isabella of Spain that the quickest route was to the west. He believed that the world was round and that Spain and India were on the same parallel on the sphere. Columbus had no way of knowing that whole continents stood between them, obscuring a direct route to the west. He even named the natives he found "Indians," thinking he had indeed been successful in winning the race to India.

Columbus didn't find the land of spices he was looking for, but his discovery was to have an even greater impact on world cuisine than anyone could have imagined. His voyage to the Caribbean islands opened the door for new food discoveries that would influence world cuisine forever. He brought back allspice, vanilla, hot and sweet peppers, tomatoes, corn, potatoes, beans, sugar cane, cocoa, and turkeys across the waters for the world to enjoy. Although Columbus might have thought these foods poor substitutes for the peppercorns and cinnamon he had risked his life for, future generations of chefs and bakers would be forever grateful.

HISTORICAL USE OF HERBS

Herbs may not have a history as romantic and adventurous as that of spices, yet their use in cooking dates back to humankind's earliest culinary endeavors. Compared to spices, herbs' availability throughout the world made them more convenient and less expensive to use.

The development of agriculture and herding, nearly 12,000 years ago, made the nomadic search for food obsolete in most of the world. Growing food from seeds and moving grazing livestock over open fields made food a more reliable resource. Hunting became less risky, and hunger was better controlled.

With a steady supply of food and the fear of hunger subsided, variety and flavor began to play a greater role in cooking and eating. Herbs and spices became regular ingredients in a multitude of recipes from cultures around the globe.

Most herbs grew wild and were free for the picking. Many reseeded themselves and grew back in the same locations every year; others were evergreens or grew up from root stocks. As towns began to develop, people found it easy to grow most herbs right in their own flower gardens. And they found a way to keep a supply year-round: drying herbs for winter storage. The seeds of many herbs, such as celery, fennel, dill, and mustard, could also be used for flavor. Their versatility, low price, and ease of replenishment ensured they would stand the test of time.

FLAVORING WITH HERBS AND SPICES

The *American Heritage Dictionary* defines an herb as follows: "(1) A plant that has a fleshy stem as distinguished from the woody tissue of shrubs and trees and that generally dies back at the end of each growing season. (2) Any of various often aromatic plants used especially in medicine or as seasoning." Spices include all "various aromatic and pungent vegetable substances, such as cinnamon or nutmeg, used to flavor foods and beverages." This definition segregates herbs as a subcategory of spices. The culinary definition of herbs, on the other hand, characterizes similar ingredients with similar applications. Herbs are the leaves of plants and have the greatest flavor value when they are fresh—chopped or whole—and added to the cooking at the beginning or end.

Spices are all other vegetable aromatics, including the bark, seeds, and roots of some plants. Spices usually require drying or curing to enhance flavor and are used in whole or ground form. Furthermore, they are added early in the cooking procedure to maximize characteristic flavors.

Today's culinary professionals easily obtain spices from a variety of sources. Large corporate spice companies have taken the place of the ancient Arab caravans and Venetian spice merchants. Price, quality, and availability are more consistent today than they have ever been.

Spices are adaptable to many cooking and baking procedures. Herbs that once were available only in certain regions of the world are now available throughout the globe. At the local market, fresh, dried, and ground herbs are now on hand year-round because of the shrinking global marketplace and modern greenhouse techniques that ensure perfect climate control. Chefs require fresh herbs in their culinary creations, and this demand has brought about a corresponding supply increase.

PROPER HANDLING

Like all living plants, fresh herbs require proper handling. Moisture and cool air preserve freshness. Expect herbs from quality vendors to arrive prewashed and stored in individual plastic bags. Rinse the herbs once more before refrigeration and allow some water to remain in the bag. Plastic cylindrical containers also work for storage and are best for larger quantities. Position fresh herbs stem down, as you would cut flowers, and partially fill the container with water. Cover them loosely to help retain moisture without crushing delicate leaves. Some fresh herbs are now available in sealed plastic containers where they should remain until ready for use.

Fresh herbs can be chopped prior to storage. Chop only a day's requirement at a time, and keep chopped herbs in tightly closed containers. Fresh herbs contain a lot of water; place stale bread in the containers with the chopped herbs to absorb some of the moisture released by chopping and to keep the herbs from sticking or matting together.

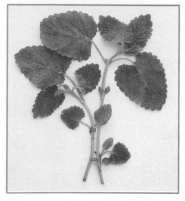

Fresh herbs offer subtle and pronounced flavors such as the lemon and mint flavors in this lemon balm.

Dave King © Dorling Kindersley

WHOLE VERSUS GROUND

Culinary professionals use fresh herbs to provide the most pronounced flavor, followed by dry leaf forms and then ground forms. Avoid using ground herbs and spices because they lose flavor quickly. Furthermore, there is no way to know how old an herb is when purchased in dry or ground form.

Containers chosen for herb storage should be in line with anticipated herb use. For example, if you use basil and oregano often, large containers are economically and practically feasible; if these herbs are needed only in a few preparations, smaller containers are better.

Whole and ground spices are available from all parts of the world. Seed and small berry-type spices can be cracked, crushed, or ground depending on the strength of flavor desired and cooking time. Longer cooking times require larger, or whole, ingredients for slow, extended flavor release. For quick cooking techniques, use ground or thoroughly crushed spices to provide quick flavor release.

CULINARY ADVENTURE

The use of herbs and spices depends on personal choice and preference. Regardless of customary practice, culinary professionals should explore new flavor combinations. Set aside traditions that prescribe rosemary for lamb, sage for turkey, nutmeg for spinach, and cinnamon for muffins. Instead, aim for a more open approach to the versatility of spices in cooking and baking. Creativity comes into play when the chef uses other combinations of herbs and spices in place of traditional ones for preparations of meats, poultry, seafood, vegetables, and baked goods.

Early cultures took full advantage of all the flavors at hand to create their food. Apicius, the great Roman culinarian of the first century A.D., had recipes calling for cinnamon and ginger as the main flavors in many meat and fish sauces. Greeks have a national dish, mousaka, that calls for layered noodles, ground lamb, cream sauce, and cinnamon. East Indians, who live in the land of spices, show no hesitation using mace and nutmeg to flavor rice and curries or cinnamon and cassia to flavor cabbage and turnips. A study of cookbooks from other countries will offer ideas for using herbs and spices in cooking. If you consider it a welcome adventure to use different herbs and spices, you can make exciting food with little difficulty.

Herbs and spices contain oils that are primary flavoring agents. These oils are released either by simmering the herbs and spices in a liquid or by frying them in fat. Nutritious cooking favors the former. Simmered herbs and spices retain their fresh taste and distribute flavors throughout the cooking liquid.

Store dried herbs and spices in tightly closed containers in a cool part of the kitchen. Air exposure weakens flavor, as do light and heat. Ground or powdered herbs and spices dissipate their flavors quickly; therefore, grind your own spices whenever possible and use fresh herbs, which contain their full flavors.

Add herbs and spices at intervals during cooking. Chefs add herbs and spices at the beginning of the cooking process, again during cooking, and one last time at the end of the cooking process to complete the flavor package. Dried herbs and spices may require up to 30 minutes to release flavors completely, whereas fresh herbs and freshly ground spices need only a few minutes.

USE A SACHET OF SPICES FOR FLAVOR

Consider employing a sachet of spices or dried herbs to flavor stocks, soups, and sauces. A sachet is a bag-infuser containing aromatics. Usually made from cheesecloth, the bag is wrapped around spices and herbs and tied with butcher's twine. Keep the twine long enough to allow the spices to settle well below the pot's liquid and long enough to reach the handle of the pot for tying. Tying the twine to the pot handle allows for easy removal at the end of cooking. Once cooking commences, toss the sachet into the pot, and allow it to simmer in the stock or sauce for 45 minutes to an hour. If you are cooking the dish for less than 45 minutes, begin with crushed spices to release the flavors quickly. Once all the flavors are released, remove and discard the sachet.

TABLE 12–1 • HERBS AND SPICES GROUPED BY PRIMARY ODORS

Pepperminty	Floral	Pungent
Mint	Anise	Thyme
Basil	Fennel	Rosemary
Marjoram	Caraway	Bay
Parsley	Celery seed	Cloves
Oregano	Dill	Cinnamon
Chervil	Saffron	Nutmeg
Tarragon	Juniper	Cumin

TOO MANY FLAVORS

Try not to confuse the taste buds by using too many opposing flavors in the same recipe. A recipe with rosemary, thyme, tarragon, and sage may produce a dish too confusing for the human palate to appreciate and leave a bad taste. Most recipes produce great dishes when they combine one or two strong-flavored spices and herbs with gentler ones. Combining rosemary and thyme with cinnamon and mace produces excellent results. Using tarragon and sage with fennel and allspice excites flavors in otherwise plain meat, poultry, or fish entrees.

MIREPOIX

A mirepoix is a selection of rough-cut vegetables used primarily as a flavoring tool. Commonly one member of the onion family (from Spanish onions to leeks), celery, carrots, and turnips are included. Chefs may also use fennel, parsnips, ginger, or garlic for a variety of recipes, creating distinct flavor combinations unique to each dish.

Chefsselect a mirepoix of vegetables when making stocks, soups, or sauces. A vegetable mirepoix is also used to lift large pieces of meat or poultry off the bottom of a roasting pan while cooking; these vegetables are used later to make a sauce for the finished item.

OLFACTORY IMPACT

Group herbs and spices according to primary shared odors. Some are pepperminty in origin, while others are floral or more pungent. Although not all herbs and spices fit neatly into these designations, the many that do set a good standard for comparison. Table 12–1 lists the most common herbs and spices grouped by primary odors.

Use selections within the same group to build complementary flavors and from different groups to build contrasting flavors.

Take advantage of the importance of smell when trying to create new flavors while cooking. Chefs interested in a certain taste may be unsure how an herb or spice will react to other flavors. Test the result before committing a whole recipe change. One way to do this is to suspend the experimental herb or spice over the product being prepared. Smell the aroma from the spice and the product simultaneously. The smells will combine in your olfactory system to offer a prelude to the actual taste. Next, take a small amount of sauce, liquid, or uncooked product and incorporate the experimental herb or spice. Cook raw samples before proceeding, and then taste the new combinations.

This test is especially important as chefs pursue nutritious cooking practices, reducing salts and saturated fats by cooking with more herbs and spices. Chefs should experiment with nontraditional taste combinations to create new and exciting flavors and test those new flavors before serving them to guests.

FLAVORING VEGETABLES

In addition to herbs and spices, cooks adopt many natural ingredients as food enhancers: bulb and root vegetables, including garlic and ginger; flavored oils; vinegars; and fruit juices. These natural flavorings contribute distinct flavors, textures, and nutrients to an assortment of hot and cold foods.

Chefs in training may feel confused initially when discussing carrots, celery, and onions in the same context as basil, oregano, and marjoram. Even though the former are not herbs, they provide many similar culinary opportunities.

It takes time to learn and appreciate the versatility of natural flavoring ingredients and the contributions they can make to recipes. Knowing what, when, and how to use these ingredients to create great-tasting foods comes with study and experience. Today's chefs are not limited to regional ingredients; they can choose from a world of flavors and textures. Ginger, once available only in dried or in powdered form, is now available fresh year-round in local grocery stores. Jalapeños are no longer restricted to pickling jars, and avocados have become a household item.

A CHANGING PALATE

The general public, with increasing awareness of the variety of available food ingredients in American markets, is accepting new flavors and culinary diversions. Publicity from chefs' associations, like the American Culinary Federation and the World Association of Cooks Societies, and the popularity of innovative chefs across the United States as well as television cooking shows, which have become one of America's passions, have all contributed to this increase in public knowledge.

Americans are willing to experiment with new foods in their own homes. They see TV chefs using innovative ingredients, and they can taste the great results by visiting restaurants and bakeries that follow culinary trends.

American consumers are discovering there is more to mushrooms than the common white mushroom *Agaricus brunnescens* and more to onions than Spanish and Vidalia. Grocery store managers, eager to please, set aside entire produce sections for new and exotic foods. Previously unheard of portabella, crimini, and enoki mushrooms; celeriac; leeks; and ginger now mingle comfortably with familiar white button mushrooms, spring onions, lettuce, and tomatoes.

Chefs who study these "newer" foods and how to use them in cooking and baking help raise consumer awareness. They transform traditional recipes into new creations.

Commercial vendors understand this trend and work to keep restaurants stocked with seasonal local produce, exotic vegetables, fresh herbs, and other natural flavorings. If a vendor doesn't already carry something a chef requires, purveyors can get it with little effort.

Cooks who take the time to learn their craft well discover that vegetables and other natural flavoring foods are as much tools of the trade as they are food for the table. Learning about these specific tools requires study, experimentation, and, most importantly, a

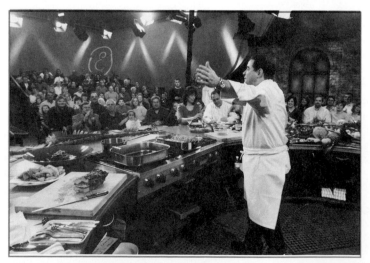

Emeril Lagasse chef and TV celebrity, helps raise awareness about foods form around the world.
AP Wide World Photos

willingness to abandon the idea that traditional foods restrict creativity. In fact, traditions and culinary foundations enhance creativity.

Experience tells cooks what combinations of foods, flavoring vegetables, and seasonings work best in many traditional cooking procedures. Chefs come to understand that low-fat sour cream can transform a basic brown sauce into a sauce fit for stroganoff, and that celery and onion can turn stale bread into a magnificent turkey stuffing. They imagine what dried plums can do for duck sauce, or raisins and almonds for rice pilaf. And they experiment continuously.

A sense of adventure, for the sake of good taste, encourages cooks to use their knowledge and appreciation of fine foods to look beyond recipes and single ingredients in their quest to satisfy educated palates and to stimulate kitchen creativity. The art of nutritional cooking uses natural flavors and natural ingredients in low-fat and controlled-salt preparations to provide healthy foods. It combines a thorough knowledge of discriminating and complementary flavors from natural food sources with the use of proper cooking techniques to create great-tasting, nutritional foods balanced by nature.

A trained and knowledgeable chef uses natural food flavors to overcome the flavor deficits associated with strictly nutritious low-fat foods, creating dishes as exciting as any traditionally cooked preparation.

THE ONION FAMILY

Creative chefs embrace many varieties of onions as seasoning vegetables in their recipes: the round bulb types, which include Spanish onions (yellow), white onions, red Bermuda onions, shallots, and pearl onions; and the elongated bulb varieties, which include green onions, leeks, and chives. Garlic is also a member of the onion family but is treated more like an herb or spice than a vegetable because of its high flavor concentration.

Onions have varying amounts of cysteine derivates. Cysteine is a sulfur-laden amino acid responsible for an onion's distinct taste. The onion's cells store cysteine compounds in a relatively stable state until those cells are broken by cutting or chopping. The breakdown of these compounds results in a mixture of ammonia, pyruvic acid, and organosulfur, which is later broken down into diallyl disulfide, the precursor of the smell of garlic.

The sharp and biting taste of onions and garlic is most prevalent in the raw, chopped state and is lost slowly during cooking. Chefs make onions milder by incorporating them in whole or large-cut form. Furthermore, dry cooking (sautéing, panfrying, grilling, or roasting) caramelizes natural onion sugars and creates a sweeter, lighter, more delicate onion flavor.

These three distinguishable taste variations—sharp and biting, mild, and sweet—help chefs vary their cooking and baking with minimal additions. An example is the production of many of the small sauces (derivatives of the five basic, or mother, sauces). To make stocks, large pieces of onions are used for the blending quality of their characteristic taste; but for flavor excitement, professionals add finely chopped shallots in final sauce preparation. The cooked onion taste in the stock, which has blended with the other vegetables, and the sharp, biting taste of the shallots in the final cooking step contribute relative yet distinct flavors to the product.

A wide range of flavors and smells exists within each variety of onion depending on where it was grown and time elapsed since harvest. Each type of onion has a distinct flavor and may lack compatibility with all recipes. The Spanish onion usually has the strongest onion flavor (depending on the time of year, storage time, and geographic growing location) and the spring onion the slightest. White onions, including the pearl onion, the Vidalia

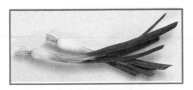

Onions come in many different varieties, each with a very different flavor profile.
Steve Gorton © Dorling Kindersley

onion (from Vidalia, Georgia), and the Bermuda onion, lean toward a sweeter taste—even when raw—and caramelize well.

Some chefs experiment with a variety of onion types in the same recipe. Three-onion quiche and veal sauté with three-onion soubise (cream sauce highlighted with onion essence) are two examples. Combinations of related yet distinct flavor ingredients add depth to the finished dish.

The following are among the most popular onion varieties:

Bermuda onion: A sweet-flavored bulb variety in white and burgundy colors. Used primarily in salads and sandwiches.

Garlic: Technically not an onion but related to the onion family, garlic is composed of several individual bulbs, called *cloves,* each protected by a thin dried leaf base with a thick, fleshy body that contains the bud for next year's growth. This collection of tiny bulbs is itself referred to as a bulb. Elephant garlic gets its name from its enormous cloves and collective bulb size. Each grows as large as 1 pound and contains five to seven huge cloves. Elephant garlic is much milder than its smaller relatives. Garlic flavor, like onion, changes slightly depending on where it is grown. Southern and western varieties are spicier than northern or eastern versions.

Green onion: Also called *scallions*, *spring onions*, *bunching onions*, and *multipliers*, these onions have slender, straight-leaf bases that never form true bulbs and green tops. Both the white portions and the green tops are used in cooking. Green onions are primarily added to salads for their subtle, sweet flavor and crisp texture. They are popular in Pacific Rim and Asian styles of cooking.

Leek: The largest nonbulb onion, leeks look like oversized green onions and are the sweetest members of the onion family. The white parts are very tender while the green tops add flavor to vegetable stocks.

Pearl onion: A very small white-skinned, white-fleshed onion with a mild flavor, pearl onions are ideal for stews, for roast meat dishes, and for pickling.

Shallot: A small reddish brown-skinned onion with pinkish white sweet flesh. Sweeter than scallions, shallots hold up well in cooking applications and are used to flavor many sauces and sautés.

Spanish onion: Bulbous onion with pale, straw-colored outer skin and white flesh. The flavor of Spanish onions lies somewhere between those of Bermuda and yellow onions.

Vidalia onion: The namesake of Vidalia, Georgia, Vidalias are believed to be the world's sweetest bulbous onion.

Yellow onion: This is the strongest onion. It has yellowish brown skin and slightly off-white flesh. The Texas onion is an extra-large yellow onion.

FLAVORING STALK, ROOT, AND TUBER VEGETABLES

Stalk, root, and tuber vegetables contribute flavor to many dishes, both hot and cold. Most of these vegetables are excellent choices when served as individual accompaniments to meals. The art of nutritional cooking examines their flavors and textures more closely and uses them to replace the flavors lost by reducing or eliminating fats and sodium.

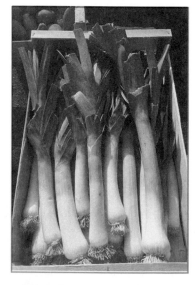

Fresh leeks offer yet another great onion flavor dimension.
Andrew Holligan © Dorling Kindersley

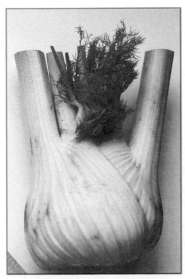

Fennel is a sweet flavoring vegetable with a taste similar to celery and anise.

Philip Dowell © Dorling Kindersley

The following, served individually or as flavor and texture additives, are the most popular stalk, root, and tuber vegetables:

Carrot: Originally, red, purple, and black carrots were common table food. The familiar orange variety, rich in beta-carotene, was developed in Holland in the seventeenth century. Brought to the United States by colonists, the carrot became one of America's most popular vegetables. Carrots are eaten raw and cooked and are used in many recipes, including salads, relishes, soups, and desserts.

Celeriac: A relative of the popular vegetable stalk celery, celeriac shares celery's distinct flavor yet is more concentrated with a slight hint of parsley. Although its common name is celery root, celeriac is not a root but rather a mass of swollen stalks that grow below ground and take the form and texture of a bulbous root. Celeriac is generally shredded and eaten raw in salads and slaws, but its versatility pairs well with soups and stuffing and as a vegetable accompaniment to veal, seafood, and poultry dishes.

Celery: A member of the carrot family, celery is grown for its fleshy leaf stalks and used in varied culinary applications. It is favored as a flavoring vegetable in soups, stews, and salads and is also regularly found raw in salad bars and relish trays. Celery has a cool, sweet, crispy taste and texture. Outer stalks contain stringy fibers that should be removed (with a vegetable parer) if the vegetable is intended for the table, whether cooked or raw.

Daikon: Also called *Oriental radish,* this long cylindrical-shaped white radish has a spicy, mustard-like flavor. A relative of mustard, the Daikon radish can grow as large as 50 pounds, but it is generally harvested in sizes from 1/2 pound to 2 pounds.

Fennel (finocchio): Adored in Italian cuisine for its sweet, subtle flavor, fennel leaves, like those of dill, are fragrant; its seeds, like anise, are sweet; and its fleshy stalks, like celery, are used for flavor or as a vegetable in their own right.

Horseradish: A member of the mustard family, this root vegetable is more often used as a condiment than as a vegetable. Purchase horseradish in grated form or grate your own, but beware of its effervescent aroma, which may sting your eyes and nose. Shave horseradish into very thin strips or slices and serve it with roasted meats and other highly flavored foods.

Jerusalem artichoke: Actually not an artichoke but a member of the sunflower family, the Jerusalem artichoke was not originally cultivated or sold in Jerusalem. In fact, it is native to North America. A tuber of a flowering plant with bright yellow blossoms, the Jerusalem artichoke looks much like an oversized pale-colored ginger root with smooth skin and lumpy, bulbous growths. Its flavor resembles that of artichoke hearts and salsify, and its texture is much like that of water chestnuts.

Kohlrabi: Like celeriac, kohlrabi is actually a collective mass of swollen stems rather than a root, but it is treated in much the same way as other root vegetables. Kohlrabi has both the wild turnip and wild cabbage as its ancestors and has a flavor reminiscent of both. The swollen stem mass that makes up the bulb and the greens are used in culinary applications.

Parsnip: A member of the carrot family, parsnips have a creamy white color and distinctively sweet flavor, especially when harvested after the first frost. Serve parsnips baked, braised, simmered, fried, or raw. They are a versatile vegetable used in the cuisines of cold-climate countries like Germany, Russia, Poland, and Canada.

Radish: A member of the cabbage family, radishes come in many varieties: pink, red, white, and black; round and long; small and large (as small as marbles or as large as grapefruits). Radish flavor varies, although they are always on the spicy side. Black radishes, a common vegetable for Russians and Poles, may be as spicy as horseradish and are treated in the same way.

PEPPERS FOR FLAVOR

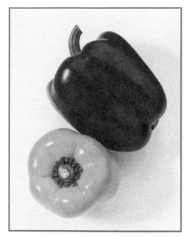

Sweet bell peppers provide great nutrients, color, and flavors.
Dave King © Dorling Kindersley

The family of capsicum peppers includes sweet bell peppers, pimentos, and hot varieties like jalapeños and cayenne. Their temperature ranges from sweet and mild to extremely hot, determining the particular fruit's culinary applications.

Sweet and mild varieties like bell peppers, pimentos, and sweet banana peppers provide flavor, texture, and color to the final dish. Their touch of sweetness balances acidic, bitter, or naturally salty foods. Red, yellow, purple, and green sweet peppers are now available annually.

Hot peppers are used for their spicy, distinct flavors. Remove part or all of the internal seeds and membranes to mitigate spiciness. Hot pepper seeds and membranes are up to 400 times as hot as the pepper pods themselves.

The following are the most common peppers from the capsicum family:

Anaheim: A mild green chili pepper up to 8 inches in length; used in chili relleno (a stuffed pepper from Mexican cuisine).

Ancho: Called *poblano* when fresh, *ancho* when dried; heart-shaped and slightly milder heat than jalapeño.

Banana: A sweet chili pepper whose name originates from its long tapered shape and bright yellow color; turns green and then red when fully ripe.

Bell: Named for its shape, this sweet pepper comes in colors ranging from green to yellow, red, and black (actually dark purple). The color does not affect flavor or spiciness.

Cayenne: A fiery red slender pepper that grows 5 to 8 inches long. Dried cayenne is called *red pepper*.

Cherry: A mildly hot green pepper that turns red when ripe. Its name derives from its resemblance to the fruit with the same name.

Habanero: One of the hottest peppers in the world, this shriveled bell-shaped fruit turns fiery orange-yellow when fully ripe.

Hungarian wax: A spicy yellow pepper that grows 6 inches long. A red color signifies maturity.

Jalapeño: A spicy pepper that grows 3 to 4 inches long. It is harvested green yet turns red when fully ripe.

Pimento: A heart-shaped chili pepper ranging in spiciness from sweet to mildly hot. Fruits turn from olive green to scarlet red when ripe.

Relleno: Commonly called *green chili* and most widely used in Mexican and Southwest American cuisine; a mildly hot chili.

Serrano: Slender 1- to 2-inch-long fiery-hot fruit.

MUSHROOMS FOR FLAVOR

Mushrooms, or edible fungi, are a class of vegetables. Fungi are one of the simplest life-forms on earth today. Mushrooms are extremely flavorful and are used in many cold and hot culinary dishes. Either raw or cooked mushrrooms work well, but cooking mushrooms passes full mushroom flavor on to the other ingredients of the dish.

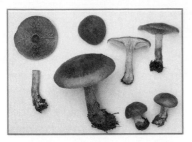

Mushrooms have simple or complex flavors depending on the variety used and the cooking technique that is applied.
Neil Fletcher © Dorling Kindersley

The mushroom is the one class of vegetable that does not lend itself to genetic alteration. The same mushrooms available today were gathered and eaten thousands of years ago by our ancestors. Over a quarter million mushroom varieties exist, but only about thirty thousand are edible ones, of which only a few dozen have been successfully cultivated. Poisonous mushrooms range from slightly poisonous to hallucinogenic to deadly.

Picking wild mushrooms is a science practiced in most of Europe, Asia, and the Far East. Novice mushroom pickers who consume wild mushrooms may find themselves in danger. If you are determined to pick wild mushrooms, learn a few easily recognizable varieties and harvest only these. Some poisonous mushrooms look like edible varieties when immature, and there are no straightforward rules for distinguishing delicious from deadly.

The following are some of the most common varieties of mushrooms, both raw and dried. They are found in many neighborhood grocery stores or are readily available from any good produce company:

Agaricus bisporus: The common white mushroom, agaricus is the most familiar mushroom in the United States because it grows well in controlled environments. Grilled agaricus mushrooms offer a mild flavor; raw ones are suitable in salads. Larger agaricus caps are sometimes stuffed and baked. Farmers harvest agaricus mushrooms with caps 1 to 4 inches in diameter.

Chanterelle: The most readily available chanterelle is a golden yellow trumpet with a spicy, almost fruity, flavor.

Crimini: Similar to the common white mushroom except with a brown cap and stem and a stronger flavor.

Enoki: Long-stemmed mushroom with small caps and a sweet fruity flavor. Used raw in salads and sandwiches.

Morel: The most familiar cup-shaped mushroom offering a sweet, earthy, and slightly nutty flavor. Grows 2 to 5 inches long throughout the United States and France.

Oyster: Found on living trees in the wild, but cultivated on fresh straw or hardwood sawdust and compost. The flavor resembles that of the familiar mollusk from which they get their name.

Porcini: One of the many edible boletes; also called *cepes* in France. Porcini have caps as large as 8 inches across but are usually harvested at 2 to 4 inches in diameter. They appear brown with slightly swollen, almost bulbous stems. Boletes have pores instead of the gills common to other mushrooms.

Portabella: A meaty, large-capped gill mushroom related to crimini; excellent grilled because of its size and firm texture.

Shitake: Originally grown in China, more shitakes are now grown in Japan than in any other country. Shitakes are grown on teak or oak logs or in hardwood sawdust in a controlled environment. They are buff brown with a shaggy, rolled-in cap and pronounced flavor.

Straw: Grown naturally on the decaying straw of rice plants in China and Japan, these mushrooms have small grayish brown caps and short stems.

Truffle: An underground fungus grown in clusters attached to the roots of fir, oak, and beech trees 3 to 12 inches below ground. There are two major varieties of true truffles, the French black truffle and the Italian white Piedmont truffle. The white truffle is more pronounced in flavor and odoriferous. The Oregon white truffle is not a true truffle but resembles a small puffball that grows on or just below the ground.

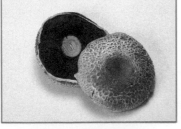

Portabella mushrooms have gained a lot of popularity over the past several years because of their large size, firm texture, and complex flavors.
Pearson Education/PH College

The Natural Flavor of Foods   **241**

OILS: HEALTHY AND FLAVORFUL

If it is confusing to think of using fats and oils for flavorings in nutritionally prepared foods, it is because of old habits and unqualified traditions. Chefs can use fats and oils in cooking for the media they are and for the flavors they impart when used moderately.

Choose from many different oils and fats depending on cooking temperature and desired flavor. Whole butter, for example, burns easily when heated, whereas peanut oil consistently withstands temperatures over 350°F. Fats that present the strongest flavors are sesame and olive oils, any of the nut oils (hazelnut, walnut, etc.), butter, and then margarine.

A stir-fry dish that uses a small amount of sesame or walnut oil accentuates the taste of the other ingredients, allowing chefs to reduce the amount of soy sauce (a fermented sauce high in sodium) or other flavor enhancers, such as MSG, without sacrificing flavor.

Sautéed dishes or pan-fried items take on new character when cooked in olive oil. Even omelets cooked in a small amount of this ancient oil take on a different characteristic. Olive oil provides an exciting flavor break with virtually no difference in cooking.

Some chefs shun these highly flavorful oils in their cooking. They believe that if they use enough of these oils for proper cooking, the oil's flavor will dominate the dish (sesame oil has an extremely strong flavor; virgin olive oil a close second). View these oils as seasonings rather than frying media. In a recipe that calls for a fat to stir-fry, sauté, or pan-fry, use an oil with little or no dominant flavor, like canola, soybean, or sunflower. Select a flavorful oil as only a portion of the frying medium. When used in this fashion, sesame, walnut, or olive oil function more like a spice to accent the flavor of the final product.

Flavored Oils

Flavored oils allow chefs to give recipes complex taste by utilizing flavor extraction techniques and the cooking medium to disperse flavors evenly throughout the entire dish. Chefs make flavored oils by infusing the essence of their favorite herbs and spices into any of the pure cooking oils regularly used in their operations.

Create garlic-tarragon oil, for example, by combining safflower or soybean oil with crushed garlic cloves and fresh tarragon sprigs (approximately four cloves of garlic and two full sprigs of fresh tarragon per quart of oil). Use the oil creation to sauté or pan-fry, or in a marinade or salad dressing, to give the final dish a signature taste.

The procedure of making flavored oils could create ideal conditions for botulism and should be handled carefully. *Clostridium botulinum*, a spore-forming bacterium, is found in the soil and may be present on fresh garlic cloves. The bacteria thrives in oxygen-free environments, such as in canned foods and foods immersed in oil. Prevent this problem by making only small quantities for near-immediate use and by keeping the oils refrigerated.

Some restaurant chefs maintain chopped garlic and chopped shallots as part of the hot line *mise en place* and cover the chopped bulbs with fresh oil. If the recipe calls for a stronger garlic or shallot taste, they have access to the actual chopped product. When chefs require just a hint of these flavors, they merely incorporate a tablespoon of oil during cooking. Then they replenish the oil at the end of the shift for later use.

Fresh herbs and cracked whole spices are best suited for this type of oil infusion because their fresh flavor stands out. Use olive oil and other flavorful oils for these herbal infusions. Strong natural oil flavors add greater dimension to the infused taste.

Chefs may develop their own herb-oil blends. Employ these blends for many cooking procedures. Just like a chef's own restaurant blend of spices, these oil blends offer character and depth to the simplest applications.

RESPONSIBLE BUTTER USE

Many people are concerned with the amount of cholesterol and saturated fats in their daily diets and want to reduce intake accordingly. Nutritious diets do not dictate total elimination of these fats (10% of the total daily caloric intake should consist of saturated fats) but simply reduction.

Avoid butter and margarine as cooking media, because the same results can be achieved effortlessly by using liquid oils. Regarding flavor, though, nothing tastes the same as fresh whole butter. Margarine, on the other hand, is hydrogenated vegetable oil that is solid at room temperature. Some products today provide an artificial butter flavor without the cholesterol.

If your recipe calls for the taste of butter, think of butter as a seasoning. Add a small amount at final cooking to provide the taste. If the recipe calls for butter as the cooking medium, replace it with a combination of a nonflavored oil and a smaller amount of butter.

Compound Butters for Flavor

Compound butters are flavored butters incorporated as seasonings for a variety of sautéed, roasted, grilled, poached, or broiled preparations, including vegetables, poultry, beef, fish, and veal.

Compound butters are a combination of fresh sweet butter, herbs, spices, and other highly flavored ingredients. When combined, rolled into cylindrical shapes, and refrigerated, compound butters can be used easily and quickly. Slice off an appropriate amount and add it to the cooked item just before service.

The advantage to using compound butters is their high flavor concentration. One thin slice, less than a teaspoon (which contains approximately 36 fat calories), significantly alters the taste of a food item without exceeding nutritional guidelines for fat.

Compound butters derive their concentrated flavors from the other ingredients that make up each individual formula. Maître d'hotel butter, perhaps the standard to which other compound butters are compared, is a mix of fresh sweet butter, fresh chopped parsley, lemon juice, salt, and pepper. Other compound butters might include additional herbs and seasonings, finely chopped shallots or garlic, or even ground shellfish, like shrimp or lobster. A shrimp-flavored compound butter is an excellent accompaniment to poached, grilled, or broiled fish, whereas a garlic, chive, and thyme compound butter pairs well with grilled chops or steaks.

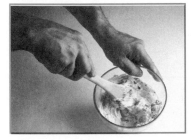

Compound butters are a way of adding a small amount of fat and extra flavors to grilled items.
Jerry Young © Dorling Kindersley

ACIDIC FLAVORINGS

Sour is one of the five true tastes. Distinguishable from the other tastes, sour acts as an influencing flavor over other flavors. Just as salt heightens the taste of many recipes, additional acid has the same stimulating effect without the sodium. In some cases, acid use eliminates salt requirements.

There are many forms of acid products, including citrus juices from lemons, limes, and oranges; tomato products; vinegars; and sour cream and yogurt. Each of these gives chefs great flexibility in preparing the finest recipes. Chefs who create recipes take advantage of the versatility these products provide, bringing excitement to the simplest preparations.

Sour cream, for instance, is the exciting ingredient that elevates beef stroganoff beyond elementary beef stew status. Flounder meuniére is a fantastic variation of sautéed flounder that has a few drops of lemon juice added, which makes all the difference. Seasoning with acid products transforms average to gourmet.

Flavored vinegars have become very popular in professional kitchen larders. Not only can they impart a sour taste to balance flavor profile, they also add flavor of their own.

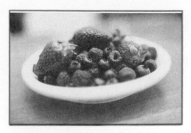

Fresh berries are often used to flavor vinegars and add a slight twist to their natural acidic punch.
© *Dorling Kindersley*

Tarragon vinegar, for example, adds sour from the vinegar and a strong tarragon flavor with only a few drops.

Flavored vinegars are simple to make. Infuse herbal and spice essences into a favorite vinegar; fresh herbs and cracked whole spices produce the best results. Rosemary-thyme white vinegar, for example, delivers extra definition to seafood marinades, whereas dill-garlic vinegar gives character to cucumber, potato, and pasta salads.

Fruit-flavored vinegars are gaining popularity for salad dressings and marinades. These vinegars use crushed berries or chopped fruit for flavor; once the fruit flavor has been fully steeped out (three to four days), strain the vinegar off the fruit residue and store it indefinitely. Culinary professionals use finely puréed fruit and add some of the fruit to the dressing to make fruit vinegars more rapidly for quick service. The presentation will be quite different, however, and the versatility of use not as great.

In choosing the base for a flavored vinegar, consider white, red, red wine, cider, and balsamic vinegars. The resulting flavors depend on the base vinegar.

To make a fruit-flavored vinegar like raspberry vinegar, add 1 pint of whole and broken raspberries to 1 quart of vinegar. Steep the mixture for at least 48 hours to allow the berry flavor to permeate the vinegar. To spice it up even more, add 1 tablespoon of cracked black pepper per quart for raspberry-black pepper vinegar. Make peach vinegar by adding 1 pint of cut whole peaches or 1 pint of peach nectar to 1 quart of cider vinegar. The combination of fruit flavors creates an excellent vinegar blend.

Refrigerating flavored fresh fruit vinegars prevents them from becoming rancid. Straining fruit out of the vinegar after steeping enhances the shelf life of the flavored product.

ALCOHOLIC BEVERAGES

Alcoholic beverages provide another flavor enhancement to foods. Humans have enjoyed alcohol drinks for thousands of years; but professional chefs also utilize alcohol to impart unique tastes to cooked foods or pastry.

Many different kinds of alcoholic beverages may be used to flavor foods and pastries before, during, and after cooking or baking. Wines, beers, ales, brandies, and various liqueurs have been used for centuries to flavor some of the most common and exotic foods and pastries.

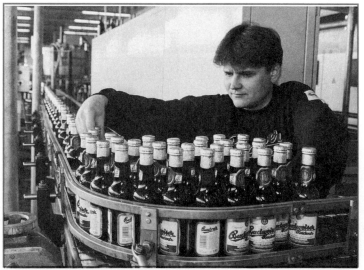

Wines and other alcoholic beverages can add complex flavors to the simplest dishes.
AP Wide World Photos

Alcoholic beverages represent an entire spectrum of flavors that can blend in or dominate any particular dish, giving character to the final presentation. When enhancing flavors in food, chefs cannot afford to overlook the versatility these liquid flavor enhancers provide.

As cooking and baking developed, use of these natural flavor enhancers developed too. Brandies and liqueurs, for instance, offer extraordinary distinction to otherwise simple tastes. These liquids impart character and excitement to the easiest of preparations without fat or other unhealthy components.

Not only do wines, beers, brandies, and liqueurs confer flavor, but many add to the nutritional value of a finished product. Alcohol itself, as well as protective phytochemicals in darker alcoholic beverages, contributes healthful properties. Some wines contain potassium, calcium, phosphorus, magnesium, and iron. Most other wines aid in the absorption of these minerals as well as zinc when made part of a meal. Research is under way to investigate correlation between moderate consumption of wine and other alcoholic beverages and high-density lipoprotein (HDL, or the "good" cholesterol) improvement. If true, moderate alcohol consumption (one drink per day for women; up to two for men) may reduce risk for heart attack and stroke.

Beers contain traces of protein or amino acids, fats, and some B vitamins that remain in the bottle or can from yeast used in fermentation. Liqueurs are often flavored with the essences of herbs and spices and were originally created as medicinal cures. Their contribution to health is open for debate but not totally deniable.

Culinary professionals use alcohol to flavor food. Depending on the recipe and the desired flavor, the flavor of some dishes is greatly enhanced by the addition of wine, beer, or spirits.

Wines

Chefs use all of the four wine classifications—table, sparkling, fortified, and aromatized—in cooking and baking. Each imparts its own special quality and flavor.

Table wines, or still wines, are wines whose fermentation has completely ceased before bottling. Table wines are named after the particular variety of grape (cabernet sauvignon, merlot, etc.) from which they are made, or they may consist of a blend of various types of grapes and be identified simply as red, white, rosé, or blush table wines.

Sparkling wines undergo a second fermentation process after bottling. This traps yeast-produced carbon dioxide inside the bottle, which creates bubbles (the sparkle) when the bottle is opened. Only sparkling wines produced in the French region of Champagne are allowed to carry the family nomenclature, although many champagne-type sparkling wines appear throughout the wine-producing world.

Fortified wines have had brandy added before bottling to help raise the alcohol content of the wine. Familiar types of fortified wines are Madeira and Marsala.

Aromatized wines, sometimes fortified, are flavored by herbs, spices, or both. Primarily used as aperitifs, some aromatized wines also make excellent cooking wines. Aromatized wines are almost always fortified with brandy.

Vermouth is perhaps the most popular aromatized wine used in the kitchen. It is made from white wine grapes. Vermouth is aromatized with 20 to 50 different herbs, plants, roots, seeds, barks, flowers, and citrus fruit peels. Using vermouth in the kitchen in place of white wine adds the flavor of a well-developed spice blend. Vermouth is produced in dry and sweet versions; each has different culinary advantages.

Other aromatized wines that may have a place in the kitchen pantry include French Dubonnet, which is excellent for dessert sauces and currant pies; Campari from Italy, which can accent salad dressings or chutneys; and Cynar, whose flavor comes from artichokes and adds softness and elegance to a variety of cream sauces and vegetable dishes.

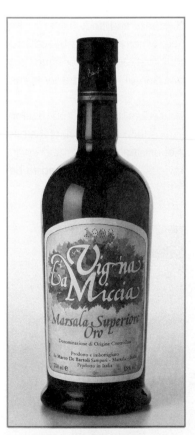

Marsala is a fortified wine, made stronger with the addition of brandy.
Clive Streeter © Dorling Kindersley

Use wines for cooking or baking that would be suitable for drinking as well. Often, chefs use inferior wines in the kitchen as a money saver, not realizing that they are also sacrificing taste and quality. The opposite, however, is not necessarily true—using only the most expensive wines does not always produce a better product.

Many young chefs make the mistake of substituting a similar yet inferior wine for a specific wine in a recipe. In more than a few restaurants, staff use two- or three-day-old opened bottles of wine from the bar for cooking. This practice naturally dictates the substitution of many types of wines as long as they are similar in color (red versus white) and in the degree of sweetness or dryness. But there are so many other discriminating differences between varietal wines (those primarily from a single variety of grape), even between similar varietals produced in different regions or countries, that this practice leads to inconsistency in taste and quality. Select the right wines for the right dish.

Other Fruit Wines

Grapes are not the only fruit whose juices make wine. Apples, pears, cherries, plums, and various berries are all capable of producing some fine wines. These specialty wines do not contain the tannins and other acids of grape wines and usually are consumed while still very young. They are usually fortified with brandy made from a similar wine (for example, pear wine is fortified with pear brandy). Usually sweet, these wines are excellent flavoring liquids for fruit sauces, soups, and desserts.

Beers and Ales

Beers and ales are fermented beverages that use grains instead of fruit to feed alcohol-producing yeast. Beer is produced in varying degrees of lightness and body. Lager is the clearest and lightest of the beers. Lagers have effervescence, which is caused by artificial carbonation before bottling. Most American beers are lagers. Stout, on the other hand, is a dark beer that takes its color from roasted malt and the addition of roasted barley to the brew. Stout is slightly bitter tasting with no effervescence.

Before mass beer production, beer and ale were used in cooking and baking throughout Europe, but not as much as wine or brandy. Perhaps this was a result of the bitterness in beer; most beer was home brewed and lacked consistency in taste and color. Beer made in the traditional manner does not age, as do wines, and therefore had to be

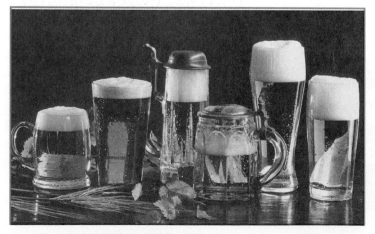

Beers have been used to cook foods for centuries; many different varieties are available today.
Photo Researchers, Inc.

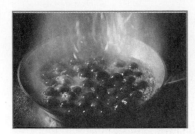

Brandy adds not only flavor but pizzaz to this table side cooking technique.

Jerry Young © Dorling Kindersley

drunk or used right away. Beer production has become more scientific today, and manufacturers can guarantee consistency in its taste, body, and color.

Some European chefs like to use the darker ales and stouts for cooking and baking. Chefs transform several of the most flavorful roasts and stews by adding a good ale to marinades or sauces. Sauerbraten, the German version of potted roast beef, can be accentuated with a bottle or two of dark malty ale.

Barley wine is a style of ale with an alcohol content that approaches 9% to 14% by volume. Aged for up to two years, barley wines have a deep, well-developed flavor that serves as an excellent food enhancer. A popular brand is Young's Old Nick, made in London.

Beer is also excellent as part of the poaching liquid for highly seasoned meat sausages and blood puddings and for steaming strong-flavored vegetables, such as cabbage, mustard greens, and kale.

In bread baking, beer contributes taste and color and aids in the dough's fermentation. In fact, no one knows for sure which discovery came first, raised bread or fermented beer. More than likely, the discoveries were simultaneous.

Brandy

Brandy is a beverage distilled from a variety of host wines. Although distillation science dates back thousands of years, the art of commercial brandy making was not realized until the sixteenth century.

Brandy can be made from any of the fruit wines—grape, apple, pear, or even berry. Brandy retains some of the characteristic flavor of the base wine and can be a great flavoring liquid in cooking. Because of its high alcohol content (from 80 to over 100 proof), brandy burns off its alcohol quickly, leaving behind a distinct flavor in just a few seconds.

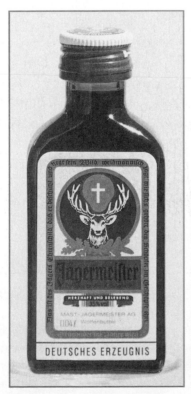

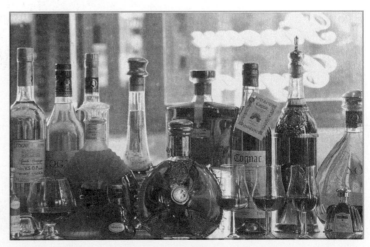

Liqueurs are made from a variety of flavoring ingredients including fruits, herbs, and spices.

AGE Fotostock America, Inc., and Dorota and Mariusz Jarymowicz © Dorling Kindersley

For example, add brandy directly to the sauté pan just before plating. Once the brandy has flamed (burned down), the sauce finishes quickly. This is why brandy is the perfect liquor to use for table side cooking presentations. The high alcohol content flames up fairly easily, giving the customer an exciting show, and what remains is excellent flavor in the sauce.

Liqueurs

During the Middle Ages, alchemists invented liqueurs—distillations flavored with all kinds of herbs, seeds, roots, and other spices—to help prolong life. Often, they were prescribed as medicinal cures and even love potions.

Liqueurs are sweetened with one or more types of sugar and then laced with brandy. Liqueurs contain anywhere from 2.5% to 35% sugar by weight; therefore, use them sparingly in cooking.

The following are some of the more widely used liqueurs and their flavoring agents:

Amaretto: Almond flavored; used in desserts and dessert sauces.

Anise or anisette: Aniseed; used in Italian cookies and candies.

Benedictine: Perhaps the oldest known liqueur, developed in the early sixteenth century; made from 27 different herbs with a cognac brandy base.

Coffee liqueur: Based on the coffee bean; Kahlua and Tia Maria are two types.

Creme de cacao: Flavored with cacao and vanilla beans.

Creme de cassis: Black currant–flavored liqueur.

Creme de menthe: White or green (color added); flavored primarily with peppermint.

Creme de noyaux: Also almond flavored; derived from crushed fruit stones (pits).

Curaçao: Flavored with the fresh peel of green oranges; comes from the island of Curaçao.

Drambuie: Made from old Highland malt Scotch whiskey and heather honey in an area of Scotland known as the Highlands.

Galliano: Italian liqueur made from flowers and herbs.

Gran Marnier: Orange curaçao liqueur with a cognac brandy base.

Kummel: Caraway-flavored liqueur; made in Germany.

Pear liqueur: Made from fresh pears.

Peppermint schnapps: Mint-flavored liqueur, usually with a higher proof than creme de menthe.

Sambuca: A licorice-flavored liqueur infused with the flavors of star anise and elderberries.

Sloe gin: Considered a flavored gin; a sweetened liqueur flavored with sloes.

Triple sec: A white, orange-flavored liqueur.

SUMMARY

There's a World of Flavors out There

Herbs and spices have long been used to add taste and flavor in cuisines around the world. Used since ancient times, they have a long history of intrigue, suspense, and adventure. Once worth their weight in gold, they are now readily available year-round for the average consumer and cook.

Herbs are the leaves of plants and have the greatest flavor value when they are fresh—chopped or whole—and added to the cooking preparation at the beginning or end.

Spices are all other vegetable aromatics, including the bark, seeds, and roots of some plants. Spices usually require drying or curing to enhance flavor and are used in whole or ground form. Furthermore, they are added early in the cooking procedure to maximize characteristic flavors.

In addition to herbs and spices, cooks adopt many natural ingredients as food enhancers: bulb and root vegetables, including garlic and ginger; flavored oils; vinegars; and fruit juices.

The general public, with increasing awareness of the variety of available food ingredients in American markets, is accepting new flavors and culinary diversions. Publicity from chefs' associations, like the American Culinary Federation and the World Association of Cooks Societies and the popularity of innovative chefs across the United States as well as television cooking shows, which have become one of America's passions, have all contributed to this increase in public knowledge.

CASE RESOLUTION

There are two points worth further investigation: (1) How much alcohol, if any, remains after the cooking process? (2) Are there any ethical considerations to serving recipes that may contain alcohol?

The wisest move would be to consider alternative flavorings to alcohol. Examples include substituting ginger ale or apple cider for white wine and nonalcoholic beer for regular beer.

REFERENCES

Freeland-Graves, J. H. 1996. *Fundamentals of Food Preparation,* 6th ed. Englewood Cliffs, NJ: Prentice Hall.

The American Heritage Dictionary, Second College Edition. 1985. Boston, MA: Houghton Mifflin Company. pp. 606, 1176.

REVIEW QUESTIONS

1. For the most pronounced flavor, what form of an herb should chefs use in cooking?
2. Explain the difference between herbs and spices. Consider culinary applications in your explanation.
3. Describe how to properly store fresh herbs.
4. Identify three herbs or spices customarily used with certain foods or recipes. (Hint: Think of traditions.)
5. What is a sachet, and when would a chef use one?
6. Describe two popular onion varieties.
7. How can someone know if a wild mushroom is raw or poisonous?
8. Name one ideal alcohol for demonstration cooking.
9. Define mirepoix. Explain its cooking applications.
10. Why is botulism a concern with canned foods or with foods immersed in oil?

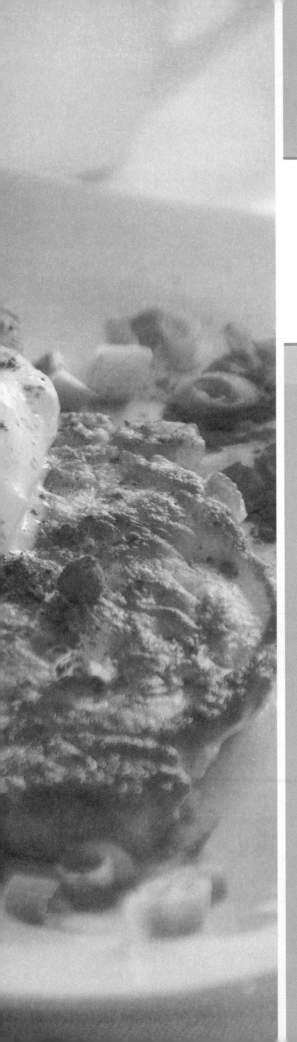

13

Building Recipes for Healthier Meals

KEY CONCEPTS

- When every food item served meets high culinary standards, the diner is more likely to eat healthful foods in the proper amounts.
- The first step in transforming an existing recipe to meet recommended nutritional values is to evaluate its present nutritional worth. Then determine how the dish can be improved without jeopardizing its integrity.
- The calorie, cholesterol, and sodium content of foods served is just as critical as their fat, vitamin, and mineral content.
- Complete substitutions sometimes make too great a change in existing recipes. Partial substitutions may be more practical while still resulting in lower fat for the whole plate.
- The nutrients in vegetable, grain, potato, sauce, and other plate accompaniments are as important as those in the main course item when trying to serve healthier meals.
- A great way to reduce the fat used in cooking is to measure the amount of fat that is needed accurately instead of pouring it into the pot or pan.
- Nutritional recipes need to be based on measurable information, not guesswork. Controls should be put in place during the entire process of ordering, preparing, cooking, and serving the foods to ensure that nutritional goals are achieved.
- Kitchen and wait staffs must be trained to deliver healthier foods to the customers. Interpretations and guesswork can cause serious problems for guests and the operation.

Whether transforming an existing recipe to meet modern nutritional guidelines or designing a completely new recipe that meets nutritional standards, the knowledgeable and creative chef has many choices of ingredients and cooking techniques to make the dishes he or she serves more nutritious. Healthier food choices, nutrient-retentive preparation procedures, and low-fat cooking methods with flavorful herbs, spices, vegetables, wines, or brandies can make the most nutritious meals unforgettable.

For example, using meat, poultry, and fat substitutions can transform many standard recipes into healthier dishes without sacrificing flavor, texture, or eye appeal. Adding vegetable and starch accompaniments can balance the plate with other nutrients, colors, and textures. Serving a sauce made from natural meat or poultry drippings combines culinary art and the science of nutrition to create a healthy recipe that looks great and tastes even better.

Proper planning, experience in cooking, and complete nutritional cooking knowledge enable chefs to make satisfying, attractive, and nutritious meals without compromising USDA standards for lower meat and poultry portion sizes or excessively increasing the total caloric content of the food. By learning the nutritional composition of foods, using proper cooking techniques, and controlling portion sizes, cooks and chefs can serve healthier foods to all of their guests and customers. These are the true foundations of the art of nutritional cooking.

THINK ABOUT IT

With your existing knowledge of food and cooking, in addition to your study of nutritional cooking, picture re-creating every recipe or formula that you know in the light of modern food sources and culinary trends. Now imagine the same new foods designed to meet nutritional guidelines of balance, variety, portion control, low fat, low sodium, and high fiber. What do you think they will be and how will they taste?

CASE STUDY

The Story of the Missing Flavors

Chef Mike has been asked to prepare a variety of low-fat and low-sodium meals for convention visitors at a hotel where he works. Knowing a little about nutritional cooking, Chef Mike easily cut out the saturated fats, reduced total fat, reduced sodium, and increased fiber by adding whole-grain foods to each preparation. He was proud to serve his new creations to his guests.

Luckily for Chef Mike, his practice is to have his staff taste the foods before serving them to the guests. One of his cooks asked, "What is this supposed to taste like?"

Chef Mike was surprised. But should he have been? What could he have done to ensure good flavor in nutritionally controlled menus? *The resolution for this case study is presented at the end of the chapter.*

THE CHALLENGE

Cooks and chefs often are asked to make existing recipes more nutritious. Whether the request comes from individual customers or corporate offices, the challenge facing the chef is to make a healthier plate of great-tasting, satisfying food without compromising the integrity, or main concept, of the original recipes. If the integrity of a recipe cannot be

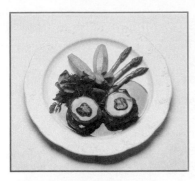

Tournedos Rossini.
Pearson Education/PH College

protected, it is better to design a completely new recipe and give it a new name and presentation.

Tournedos Rossini, for example, is a classic dish made from lightly sautéed beef tenderloin, placed on top of a toasted bread crouton, and crowned with a slice of foie gras, sliced truffles, and sauce Madeira. How could this recipe be nutritionally improved without changing its basic concept of a beef tenderloin preparation with crouton, foie gras, and roux-thickened brown sauce?

Replace the sautéed tenderloin with braised beef short ribs, and its concept totally changes; it now can no longer be called *Tournedos* Rossini (tournedos are by definition small fillets of beef). Substitute a grilled portabella mushroom for the foie gras, and the name *Rossini* no longer fits, for it is defined by the ingredients of the garnish. Serve a sautéed filet mignon on a bed of braised endive, sweated spinach, or brown rice pilaf, and it has become a totally new recipe.

The resulting foods may be healthier to eat compared to the original concept, but they vary so far from the integrity of the original concept that they should not be called by the same name. Instead, prepare healthy recipes with different names that are new healthy creations and not poor substitutions for classic or popular dishes.

If a particular recipe gets its name from the ingredients used or for a specific cooking and presentation technique, such as Tournedos Rossini, a nutritional compromise may not be possible. Even a smaller portion of tenderloin or a thinner crouton could not adequately transform this classic dish into a healthier presentation. The fat and cholesterol content found in the foie gras alone is enough to keep this recipe out of nutritional cookbooks.

A dish like Prime Rib that gets its name from a single item, roasted beef rib loin, can be part of a nutritious and balanced diet without compromising the original concept of the dish. The beef entree itself can be prepared more nutritiously, smaller portions can be served, and flavorful nutrient-rich vegetables and sauces can accompany the entree on the plate for complete balance.

Here are the steps to serve Prime Rib as a nutritious menu item:

1. Purchase select grade beef (naturally lower in fat than choice and prime grades of beef).
2. Trim the loin of most excess fat, especially the lip (the tapered end).
3. Roast it slowly at low temperatures to reduce shrinkage and moisture loss.
4. Serve only 6- to 8-ounce portions.
5. Use the drippings from the roasting pan as an accompanying sauce.
6. Prepare multiple nutrient-rich accompaniments to fill the plate.

One of the primary factors in determining USDA grades of beef is the animal's fat-to-lean ratio. Prime beef contains the highest amount of exterior and interior fat (marbling). Choice and select grades of beef have significantly lower amounts of fat in descending order respectively, while the nutritional values of the meat remain extremely high. Using select and choice grade meat for nutritional cooking will reduce the total fat on the plate and provide needed nutrients and excellent quality protein. Table 13–1 lists the fat content of common retail cuts of meats, which can help a chef choose a less fatty cut for their next menu.

One problem in cooking and serving lean meats is that they are drier in taste and texture than are fattier varieties. Roasting the rib roast slowly to preserve moisture and serving it with a reduced beef essence or stock in place of fatty gravy can return flavorful moisture to the finished plate.

The U.S. government does not allow food manufacturers or producers to advertise foods as healthy choices (low-fat and low-cholesterol, especially) unless they meet the

TABLE 13–1 • FAT CONTENT OF TYPICAL RETAIL MEAT PRODUCTS

Selected Meat Products (3 ounces)	Total Fat (grams)	Saturated Fatty Acid (grams)	Cholesterol (milligrams)	Calories (kilocalories)
Beef Eye of Round, Roasted, 1/4″ Trim				
Lean Only				
USDA select	3	1	59	136
USDA choice	5	2	59	149
Lean and Fat				
USDA select	10	4	61	184
USDA choice	12	5	62	205
Beef Rib Eye Steak, Broiled				
Lean Only				
USDA select	7	3	68	168
USDA choice	10	4	68	191
Lean and Fat				
USDA select	17	7	70	242
USDA choice	19	8	70	265
Ground Beef Patty, Cooked				
Extra lean	14	5	71	215
Regular	17	7	76	245
Pork Center Loin, Roasted				
Lean only	8	3	67	150
Lean and fat	11	4	68	180

Source: U.S. Department of Agriculture. http://www.ams.usda.gov/howtobuy/meat.htm

nutritional standards established by the USDA. The Nutrition Labeling and Education Act of 1990 mandates that all nutritional claims for prepared foods be verifiable through nutrient evaluation and comparison to nutritional standards. Chefs and owners must not falsely advertise health benefits for a plate of food that does not meet the same high standards that manufacturers must follow. Merely serving small portions of foods or foods with slightly lower fat or cholesterol content is not enough to satisfy these strict requirements.

Improving the nutritional value of more complex recipes requires a thorough evaluation of each of the recipe's ingredients and preparation procedures, increasing the challenges for the chef. Ingredients can be replaced with substitutes, healthy ingredients can be added, fats can be manipulated, and preparation and cooking techniques can be modified to improve nutrition, but the flavors, textures, and eye appeal must also be protected.

RECIPE TRANSFORMATIONS

The first step in transforming a recipe to meet recommended nutritional values is to evaluate its present nutritional worth. Then you can determine which factors can be changed without jeopardizing the integrity of the dish. The factors in a recipe that affect nutritional values are:

- The main ingredients: the meat, poultry, and seafood choices
- The amount and types of fats present or used in cooking
- The amount and variety of flavoring ingredients used including vegetables, herbs, and spices
- The cooking methods and preparation techniques
- The sauce and other specified accompaniments

Ask the following questions:

1. Are the main food items heavy in fat? If they are, can they be trimmed or can other less fatty substitutions be made?
2. What are the portion sizes of the entree and accompaniment(s)?
3. What fats are used for marinades, dressings, and cooking? Can they be eliminated or replaced with oils that contain less saturated fatty acids?
4. What flavors from vegetables, herbs, and spices could be used to enhance the natural flavors of the other ingredients?
5. Can a low-fat or no-fat cooking method replace the cooking methods specified and still create foods similar in taste and eye appeal to the original recipes?
6. How are the sauces and accompaniments made? Can they be replaced with healthier versions, considering the variety of other foods on the plate?
7. What flavors would be lost, if any, due to ingredient substitution or elimination? What could be added to return distinguishable flavors to the dish?

Answering these questions through the entire recipe transformation process will help you make great-tasting and satisfying healthy foods out of high-fat, high-calorie, and otherwise unbalanced meals.

Let's apply the questions to a standard appetizer recipe commonly referred to as "popcorn shrimp." These are typically under 100 count pink shrimp (100 shrimp to the pound, very small) that are batter dipped and deep-fried in hot grease until golden brown. Popcorn shrimp often are served with a piece of curly endive, a green leaf lettuce garnish with sliced tomatoes, or cut carrots and celery. They also usually come with cocktail sauce or tartar sauce as accompaniments.

The fat in the batter-dipped and deep-fried shrimp far outweighs any possible benefit of eating the vegetable garnish, even if the customer were interested in eating the garnish. The sauces are likewise poor choices for a healthy plate of food. The cocktail sauce is full of sugar and sodium (from prepared catsup), and the tartar sauce is laden with fat from its mayonnaise base.

The following shows the analytical process of transforming a typically fatty menu item into a healthy choice as it is applied to a batter-fried shrimp appetizer:

1. Are the main food items heavy in fat? If they are, can they be trimmed or can other less fatty substitutions be made?

    Answer: Shrimp by themselves are not overly fatty; they are a healthy seafood choice. The shrimp selected are usually small, so when they are battered and fried,

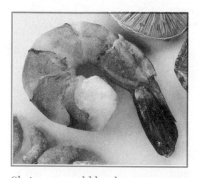

Shrimp are sold by the count per pound.
Clive Streeter and Patrick McLeavy
© Dorling Kindersley

they appear about the same size and shape as popped corn, thus the name "popcorn shrimp." They are often double-battered to give an even larger presentation. However, the excessive amount of fried batter created and the fat it absorbs from the deep-fat fryer end up in the food that is served. More than half of every bite of food is batter, an unhealthy proportion compared to the amount of shrimp and other healthy ingredients.

Increase the shrimp size to reduce the amount of batter used to coat and fry them, the amount of fat the batter might absorb, and the amount of carbohydrates and calories. A small shrimp is still required to preserve the integrity of the dish, but there are many choices larger than under 100 count to choose from. A size of shrimp slightly under 70 count per pound can still create the "popcorn" effect (small puffs of batter-fried shrimp), but with less batter overall. This will increase the proportion of shrimp to batter in every bite.

2. What are the portion sizes of the entree and accompaniment(s)?

Answer: Common recipes for this type of appetizer prepare 4 to 6 ounces of fried shrimp per serving. The shrimp are usually served alone or with a simple vegetable garnish. Instead, use only 2 ounces of shrimp per portion and serve them with 3 to 4 ounces of low-fat vegetable or fruit accompaniments for a healthier appetizer portion. The customer will still get 6 ounces of food as an appetizer, which is more than adequate, but will be encouraged to eat everything on the plate, thus consuming a balanced meal with great taste and substance.

3. What fats are used for marinades, dressings, and cooking? Can they be eliminated or replaced with oils that contain less saturated fatty acids?

Answer: Use canola oil for deep-fat and pan-fried applications. Canola oil does not last as long in the frying process as do hydrogenated fats and other vegetable oils, but it has less saturated fat than any other commonly available oil. Corn oil is another good choice, with peanut oil as a close third. Also, eliminate the tartar sauce and cocktail sauce; substitute any variety of low-fat sauce or salsa.

4. What flavors from vegetables, herbs, and spices could be used to enhance the natural flavors of the other ingredients?

Answer: In the original recipe, the only vegetables were sliced tomatoes, leafy lettuce, and chopped carrots and celery. These are healthy foods, but their simple

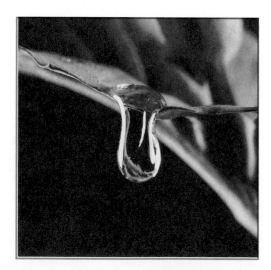

Canola oil is a healthy substitute.
Photo Researchers, Inc.

presentation does not encourage their consumption. Some customers may even request salad dressing (another high-fat item) to dress the garnish and eat it as a small side salad.

Instead, serve a freshly made, low-fat vegetable slaw or a lightly dressed julienne or brunoise vegetable salad on a piece of red curly leaf lettuce or romaine lettuce as an exciting, flavorful, and satisfying accompaniment. The vegetables will add crunch (texture), color to the plate for eye appeal, and healthful vitamins, flavonoids, and minerals.

5. Can a low-fat or no-fat cooking method replace the cooking methods specified and still create foods similar in taste and eye appeal to the original recipes?

Answer: Unfortunately, no, for this particular dish. Steamed or poached shrimp can be served as a healthier appetizer, but this is too far removed from the original concept to still be called "popcorn shrimp." However, you can use cooking oils low in saturated fats, like canola, for the deep-fat fryer, heat clean oil to temperature before adding the shrimp, and cook only small portions to cook them quickly. Overall, these steps can reduce the amount of fat absorbed by the batter and the shrimp to acceptable levels.

6. How are the sauces and accompaniments made? Can they be replaced with healthier versions, considering the variety of other foods on the plate?

Answer: You can easily add more nutrients to this type of appetizer presentation, starting with the batter and finishing with the accompanying sauces.

Instead of using a typical tempura-type batter (flour, egg, and water) to coat the shrimp, use a cornmeal batter for added texture, fiber, color, and nutrients.

Replace the tartar sauce (usually made with mayonnaise) with a low-fat sour cream and cucumber relish or some other low-fat condiment. Although cocktail sauce is low in fat, the processed catsup in it is full of refined sugar and contains large amounts of sodium per serving (190 milligrams per tablespoon). Make a fresh salsa with chopped herbs, ripe tomatoes, sweet peppers, celery, onion, and fresh squeezed lime juice (full of vitamin C) for flavor and consistency, or use some other low-fat dipping sauce to replace the traditional cocktail sauce. Adding chopped jalapeño peppers or freshly grated horseradish to the fresh salsa could give it extra spiciness to help round out the overall flavors on the plate.

7. What flavors would be lost, if any, due to ingredient substitution or elimination? What could be added to return distinguishable flavors to the dish?

Answer: In this case flavors were not lost. They were automatically replaced with the more exciting flavors and textures of cornmeal, vegetables, and herbs.

The resulting dish transforms the original simple appetizer preparation from a food item typically high in fat and calories into a new healthier version. Multiple textures, colors, and flavors are presented in a balanced manner to please the palate, the eye, and the discriminating demands of customers.

The original recipe must also be evaluated for its calorie, cholesterol, and sodium content in order to properly convert it to a healthier version. The final re-creation also must be evaluated to ensure that the transformation worked and that calories, cholesterol, and sodium are reduced. It would not be a healthier recipe simply because the fats were reduced, especially if its cholesterol, sodium, or calorie content remains high. Likewise, foods richer in vitamins and minerals served together with high-fat foods may not create a completely healthy meal either. Balance is the key to healthy eating. The consummate challenge for cooks and chefs is to encourage the customer to eat everything on the plate and enjoy the benefits of healthy cooking.

The following food charts can be used to determine the nutrient values of existing and transformed recipes; they are available free from the USDA:

- USDA National Nutrient Database for Standard Reference, Release 16
- Nutritive Value of Foods, Home and Garden Bulletin, Number 72

These charts, however, are labor intensive to reference, difficult to cross-check for a variety of foods at the same time, and may not include all the food ingredients in a particular recipe.

Many computer software programs are now available that will conduct nutrition analysis for cooks and chefs. These computer programs sometimes contain large databases with the nutritional values of thousands of different food ingredients. The chef enters the recipe's ingredients and cooking methods into the program, including the main items, all sauces, accompaniments, and garnishes, to determine the recipe's overall food value. Then the computer automatically calculates the amount of nutrition per serving, based on a stated portion size (in weighted ounces or volume measures).

Computerized nutritional assessment programs also enable cooks or chefs to immediately measure the effect of making certain substitutions for meats, fats, and other ingredients in a recipe by recalculating the collected nutritional information based on the substitutions. The cook can determine right away whether the substitution creates the desired results, or can select another substitution and repeat the process. The cook, in just a few minutes at the computer, can repeat the same process until healthy results are achieved. Searching through manuals and online databases would take much longer.

SUBSTITUTING MEATS AND POULTRY FOR HEALTHIER COOKING

Many traditional recipes call for meats that are high in saturated fat, like beef and pork. These dishes can be made with a more nutritious meat substitute without sacrificing flavor, texture, and appeal. Turkey, chicken, and game meats like venison and rabbit are good choices for healthy substitutions.

In some cases, an entirely different type or cut of meat can replace another in a particular recipe and still produce a quality dish. For example, you can replace the fattier chuck roast with lean flank steak to prepare a healthy version of Beef Bourguignonne that can be named *Flank Steak Bourguignonne*.

To make this substitution work well, slice the flank steak very thin and manually tenderize it with a meat mallet. Then roll the flank steak into roulades and braise them in full-flavored lean beef broth. When done, finish the braising liquid by adding a cornstarch slurry (cornstarch dissolved in cold water or lean broth), which will thicken the sauce without using traditional fatty rouxs (fat and flour blended together). To preserve the Bourguignonne presentation, add caramelized pearl onions and cooked sliced or button mushrooms to the finished sauce.

Other healthy meat substitutions for traditional preparations could include Chicken Chasseur, Chicken Roulade Florentine, and Beef Brisket Montmorency. All of these are healthy meals that can be served while maintaining the integrity of the Chasseur, Florentine, and Montmorency preparations.

Some recipes can have a portion of the meat replaced with a healthier choice and still maintain the integrity of the dish. Much like milk, which can be purchased as whole milk

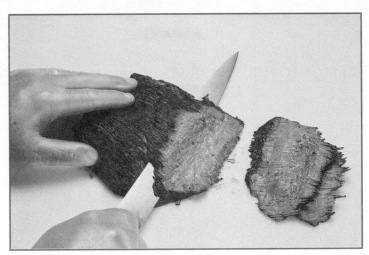

Lean flank steak makes a healthier choice.
Pearson Education/PH College

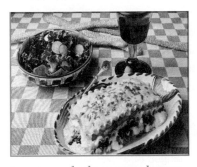

Lasagna and other casserole-type dishes work well using a mixture of lean ground meats because the other flavors help balance the taste of the whole dish.
Getty Images, Inc.—PhotoDisc

and in less fatty forms, and coffee, which can be purchased in regular and decaffeinated forms, some meat recipes allow the substitution of lower-fat meats to offer a more balanced, nutritious meal. Customers then can eat their favorite meals with many of the traditional flavors they enjoy but with less fat.

Casseroles, stews, sausages, stuffing, and many meat sauce recipes can use meat substitutions with little effect on overall taste. If complete substitution makes too great a change, partial substitution may be more practical yet still provide a lower-fat meal. For example, you can use a mixture of 25% to 50% ground turkey and 50% to 75% ground lean beef to make healthier versions of chili, lasagna, meatloaf, hamburgers, and any other recipe that calls for ground beef. The end result will have significantly less fat and cholesterol and still be loaded with great flavors and textures.

Less fatty cuts of meat and poultry can substitute for the more traditional fatty meats in many everyday recipes, drastically reducing the fat in the served foods. For example, Turkey Parmesan uses thin sliced turkey breast in place of the scallopini of veal in Veal Parmesan; Turkey Chili replaces part or all of the beef in regular Beef Chili with lean ground turkey. These recipes are healthier versions of their named counterparts simply because of the meat substitutions. (Transformed menu items should be appropriately renamed, as with the Turkey Chili and Turkey Parmesan examples here, so as not to confuse the guests on what is being served.)

Turkey is one of the best meats for substitutions. It is naturally low in fat and is suited to most cooking procedures and taste combinations. Ground turkey is the most versatile form to use; it is easily incorporated into a multitude of ground beef, veal, and pork recipes. Ground turkey is readily available through most meat purveyors, or it can be ground in-house.

Thinly cut and flattened turkey breast meat is also a good substitution for chicken, pork, or veal in many cutlet dishes. Turkey Parmesan (breaded breast cutlet baked with tomato sauce and cheese), Turkey Florentine (with whole leaf spinach rolled inside a thin cutlet or served on the side of the finished dish), Turkey Chasseur (with fresh tomatoes, mushrooms, and herbs) and Turkey Marsala (with Marsala wine and mushrooms) are just a few examples of what re-creations are possible using this versatile, lean meat as a healthy substitute.

Venison and other game meats, which are naturally leaner than most domesticated animals and birds, also make excellent substitutes for fattier beef and poultry entrees. Game meats can be purchased from many local meat purveyors in a variety of cuts including venison top rounds, ground venison, wild boar rib steaks, pheasant breasts, and whole squab.

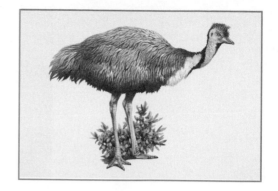

The emu is a flightless bird that offers very lean red meat similar in texture to beef.
Kenneth Lilly © Dorling Kindersley

Game purchased through registered meat purveyors consists of farm-raised animals and birds, which are characteristically lean but less "gamey" than their wild counterparts. Although game is more expensive than beef or pork, its nutritional benefits and distinguished flavors are worth consideration.

Many customers may willingly pay more for healthier game meat entrees if the recipes are well designed and the taste and presentation are top quality. For budget-minded customers, the chef can combine smaller portions of game meats with vegetables, potatoes, pasta, or dough into a complete single meal to reduce the cost of the finished plate.

Emu and ostrich are other lean choices for meat substitutions. The emu and ostrich are flightless birds, and both have red colored flesh that is like beef. The edible meat per pound costs typically two to three times more than beef, however, so consistently substituting either of these two birds for beef may be cost prohibitive. But new and exciting recipes that could command higher prices can be made from their lean, flavorful meat.

Meat substitutions need not always create drastic changes to deliver healthier foods. Although a substitution may not dramatically reduce total fat, it may decrease it enough to balance the other foods on the plate. The overall goal is less than 30% calorie content from fats on any given plate. Often only a slight change in the meat item or portion size is all that is required to achieve those goals (Table 13–2).

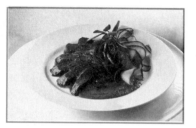

Venison is a great-tasting lean meat.
Ian O'Leary © Dorling Kindersley

TABLE 13–2 • SAMPLE NUTRITIONAL MEAT SUBSTITUTIONS

Recipe	Substitute I	Substitute II
Beef rib eye	Beef sirloin	Beef tenderloin
Beef sirloin	Beef top round	Beef eye round
Beef chuck	Beef brisket	Beef flank steak
Ground beef	Ground turkey	Ground venison
Any beef cut	Any venison cut	
Pork ribs	Lean pork chops	Wild boar rib steaks
Pork shoulder	Fresh pork ham	Fresh wild boar ham
Any red meat	Venison	Emu/ostrich
Duck	Chicken	Squab
Veal scallopini	Turkey scallopini	Venison scallopini

For example, cooks and chefs can substitute relatively lean beef tenderloin steaks for fattier rib eye steaks for slightly healthier dishes. Both steaks contain fat, but the rib eye steaks have much more fat in proportion to lean muscle than do tenderloin steaks. Likewise fresh pork hams are a healthy substitute for pork shoulder (Boston butt) and fattier pork loins in many recipes. If the ham is too large, it can easily be cut into various size pieces and even scallopini (thin slices) if needed to fulfill a recipe specification.

SUBSTITUTING PROTEIN ALTERNATIVES FOR MEATS, SEAFOOD, AND POULTRY

Vegetarianism is on the rise in the United States. An estimated 13 million Americans choose either not to eat meat or to limit their meat consumption. Cultural, ethnic, and religious practices and beliefs that promote vegetarianism have historically been the reasons why people choose not to eat meat. Today, health and diet considerations also motivate people to eat meatless entrees, salads, and sandwiches in increasing numbers.

To satisfy this growing market, food manufacturers now provide meat replacements that are constructed from vegetable compounds and made to look, taste, and feel like real meat. These meat analogs imitate real meat and meat-based products like ground meat, bologna, bacon bits, chicken nuggets, and hot dogs. Many of these products are made available through retail and commercial suppliers. Using these substitutes, consumers can still eat traditional foods yet with no animal proteins.

Many vegetarians do not want their foods to look and taste like meat. Even the idea of eating meat or meat-based products is offensive to them. For this group of consumers, completely meatless products are available that totally replace meat items on the menu. Soy burgers are now sold in college cafeterias everywhere; fine institutions, including the best hotels and clubs, offer veggie burgers; even the fast-food industry is now considering meatless burgers.

Besides using manufactured meat replacements and meatless entrees, creative chefs can also create their own tantalizing meatless entrees that contain only vegetables and vegetable by-products. Vegetable pancakes, vegetable lasagna, and vegetable stir-fries can satisfy the growing demand for meatless, vegetarian entrees and still provide good amounts of essential amino acids as part of a balanced diet.

Amino acids are necessary for good health yet are not easily found in vegetables and starches. Legumes, especially soy beans, seeds, and nuts, do contain lots of amino acids, which can be combined with other vegetables, grains, and pastas to present healthy, tasty and satisfying entrees, soups, salads, and sandwiches.

Many protein alternatives are made from vegetable sources and are used to supply essential amino acids and other healthy nutrients to vegetarian dishes. Three of the most popular protein alternatives are seitan, tempeh, and tofu.

Seitan is made from a mixture of water and flour. The flour absorbs some of the water, forming a soft ball of gluten and starch. The soft dough is rinsed to remove the starch compounds, leaving the elastic gluten behind. What remains is a type of wheat-based protein that can be flavored, shaped, cut, and cooked in a variety of preparations. Seitan has been used as a protein source for daily meals in Asia for hundreds of years.

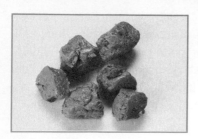

Seitan, a protein substitute, is made entirely of wheat gluten.
Pearson Education/PH College

Seitan can be made by hand, but the process is time-consuming. Commercial mixes are also available, which are quicker to regenerate and are used in cooking. Seitan is available in most health food stores under the name of seitan or "wheat meat," and in Asian stores as Mi-Tan. Fresh seitan can be stored in marinades, which impart their flavors to the gluten for tasty preparations.

Seitan cannot be consumed by people with gluten intolerances (Celiac disease). It is sold in various shapes and sizes, with cubes, strips, and cutlets being the most popular. Fresh seitan can be simmered in any flavored stock, or it can be braised in a combination of stock, vegetables, tomatoes, wine, and other flavoring ingredients. Cooked seitan (simmered until firm) can be cut into various shapes and baked, grilled, or sautéed in hot oil.

Tempeh is believed to have originated in Indonesia, where its production dates back several hundred years. It was introduced into Europe by Dutch settlers of Indonesia in the nineteenth century, yet it was not introduced into the United States until late in the twentieth century.

Tempeh is made by fermenting cooked soybeans with a particular type of mold known as rhizopus mold, or tempeh starter. Fermenting tempeh with the rhizopus mold binds the cooked soybeans together into white cakes that can be easily formed into multiple shapes and sizes for cooking. The tempeh fermentation process also creates natural antibiotic agents that protect against certain intestinal infections when the tempeh is consumed and digested.

Besides providing healthful enzymes created during the fermentation process, tempeh is a complete and healthful protein substitute. Tempeh contains all the essential amino acids needed for human health and is naturally low in fat. It contains many beneficial isoflavones and all the fiber of the soybeans from which it is made.

Tempeh cakes have a firm texture and a nutty, earthy, almost mushroom-like flavor that comes from the mold used in the fermentation process. Usually they are sliced and fried until the outer layers become brown and crisp.

Cooked tempeh can be used in sandwiches, as a topping on fancy combined salads, and as a main plate item together with other healthy vegetables. Tempeh can also be used in soups, stews, and sauces. It can also be incorporated into any other common recipe in which the texture and flavor of mushrooms are required.

Many health food stores sell the tempeh starter needed to make fresh tempeh from cooked soybeans. The starter is added to already cooked soybeans and given an incubation period of 36 to 48 hours to ferment. Premade tempeh can also be purchased from health food stores and some specialty commercial food purveyors.

Tofu is the most common protein substitute used in American kitchens. It is combined with other proteins in a multitude of Asian and American-style recipes. Tofu was introduced in the United States in the middle of the nineteenth century by Chinese immigrants who worked on the railroads.

Tofu is a type of soybean cheese. It is made by curdling a mush of cooked and mashed soybeans with a coagulant called nigari. Nigari is a natural compound found in fresh ocean water. Calcium sulfate, a naturally occurring mineral, and acids like lemon juice and vinegar can also curdle the cooked soybean mush. Other types of soy-based products are listed in Box 13–1.

Tofu is the main dietary protein in Asia and can be found in every market, even specialized tofu shops, where it is made fresh daily. It is stored in water-filled pans, in which the water is replaced every day to ensure a fresh taste. Tofu is also available commercially in vacuum packs and aseptic brick packages.

Three densities of tofu are available in American stores. Homemade tofu can have many different levels of density depending on the amount of coagulant used and how long

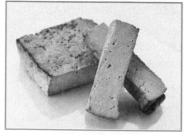

Tofu is a protein substitute made entirely from soybean curds.
Ian O'Leary © Dorling Kindersley

BOX 13-1 • OTHER SOY-BASED PRODUCTS

Miso: Fermented soybeans made into a paste ground with grains; used to season soups, sauces, dressings, and dips.

Soy milk: Made by soaking and pressing whole soybeans.

Soy flour: Ground from roasted soybeans.

Soy grits: Coarsely ground soybeans.

Soybean oil: Pressed from soybeans; contains large amounts of oleic, linoleic, and alpha-linolenic acids; oleic is a monounsaturated fat, and linoleic and alpha-linolenic are polyunsaturated fats.

Hydrolyzed vegetable protein (HVP): Soybean protein broken down by acid.

Textured soy protein (TSP): Used as a meat substitute or meat extender in traditionally meat-based items like sausage, hot dogs, ham, and ground beef.

the tofu was allowed to form. Each density has its own place as a protein substitute in cooking:

- *Firm*: Tofu is dense and solid. It holds up well in stir-fry preparations, soups, and stews. Firm tofu can also be sliced and grilled or pan-fried.
- *Soft*: Tofu does not hold its shape very well. It is often used in soups and blended recipes.
- *Silken*: Tofu, which is made by a slightly different process, is a creamy, custard-like product. It can be eaten plain, with a touch of soy sauce and chopped scallions, or in a variety of blended shakes and baked desserts.

Firm tofu can replace meat in many recipes. Tofu's texture enables it to absorb many flavors just by coming in contact with them. For example, tofu used in stews tastes like the sauce and vegetable flavors prominent in the stew base; tofu used in soups takes on the predominant flavors of the other soup ingredients.

THE WHOLE PLATE CONCEPT

In nutritional cooking, eating a balance of foods is one of the predominant tenets, and all the foods on the plate play a critical role in promoting good health. The nutritional and flavor contribution of the main item is relative to the amount of the other foods on the plate. The vegetables, fruits, grains, and sauces that make up the other foods on the plate also contribute vitamins and minerals, providing more nutrients with every bite.

Colors, textures, flavors, shapes, and mouth feel are all important factors to consider when placing only two different foods together, let alone the four or five different food items and half a dozen flavor components found in a typical recipe. Plate sauces and all plate accompaniments can complement the flavors, textures, and nutrition of the main food item when selected from a list of healthy items and cooking methods.

Plate sauces should be reduction sauces or starch-thickened sauces to lessen the amount of fat on the plate. Vegetable accompaniments should have varied textures and colors as well as flavors that complement the other flavors on the plate. The foods should be processed as little as possible (no puréed or finely chopped foods), especially when cooked.

Vegetables, legumes, potatoes, and grains can be excellent sources of vitamins, minerals, and fiber. The Food Guide Pyramid recommends at least 4 servings of vegetables and 6 to 11 servings of grain products and starch-based foods every day to obtain the needed nutrients.

There are hundreds of varieties of these foods to choose from and thousands of ways to prepare them using nutritional cooking guidelines. Either by themselves or combined in myriad flavors and textures, vegetables, legumes, potatoes, and grains play an integral role in the human diet.

Follow these guidelines to retain nutrients and expand your skills in preparing exciting vegetable, legume, potato, and grain dishes and accompaniments:

- Purchase only the freshest products available.
- Purchase locally grown vegetables whenever possible to decrease shipping and storage time.
- Store all products properly, whether fresh, frozen, or dried.
- Prepare products as close to cooking time as possible.
- Never store cut vegetables or potatoes in water for long periods of time.
- If blanching is part of the cooking process, shock vegetables quickly and remove them from the water/ice bath as soon as they have cooled.
- Steam blanching retains more nutrients than blanching vegetables in water. Be careful not to overcook the vegetables.
- If combining ingredients, learn the different cooking times of leaf, root, stem, flowering, and fruit vegetables.
- Cook vegetables that take the longest amount of time first and those that take the least amount of time last.
- Cook and serve vegetables with as little processing as possible. Avoid puréed or finely chopped vegetable preparations.

Serving healthy vegetable accompaniments is an important goal. Making them tasty and satisfying takes a little more planning. Common vegetable accompaniments like candied carrots, broccoli with hollandaise, and the infamous vegetable medley are either loaded with unnecessary calories, fat, and cholesterol (brown sugar and butter for the candied carrots, and eggs and butter for the hollandaise) or are simply not interesting enough to tempt the diner to consume them.

Getting guests and customers to eat all of the accompaniments on the plate so they walk away satisfied after a complete meal full of flavors, textures, and nutrients is a challenge. Fortunately, vegetable cookery has kept pace with innovations in meat and seafood cookery. Today, vegetables can be a major and gratifying part of the dining experience with some creative thinking and a mind open to flavor combinations and cooking techniques.

In single vegetable presentations like Creole Cauliflower, the prominent vegetable should be cooked so as to ensure full flavor, attractive appearance, and proper texture in the final preparation. If steaming is the method preferred to retain the vegetable's color, shape, and nutrients, then cook the remainder of the recipe (the Creole sauce) separately and add steamed cauliflower at the end. Do not cook the cauliflower with the sauce ingredients at the same time in a single pan; the results will not be satisfying. The flavors and nutrients might remain (if all the accompanying sauce is also consumed), but the presentation will be lacking.

In combined vegetable accompaniments like vegetable medleys, each ingredient must be properly cooked to allow its individual flavor and texture to remain in the combined presentation. Either steam blanch each vegetable separately and then add them together in the final presentation, or add the vegetables one at a time depending on the amount of time required to properly cook each vegetable. When all the vegetables are finished cooking, season them all together to finish the dish.

Use seasoning vegetables like celery, celery root, onions, garlic, fennel, bell peppers, parsnips, and turnips in addition to herbs and spices to season vegetable, grain, and starch

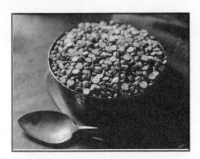

Split peas make an excellent puréed vegetable sauce.
Getty Images, Inc.—Photodisc

dishes. These flavoring vegetables and ingredients add great flavors as well as many nutrients, textures, colors, and shapes depending on how each ingredient is cut and then cooked.

Combine multiple flavoring ingredients together to present an accompaniment with a full complement of textures, colors, and flavors. Balanced textures (crunchy and soft), colors (red, purple, orange, green, white, and yellow), flavors (sweet, salty, sour, astringent, and umami), and aromas (pepperminty, floral, and pungent) make every mouthful exciting, which helps stimulate the appetite and satisfy hunger.

If you are serving a vegetable accompaniment with a sauce, make a vegetable-based reduction sauce with nothing more than rice, split peas, or some other vegetable thickener. Produce only as much sauce as is needed to serve the accompaniment; excess sauce wastes good flavors and nutrition.

Creating vegetable and starch accompaniments that stimulate the senses of sight, taste, smell, and touch (texture) while retaining nutrients can be challenging and fun. Replace traditional or common vegetable preparations with exciting and satisfying healthy creations.

NUTRITIONAL SAUCES

Sauces have played such a critical role in classic cooking that it is hard to imagine serving some foods without them. Traditionally, sauces have been used to mask the "off" flavors of aged meats and moisten dried, salted, or overcooked meats, poultry, and seafood. Modern farming and herding practices together with refrigeration and freezer storage that extend the shelf life of foods have made this use of sauces an outdated practice. It is best to serve foods prepared fresh, properly cooked to allow the natural juices and flavors to keep the food moist in the mouth.

In modern cooking, the sauce is used to add flavors to a dish, not to hide existing flavors. Adding a fat-laden sauce to healthy meats and vegetables, however, detracts from the total nutritional value of the meal. Low-fat or no-fat sauces are ideal for nutritional cooking techniques.

Many traditional and classic European-style recipes use roux-based sauces (fat plus flour) or emulsified sauces (egg yolks, butter, and vinegar/wine). These heavy sauces were often used to mask the flavors of the foods they accompanied. Fresh meats and seafood were not readily available, and the aged meats that were available had a strong, pungent flavor. Aged meats benefited from the heavy flavors and thick textures of roux and emulsified sauces. Nutritional cooking, however, which uses the natural flavors of foods to stimulate appetites and please palates, dictates that sauces and all accompaniments must enhance and complement the flavors of other foods, not hide them.

The wines and brandies used in traditional sauce preparation can still be used in nutritional cooking. Using them in various cooking and baking applications is a great way to build complex flavors with no fat. The alcohol either evaporates when cooked or is so low when the cooking is complete that it does not affect the overall caloric or nutritional values of the dish.

We have so many ways of thickening stocks to make sauces today that the traditional roux could be permanently retired from a cook's repertoire. For nutritional cooking, the options are unlimited. A lot of traditional sauces, like velouté, béchamel, and espagnole and all their derivative sauces, can be thickened by using arrowroot, cornstarch, and other refined starches in place of the roux.

Never add dried starch to liquid, for it will clump together. Place dry starch in a cup or container and then add enough cold liquid to thoroughly dissolve the starch. Once the starch is completely dissolved into a slurry, pour it into simmering stock to create the sauce.

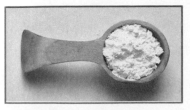

Cornstarch helps thicken sauces without the use of any fat.
Dave King © Dorling Kindersley

Add flavoring ingredients like wine, shallots, herbs, spices, and vegetable garnishes just as you would for roux-thickened sauces to make a variety of healthy sauce recipes.

The thickening process for sauces is not the only factor that affects nutrition. The stock or other flavored liquid that is used as the body of the sauce can contribute large amounts of vitamins, minerals, and flavonoids to the finished plate if prepared with nutritional goals in mind.

Make chicken, beef, and seafood stocks using additional flavoring ingredients in the mirepoix besides the traditional carrots, celery, and onion. Add other root vegetables like turnips, rutabagas, and golden beets to the traditional choices to contribute a greater variety of nutrients. Fresh parsley and other fresh herbs add several beneficial vitamins and minerals to stocks and the sauces that are derived from them; use these freely in the last hour of cooking the stock.

Bone and marrow fat used in stocks naturally floats to the top as the stock cools. Remove as much of the fat as possible before making sauces; lean stocks make for healthier sauces.

A lot of sauce recipes call for additional mirepoix to be sautéed in fat and floured to make a roux. In nutritional cooking, increase the mirepoix to include a variety of ingredients. Dry sauté the mirepoix in a hot pan (with no fat) until the edges turn brown, for brown sauce, or in a pan with additional stock to sweat them for a more natural color, appearance, and flavor.

Do not strain out the extra cooked vegetables in these preparations, but purée them together with the thickened sauce to create a full-bodied sauce. The finished sauce will be lighter in color with a coarse texture and mouth feel, but it will provide greater nutrition than it would if you threw out the cooked flavoring vegetables.

Arrowroot and cornstarch thicken stocks, milk (for béchamel), and other flavored liquids to a similar consistency as those thickened by rouxs. Arrowroot tends to leave the finished sauce or dressing clear or opaque and is preferred when thickening salad dressings and pie fillings. Cornstarch works well for brown sauces, velouté, and béchamel-based sauces.

Rice, potatoes, dried beans (legumes), and peas (split peas) are other healthy choices as thickening agents for soups and sauces. Rice was the original thickening agent in classic bisque preparations before roux became popular. Simply cook the rice, potatoes, beans, or peas directly in the liquid to be thickened. When done, purée all the ingredients together for a lightly thickened sauce or soup.

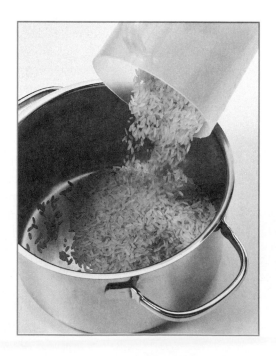

Rice was one of the original thickening agents used for soups and sauces.
Dave King © Dorling Kindersley

The starch from the rice, potatoes, beans, and peas helps thicken the liquid with no added fat. Add cooked vegetables or some other garnish to the finished sauce after purée-ing the thickening agent.

Match the color of the vegetable thickener with the desired color of the finished sauce. Unlike rouxs, which change color from white to brown depending on how long they are cooked, vegetable thickeners do not. White rice, potatoes, and beans are the best thickeners for light-colored soups and sauces since they too are light in color. Brown rice and pinto beans are best suited for darker-colored soups and sauces.

Asian, African, Middle Eastern, and Latino foods do not largely depend on rouxs, eggs, or butter for sauce preparation but rely on starch-thickened (cornstarch) and reduction-style sauces for their dishes. Neither butter fat nor animal fat (lard) were readily available to these cultures, so they relied on the natural thickening properties of vegetables and starches to make accompanying sauces when developing their characteristic cuisines.

Today, many of those traditional sauces remain popular. These include chutneys, salsas, and puréed seed, nut, and legume dipping sauces and spreads; they already meet high nutritional values and do not need to be replaced to improve nutrition.

Reduction sauces are also a good nutritional accompaniment since they contain little or no fat. They are poor substitutes for classic or traditional sauces but are excellent choices when creating new recipes.

Reduction sauces are stocks and other flavoring ingredients like wine, shallots, herbs, and spices that are cooked together over an open flame to reduce the liquid content. As the water evaporates from the stock, the sauce thickens slightly. Reduced sauces will never have the same appearance and mouth feel as roux-thickened sauces, yet they do have a higher level of natural flavors to complement a greater variety of tasty foods.

SUBSTITUTING FATS FOR HEALTHIER COOKING

Although Americans should reduce all of their fat consumption, the biggest culprits are fats that contain large amounts of saturated fatty acids (butter, clarified butter, margarine, bacon grease, lard, and vegetable shortenings). Most recipes that call for these fats can be altered by making simple substitutions that reduce unhealthy saturated fats and still provide great flavor and taste.

Before making substitutions, determine the purpose of using particular fats in recipes. Are they used as cooking media, to keep foods from sticking to hot pans or grills, for flavor only, or for a combination of cooking method and flavor? In some cases, exchanges can be made with few other recipe adjustments. In other cases, exchanges may require significant changes in the recipe to produce the same or a similar dish.

Problems arise when you try to make substitutions in an item like pound cake, which is very high in fat and saturated fat, based on levels of saturated fats only, and expect something that tastes and looks the same as before. This is an unrealistic expectation. Although there are low-fat pound cakes on the commercial market, these are made by large bakery conglomerates with all the latest scientific knowledge and skills. Such companies use technology that is not available to restaurant chefs. This technology involves microparticulated proteins and special gums that create the feel of fat in the mouth.

Other bakery items like sponge cakes, pies, and muffins can have acceptable tastes and mouth feel if vegetable oils (which are naturally low in saturated fatty acids) are substituted for butter, margarine, lard, or shortening. To offset the loss of moisture in finished

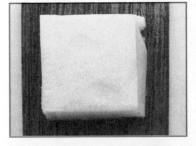

Lard is no longer considered a healthy fat.
Ian O'Leary © Dorling Kindersley

baked products, add apple juice concentrate, puréed bananas, or a variety of other fruit purées to the recipe. Neither apple juice concentrate, bananas, nor other fruit purées will significantly alter the taste of the finished product but will provide sweetness and moisture during baking and drying. Sweetness, one of the five basic tastes, stimulates the mouth's taste buds and saliva secretions. The end result will be a moist product, full of flavor and with an adequate mouth feel and much less fat.

If the baking structure, or rise, is lessened because of a reduction in eggs or saturated fats (which trap air molecules during mixing and provide solid, internal structure), the addition of whipped egg whites can help. Whipping egg whites traps air bubbles in the egg whites' albumen, ovalbumin, and other proteins, causing them to stretch and expand in volume and then stabilize so they do not break. The trapped air in meringue (whipped egg whites) helps make chiffon pie fillings light and fluffy; in baked goods, like soufflés and cakes, the trapped gases in the protein strands expand under heat, creating rise in the product.

For baking, vegetable oils are not the best substitutions in all cases. In rolled-in dough and pastries, such as puff pastry, Danish, and flaky pie crusts, the substitutions do not work. In cakes, muffins, and breads, oils work just as well as butter or shortening, but with a slightly lower volume. This difference in volume can be overcome by the addition of whipped egg whites before baking. Whipped egg whites give volume to bakery products because of the air that is trapped in their protein strands.

Replacing butter with oil is a sound nutritional choice, but taste is compromised. The lost buttery flavor should be replaced with other flavorful ingredients, such as puréed fruits, vegetables, vanilla, extracts, or liqueurs.

Vegetable oils can be substituted for butter, margarine, bacon fat, or other highly saturated fats in many dry-heat cooking methods, such as sautéing or pan-frying, either partially or entirely without significantly changing the cooking method. To reduce fats even further, use nonstick cooking pans or grills.

Another helpful way of reducing the overall fat used in cooking is to measure the exact amount of fat needed to sauté, grill, or marinate foods instead of pouring the fat into the pot or pan. Pouring fat can easily supply two or three times the amount of fat actually needed.

Cooks often use a large ladle to carry oil or clarified butter to the pan for cooking when 1 or 2 teaspoons are all that is required, since it can be cumbersome to measure this small amount in a spoon. A smaller ladle, however, is better for this purpose. Similarly, cooks often ladle a generous supply of fat across the face of a grill to make sure that enough fat remains on the surface for proper cooking and does not all end up in the grease

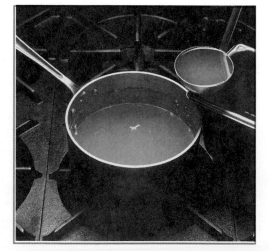

Use a ladle or other measuring device whenever adding fat to a pan or dish.
Pearson Education/PH College

tray. But simply putting the oil or clarified butter into a spray bottle and giving a pan or grill one spray at a time will distribute the fat in a fine mist (less than 1 teaspoon per spray) evenly over small and large surfaces. For easiest application, keep both oil and clarified butter spray bottles in a hot bain-marie, either on or near the stove, to keep the fat free flowing.

In recipes that call for whole or clarified butter in sautéing, use a nonflavored vegetable oil instead. Nonflavored vegetable oils include safflower, sunflower, and canola oils. These oils produce the same effect as butter in cooking (providing an even exchange of heat and a nonstick medium), but without the saturated fat.

Even though butter and lard are staples in traditional cooking and baking, new information on the use of vegetable oils makes substitution a simple and healthy process in most cases. Margarine is often substituted for butter and vegetable shortening for lard, but these hydrogenated fats have the same ill effects as saturated fats. It is better to use one of the many liquid vegetable oils whenever possible because they contain no cholesterol and low amounts of saturated fats.

Olive and sesame seed oils are ancient in origin, but some chefs today don't use them because of their pronounced flavors. Using flavored oils in moderation and in combination with nonstick pans, which require little or no oil, can produce tasty and healthier results.

New techniques in oil extraction have given chefs a greater variety of vegetable oils to choose from. Sunflower, safflower, rapeseed, corn, peanut, walnut, and sesame oils are readily available. Even the traditional oils like olive oil are now available in lighter-tasting forms. Olive oil can be purchased in extra virgin, virgin, pure, and light versions, each with a different intensity of olive flavor.

One problem with using liquid oils instead of hydrogenated oils is lower smoking points. Smoking point is the temperature at which the oil will burn and give off an unpleasant taste. For frying, a simple solution to the lower smoking points of liquid oils is to trim the size of foods and remove bones whenever possible. This enables the foods to cook quickly at lower temperatures. When it is impossible to do so, the items can be completed in a very hot oven, which will finish the cooking process and retain the desired crisp texture.

A lower smoking point also means that the fat in the oil breaks down more quickly and must be replaced sooner. A sign that the oil is breaking down is that it smokes while heating up in the fryer. Filtering the oil after each day's use will help remove food particles and keep the oil fresher longer.

Another way to replace saturated animal fats with vegetable oils and to increase taste at the same time is to marinate trimmed and naturally lean meats and poultry with a variety of tasty marinades. For meats and poultry containing a lot of exterior fat, trim the excess fat off first, which is loaded with saturated fatty acids, and then marinade the meat in flavorful liquids that contain less saturated vegetable oils.

It is the interior fat in meat that, when cooked, makes the finished product tender and juicy. Therefore, leaner cuts of meat like flank steak and first-cut brisket are naturally less tender and juicy than fattier meats. To use these leaner types of meats in quality presentations you need to create flavorful marinades that tenderize and season the tough muscle tissue or to use slow-cooking methods like braising or stewing to make the flesh more palatable.

Marinades are flavored liquids used to tenderize and impart flavor and moisture to lean cuts of meats. Lean parts of poultry, such as skinless breasts, and seafood do not require tenderization yet often are marinated for the flavors that marinades can provide. Tough meats can be softened by soaking them in acidic marinades (containing vinegar, wine, tomato, or other acidic cooking ingredients) for two to three days. Tender cuts of meat, poultry, and seafood need only a few hours to extract an appropriate amount of flavor from the marinade ingredients.

Typically oil, flavoring ingredients, vinegars, wine, or other acidic ingredients are used in marinades. Keep marinades low in saturated fats and full of flavor by using canola, olive, or corn oil; fresh chopped herbs; ground spices; and a host of flavoring vegetables like celery, onion, ginger, and garlic.

With proper planning chefs can find creative ways of serving leaner cuts of meat, such as beef brisket, flank steak, and shoulder (chuck) roasts by using marinades and slow cooking. Use the cooking liquids in the final sauces to transfer the leached-out nutrients onto the served plate.

In reducing fat, you lose some flavor. This is the area in which most nutritional recipe conversions fail: The importance of taste in a healthier recipe is forgotten. Chefs must realize that flavor must be re-created. When fat that is used in part or entirely for flavor is removed from the original recipe, other ingredients must provide an equivalent level of flavor. This practice will preserve full taste in the finished product.

If you want the flavor of butter but the health benefits of oil, sauté in oil and add butter, as you would any seasoning, at the end of the cooking process. A recipe that calls for 2 or 3 tablespoons of butter as a frying medium may be cut back to only 1 teaspoon of butter when the butter is treated as a seasoning. The delicate flavor of the butter is present in the final dish, but the benefits of cooking with oil are realized.

Using stock to sauté vegetables greatly affects the amount of fat in the finished dish. Although the use of stock is not part of the true definition of sautéing, the results are the same: the heating of prepared vegetables for table service. A carefully measured amount of butter (about 1/2 teaspoon per serving, for approximately 17 calories) added to the sauté pan after the vegetables have been heated through gives the taste of butter without all the fat.

If butter is not the desired flavor, then your choices are many. Using fresh herbs and aromatic vegetables together with the main ingredients can add great amounts of flavor to very basic preparations. Instead of sautéing green beans in butter, try sautéing them with red pimento slices and sweet basil; add some garlic or shallots if you want even more flavor. Instead of chicken breast sautéed in butter, try chicken breast sautéed with fresh thyme, lemon, and cracked peppercorns.

In place of bacon fat (used by many southern cooks to season vegetables), try using hickory-smoked turkey wings, backs, or necks sautéed lightly in vegetable oil instead. Sauté the turkey parts in plain vegetable oil for 10 minutes; then strain and reserve the oil. Using a teaspoon or two of this oil in flavoring braised cabbage, steamed Brussels sprouts, sautéed green beans, or any other bean recipe will impart a great smoky flavor without adding the saturated fat of bacon.

In grilling or broiling steaks, chops, and chicken, first remove all the exterior fat and skin from the meat. Use a knife to trim the solid fat as close to the meat as you can. Then prepare a marinade of flavored liquids, herbs, and spices that can be brushed onto the item just before cooking. This gives flavor back to the meat in which the flavor of the fat has been drastically reduced. The small amount of oil needed to keep these items from sticking to the grill can be supplied by brushing or spraying 1/2 to 1 teaspoon of oil onto the cooking surface. This method reduces the amount of fat in grilled or broiled items by as much as 60%.

To reduce the fat in other cooking and baking preparations, make the following substitutions: evaporated skim milk for heavy cream, low-fat yogurt for sour cream, and part skim-milk cheese for whole-milk cheeses. Take a careful look at the remaining flavors and make substitutions or additions that will replace the level of flavor.

The simplest way to reduce natural saturated fat in cooking is to cut exterior fat away from meats and poultry before cooking them. The visible fat on steaks, chops, and roasts can be cut away with a sharp knife easily when the food is still raw.

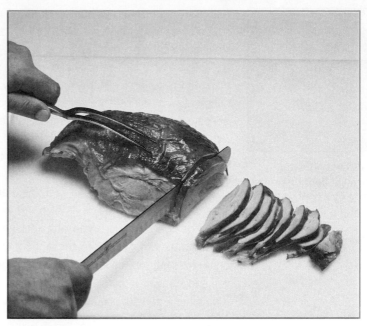

Smoked turkey makes an excellent flavoring ingredient in place of fatty bacon.
Pearson Education/PH College

PORTIONING

The proper portioning of high-fat foods is a simple way to control fat consumption. Simple answers are usually not the full story, however. Although both the ADA and AMA recommend that meat consumption be limited to 3 ounces three times per week, most Americans eat much more than that, often in a single meal. The 10-ounce filet mignon 12-ounce rib eye steaks, and 16-ounce sirloin steaks on restaurant menus across America make it difficult to follow more stringent guidelines.

Imagine a diet that starts out with a three-egg omelet in the morning, a ham-and-cheese sandwich for lunch, and roasted Prime Rib for dinner. The amount of fat in this diet, especially saturated fats and cholesterol, soars off any recommended dietary chart. The problem, however, is one of appetite: Does a two-egg omelet satisfy the consumer's hunger? Will 3 to 5 ounces of roasted Prime Rib leave the consumer wanting more?

In making omelets, some or all of the eggs can be substituted with commercially prepared egg substitutes that contain no fat and no cholesterol, but taste may be sacrificed. A two-egg omelet made with real eggs seems small and unsatisfying unless you incorporate air into the egg mixture before cooking it and serve the omelet with many varieties of vegetable fillings. Whipping air into eggs, either by hand or with a blender, will cause the omelet to soufflé during cooking. This will add height and structure to the small amount of product. Filling the cooked omelet with steamed julienne vegetables like carrots, celery, onions, fresh chopped parsley, chopped basil, or spinach will present a satisfying array of flavors and a quantity of food that will please even the hungriest of diners. Adding extra egg whites, which contain no fat or cholesterol, also increases the bulk of the final omelet.

Reducing the amount of meat in a serving will reduce the amount of fat in the diet, but if diners walk away hungry, they are likely to eat other foods later to compensate. Likewise, customers who leave restaurants unsatisfied with the size of portions are reluctant to return.

Don't reduce the amount of meat in dishes and do nothing else; add back volume by creating combination dinners like stews, stir-fries, and casseroles. A braised beef ragout

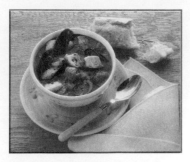

Ragouts and stews offer good nutrition through limiting protein and offering a variety of vegetables for nutrition, flavor, and texture.
© *Dorling Kindersley*

full of tourné turnips, potatoes, carrots, pearl onions, green beans, herbs, spices, and a sauce made from lean beef stock or vegetable stock limits the amount of meat consumed and satisfies the heartiest appetite as well.

Try serving beef with pasta, or chicken with rice. These combination dinners, when created with flavor as the number one priority, reduce the amount of meat the average diner consumes but still satisfy even the most discriminating restaurant guests. Don't call the dish beef stew, but Ragout of Beef Primavera, served with fresh tourné garden vegetables and a rich-flavored sauce. Instead of chicken and rice, create a new dish using breast of chicken, fresh chopped broccoli flowers, diced fresh tomatoes, cumin, and scallion tops and then call it Fricassee of Chicken Portuguese, offering a healthier, yet similar, preparation.

If reduction of fats is the goal, there are thousands of alternative solutions. Meat and fat substitution replaces foods high in saturated fats with other foods lower in saturated fats. The use of modern nonstick cooking pans and grills reduces the need for fat as a cooking medium. Measuring the amount of fat with either a spoon, a small ladle, or a spray bottle will help provide lower-fat cooked products. Portioning, with a plan to satisfy both flavor and hunger, becomes a tool the chef can use to design great dining pleasure while maintaining nutritional guidelines.

CREATE NEW HEALTHIER RECIPES

Often cooks and chefs are given the opportunity to create entirely new recipes based on nutritional standards. It is a great challenge to make healthy food taste and look good too. These recipes need to be based on measurable nutritional information, not guesswork, with controls put in place during the entire process of ordering, preparing, and cooking the foods to ensure that higher nutrition is achieved.

The first step in designing new healthy recipes is to decide the dietary goals you want to achieve. Here are some questions to ask:

1. Do you want to create an item with no fat, or is a low-fat (under 10% calories from fat) item acceptable?
2. Are you designing a high-carbohydrate or a low-carbohydrate diet; a high-protein or a low-protein diet? Obviously each requires different types of recipes.
3. Do you need to keep sodium at acceptable levels or reduce it as much as possible?
4. What total caloric content is acceptable for the meal?
5. What vitamins and minerals do you want to serve through food?

Based on your answers to the questions above, you will be able to select from a various foods and cooking methods to achieve the desired results.

Recipes do not always have to meet the highest nutritional standards possible. Healthy diets are based on balance and exercise and not on restrictions and abstinence.

Healthy recipes are those that present the most nutrients given the desired end result of the dining guest. Even a Prime Rib dinner and a fried shrimp appetizer can be presented with higher nutritional values to please the discriminating palate of customers while offering tasty, healthy foods.

The second step in designing new healthy recipes is to select the main food item (meat, poultry, seafood, or vegetable protein) to be presented and the cooking technique that you intend to use. Kitchen design, the experience level of the staff on hand to perform

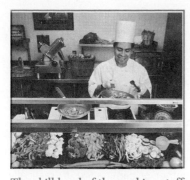

The skill level of the cooking staff is critical to the success of all menu items.
Silver Burdett Ginn

the cooking techniques, and the desired nutritional results are all factors that must be considered in this selection. You should not design new recipes calling for the braising technique if your kitchen is limited to oven space; nor should poaching become a regular recipe cooking technique if the top burner space or cooktop space is too small to keep the simmering pans cooking. Recipe development should always be based first on available equipment and second on the skill level of the staff in order to ensure the recipe's success.

The skill level of the cooking staff is critically important to the success of all menu items. Designing healthy yet complicated recipes that are difficult to execute properly will only result in poorly presented food that the customer will ultimately reject.

Provided that the staff can accommodate multiple cooking techniques and the kitchen has an ample selection of cooking equipment, selecting low-fat or no-fat cooking procedures is the best way to provide healthier foods to guests and customers.

Main plate items can be selected from a world full of animal, bird, fish, shellfish, and plant species. From many animal species, a large selection of cuts, shapes, and sizes of items helps determine the nutritional values in the final presentation. Be sure to research each food item through printed bulletins, online databases, or nutritional analysis software to ensure the item has the nutritional makeup your recipe requires.

Once you have selected the main food item and the cooking technique required to cook it properly, the portion size is the next factor to design. As discussed earlier in this chapter, portion sizes are based on two factors: the USDA recommendations for portions and the customer's expectations. So portioning is partly defined by the overall fat and caloric content you require for the nutritional goals set for that particular recipe, and partly by the demands of the paying guest. You can compromise with the customer on the portion sizes of main plate items by designing delicious accompaniments and attractive combined food presentations.

If the portion size you determine meets both customer and nutritional demands, you need to decide if it can stand alone or should be incorporated into a combined food presentation to enhance the appearance of the finished food. A boneless breast of chicken, for example, can stand alone as the main plate item for lunch but may not be enough to satisfy the hunger and expectation of a dinner guest. That same single boneless chicken breast can be made into skewers; served with rice, pasta, or a variety of farinaceous foods and by-products; or combined with vegetables in a stir-fry to appease even the hungriest diners.

Herbs, spices, and other natural ingredients should be used specifically for the taste, colors, textures, and nutrients they provide. They should be used to season main food items, sauces, and all plate accompaniments. You should incorporate seasonings into each of the cooking or preparation stages to create complex flavors that are blends and variations of the flavors used. Seasonings are typically added at the beginning of the recipe and then during the final cooking or marinating stages to ensure an intensification of flavors throughout the cooking process.

Freshly chopped herbs or freshly ground spices stirred into a dish just before service give a fresh-tasting characteristic to the finished flavors. Likewise, a small amount of wine, liqueur, or brandy laced into a soup or sauce before plating can enliven flavors without overpowering the main ingredients.

The use of low-fat meat items will greatly affect the flavor of the final dish. When these items are chosen, be sure to add something back into the recipe to replace some of the missing flavor and moisture of fat. For example, a traditional Beef Chili can become Turkey Chili with Cilantro and Sun-Dried Tomatoes, offering the guest a full-flavored menu item with less fat. The cilantro adds a contrasting flavor, which makes the whole spoonful rich with flavor, and the sun-dried tomatoes (partially hydrated by the chili's natural broth) add back moisture in every bite. Beef Stroganoff can become Venison Stroganoff with Plum Tomatoes and Fresh Yogurt; both the tomatoes and fat-free yogurt replace some of the flavors and moisture lost by substituting venison (a lean animal) for fattier beef. Many variations like these can be realized by having an open mind and using a little creativity.

Successful healthy baking also can be achieved when the same principles used to prepare flavorful and nutritious appetizers and entrees are applied to baking formulas and dessert presentations. Knowledge of the ingredients, their use in the baking process, as well as the flavors they impart and skill in manipulating ingredients according to the science of baking are the tools needed to produce healthy desserts.

The choice of baking ingredients depends on the desired final results. Baking follows a strict chemistry, and substituting one ingredient for another or eliminating it drastically changes the results. Therefore, we must look for baking and serving strategies instead of simple substitutions when designing low-fat healthy desserts.

New desserts can be designed that contain less fat and calories and more vitamins, minerals, and fiber with just as much flavor, plate presentation, and dining appeal as traditional desserts. Consider that all the parts that make up a dessert—the base, filling, icing, sauce, and garnish—are subject to nutritional concerns and that each contributes to the appeal of the final product.

Concern about nutrition and desserts centers on fat-laden icings and fillings and the large amounts of refined sugars and flours that the majority of baking formulas use. Cholesterol-rich, laden in saturated fats, and high in empty calories, traditional desserts are far from healthy. With proper planning, however, even a génoise can be used as the base of many healthy desserts designed to fit nutritional guidelines.

The following guidelines will help you prepare nutritious and tasty desserts:

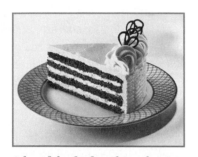

A lot of the fat found in cakes is in the icing.
Dave King © Dorling Kindersley

- Substitute skim milk for whole or low-fat milk.
- Use low-fat mock sour cream or low-fat yogurt for sour cream.
- Try egg substitutes for whole eggs.
- Replace all or part of the egg requirement with egg whites only.
- Add whole-wheat, rye, buckwheat, or oat flours to basic formulas.
- Use low-fat condensed milk or soft tofu instead of cream.
- Substitute cocoa for baking chocolate.
- Use natural condensed fruit juices in place of refined sugars.

When an ingredient is substituted for or eliminated because of fat content, flavor is also sacrificed. Prudent cooks understand this fact and make adjustments through the selection and use of other flavorful ingredients. Extracts, real fruit, fruit juices, fruit zest, honey, molasses, wines, liqueurs, and brandies are important flavor ingredients in healthful baking. A dessert with reduced fat and calories but no flavor will not be a success. The goal of nutritional baking is to follow dietary guidelines yet still create desserts that people will savor and enjoy.

STAFF DEVELOPMENT

Chefs or dining room managers may want to offer low-fat, low-sodium choices to their customers. But their plans are easily foiled if their waitstaff and kitchen staff are not properly trained to deliver such alternatives.

The wait staff are the salespersons and ambassadors for the restaurant. They must be trained to answer the questions customers will ask. Servers must know the preparation methods and ingredients for all menu items. They also must have a basic understanding of nutritional cooking so they will know what substitutions can transform a traditional recipe to a more nutritionally balanced recipe. Can the chef use oil instead of butter or no fat at all in any particular recipe? Can the flounder be broiled or baked instead of fried? Can the customer substitute a small salad for the baked potato or a vegetable for the fries? Nutritional awareness will enable the waitstaff to help customers make sensible choices. Customers will view an informed waitstaff as a valuable part of the dining experience.

Make sure all members of the waitstaff taste all new menu items, all specials, and all nontraditional menu items. They can then give their honest opinions to inquiring customers. If a waitperson does not like the taste of a dish, the chef must find out why. Customers may agree with the waitperson.

The kitchen staff must also be trained in nutritional cooking concepts so they can make alterations and substitutions within company policy and sound nutritional guidelines. It doesn't help to send out a baked flounder, requested by the customer for its lower fat content, if the cook brushes butter on top just before serving it. And if the chef has vegetable stocks available for vegetarian diners, the staff must be trained in their proper use.

Cooks and other food professionals must be trained to use their own judgment in making foods healthier to consume. They must have plenty of fresh ingredients on hand, including fresh herbs and an abundance of flavoring vegetables, to add flavor and substance. They can add these to a variety of dishes when called upon to reduce meats, fat, and sodium at the customer's request.

Waitstaff and cooks must also be trained on food allergies and intolerances. There are multiple circumstances in which restaurants and other food operations may be held liable for waiters and waitresses who give out false information to customers regarding the food composition of menu items.

Peanuts, nuts in general, gluten, dairy, onions, and shellfish are the most common food allergies. Each of these can cause serious injury, discomfort, and possibly death to some unsuspecting customers. Assumptions made by the staff can cause serious injury to a customer who has an allergy or food intolerance and can cause great legal problems for the entire operation.

Waitstaff as well as cooks therefore must learn the composition of the food they serve. When in doubt, they can be taught to ask the chef or kitchen manager for guidance. If a customer claims to be allergic to a certain food and the waitstaff recommends a menu item, problems can occur if the waitstaff is not correct.

For example, a customer may claim to be allergic to onions and unable to eat anything with onions in it. The server examines the menu and sees a lot of item descriptions that do not mention onions. On the basis of this observation, he or she invites the customer to choose one of these menu items. However, although onions seem not to be used in many recipes, in fact they are used in a very high percentage of recipes.

A trained staff knows the ingredients of every recipe. They also know the importance of checking with management when confronted with a customer who makes any kind of health or allergy/intolerance claim.

The importance of a trained, knowledgeable staff in both the front and the back of the house is critical to the success of all operations. Giving a customer good service includes providing good, accurate information on all the food on the menu and how it is prepared.

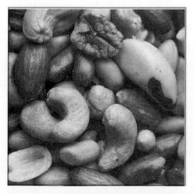

Many people who are allergic to peanuts are also allergic to other nuts.
Photo Researchers, Inc.

Trim the Fat, but Keep the Flavor

The knowledgeable and creative chef has many options when choosing recipe ingredients and cooking techniques to increase the nutritional values of the foods they serve. Healthy versions of traditional recipes should be given different names that the customers can recognize as new healthy creations and not poor substitutions for classic or popular dishes.

Improving the nutritional value of more complex recipes requires a thorough evaluation of each of the recipe ingredients and procedures, which increases challenges for chefs. Substitutions can be made for ingredients, healthy ingredients can be added, fats can be manipulated, and preparation and cooking techniques can be modified to improve nutrition, but the flavors, textures, and eye appeal of the final dish must also be protected.

CASE RESOLUTION

Chef Mike should reexamine the components of the original recipes that he used for the dinner party and determine which contained the most flavor and textures but also contributed high amounts of fat and sodium. Then he can make smart substitutions of lean meats for fatty ones; choose a variety of fresh vegetables; and add back flavors through the use of fresh herbs, spices, flavoring vegetables, and alcoholic beverages like wine, beer, and liqueurs to recreate the recipes into dishes that not only are good for his guests to eat but satisfy both their palates and their hunger.

Hillman, H. 1981. *Kitchen Science*. Boston: Houghton Mifflin.

Hodges, A. 1989. *Culinary Nutrition for Foodservice Professionals*. New York: Van Nostrand Reinhold.

The Encyclopedia of Organic Gardening. 1978. Emmaus, PA: Rodale Press.

1. What is meant by the whole plate concept when referring to healthy cooking and dining?
2. In what types of recipes would it be appropriate to make a full protein or fat substitution when transforming them into healthier versions?
3. In what ways can a cook reduce the overall amount of fat in a meal without changing any of the ingredients?
4. How can selective purchasing, proper storage, and nutritional cooking of food help ensure nutritional value from harvest to the table?
5. Why is a well trained waitstaff necessary to the success of a nutritional cooking program—whether it includes single menu items or the entire menu?

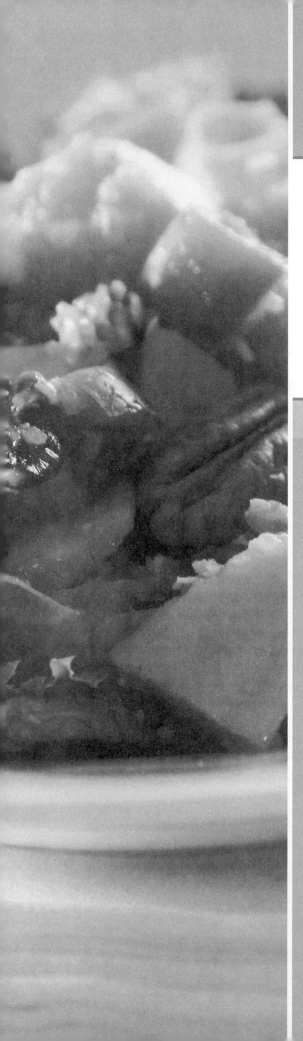

14

Menu Planning: Adding Nutritional Choices

KEY CONCEPTS

- A well-constructed menu is one that offers a variety of menu items for the adventurous, for the traditionalist, and for the nutritionally aware customer.

- Many ancient cuisines embody healthy guidelines: South Indian cuisine, Mexican cuisine, Spanish cuisine, American Indian cuisine, and Asian cuisine.

- The use of multiple cooking methods is essential to the task of supplying good nutrition to customers.

- The human body needs a regular supply of energy foods and nutrients throughout the day.

- Appetizers should be distinctive in flavors and textures, but not overpowering in style or presentation.

- Soups can supply all essential parts of a healthy meal in a single satisfying dish.

- The more complex and contrasting the flavors of the main salad ingredients, the less that dressing is needed to satisfy the guests' palate.

- The composition of the muscle(s), the amount of exterior fat, the amount of marbling (interior fat), and tenderness are all critical issues in the nutritional cooking of meat products.

- Research proves that seafood can be one of the healthiest protein items in human diets.

Preparing food to meet nutritional standards is only one concern of restaurant chefs and cooks; designing a menu that allows this flexibility without increased work or expense is of equal importance.

Nutrition is not something that is likely to disappear from the consumer consciousness. As knowledge of the relationship between health and nutrition continues to strengthen, so, too, will consumer demand for nutritionally prepared foods increase.

Successful restaurant operators and chefs try to learn the dynamics of their particular marketplace and offer products and services to attract a wide range of customers. Most restaurants offer a mix of standard and nutritionally designed menu items to appease this wide customer base. The ability of professional kitchens to meet all customer requests for better nutrition will ultimately determine the success of the operation.

Professional chefs play a crucial role in supplying nutritionally sound menu choices for otherwise standard menus. They are the technicians who must bring nutrition to the dining table either by introducing new menu items or by transforming standard menu items into more nutritionally oriented versions.

THINK ABOUT IT

How does the public perceive the notion of healthy eating? Is it something that most people strive to achieve, or is it still so abstract a concept that it is hard for the average person to grasp it and make a part of their lifestyles?

What if most, if not all, of a particular restaurant's menu items were designed to offer maximum nutrition, and yet were not labeled as nutritionally healthy? What would be the advantages and the disadvantages?

CASE STUDY

To Bread or Not to Bread?

Adrianna is a waitress for a thriving seafood restaurant in northeast Florida catering to "snow birds" (northern tourists who go to Florida during the winter and back to their northern homes for the summers) and locals who frequent the restaurant.

Recently, when the whole country was talking about the various low-carb diets that stopped everyone from wanting breads, potatoes, and pasta dishes, Adrianna was faced with a new slate of questions from her customers regarding the ingredients and cooking procedures used to prepare and serve the restaurant's extensive menu of seafood choices.

You might think that a seafood restaurant would not normally be asked these types of questions. But many of the items were breaded seafood items, so people did appear concerned over the amount of breading they would consume when eating their favorite fried fish, shrimp, or seafood platters.

One day Adrianna served a couple of customers who claimed to be from Illinois. Clearly they were one of the pairs of snow birds who came south every winter to enjoy Florida's warmer weather. They told her that, back home, a lot of the restaurants were offering and promoting low-carb menu items. Even potatoes and pastas, they claimed, were being promoted as low-carb. They did not understand how a potato or pasta could be low-carb, but the promotions and marketing made it seem logical and appropriate.

The question they had for Adrianna was whether the breading used to coat the fish before frying was low-carb, or did they have to order something else to meet their new-found nutritional concerns?

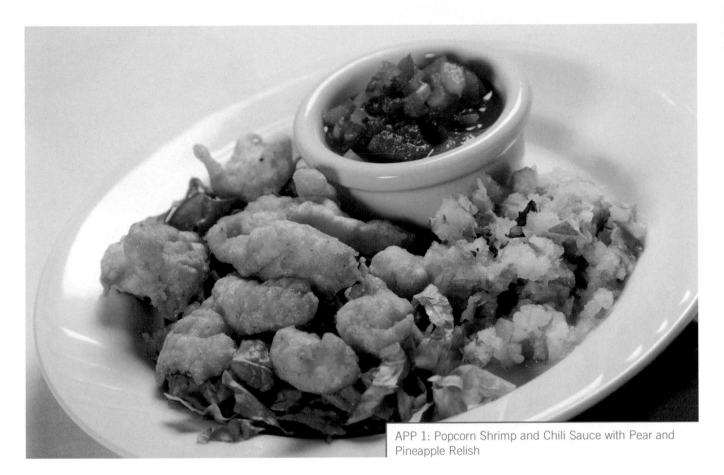

APP 1: Popcorn Shrimp and Chili Sauce with Pear and Pineapple Relish

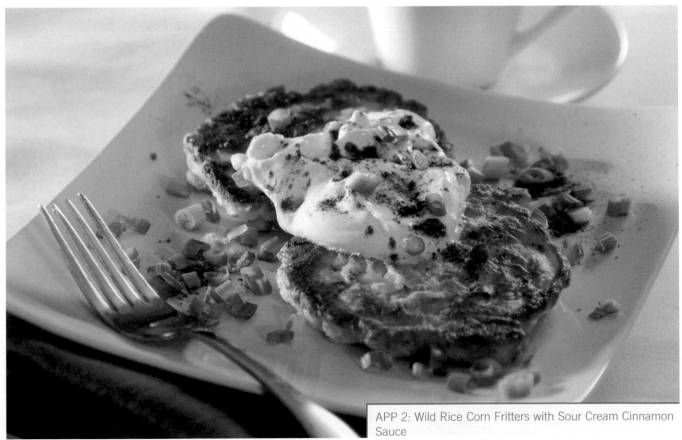

APP 2: Wild Rice Corn Fritters with Sour Cream Cinnamon Sauce

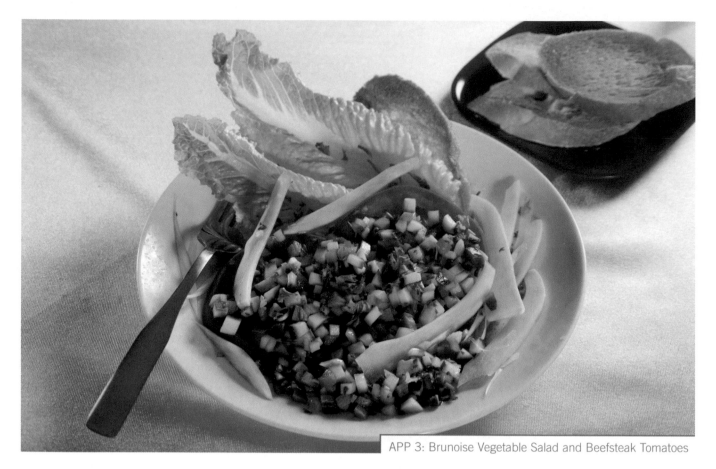

APP 3: Brunoise Vegetable Salad and Beefsteak Tomatoes

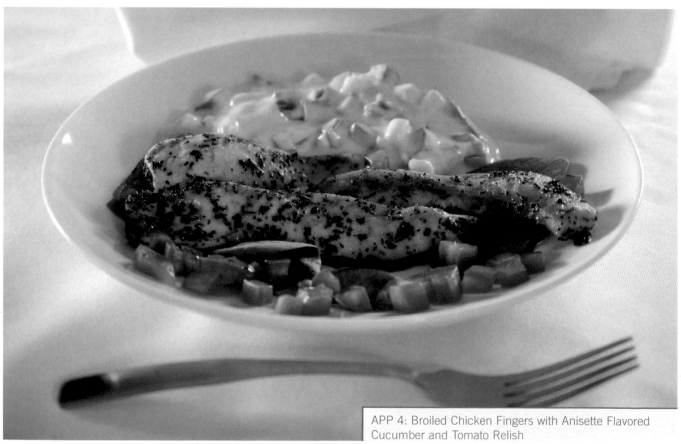

APP 4: Broiled Chicken Fingers with Anisette Flavored
Cucumber and Tomato Relish

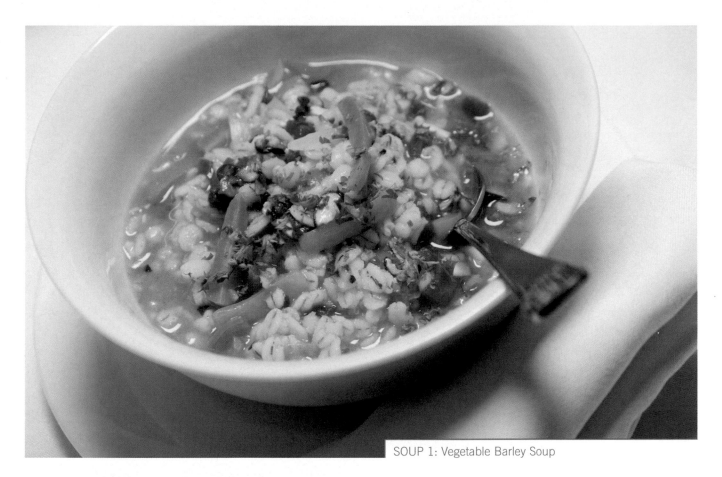

SOUP 1: Vegetable Barley Soup

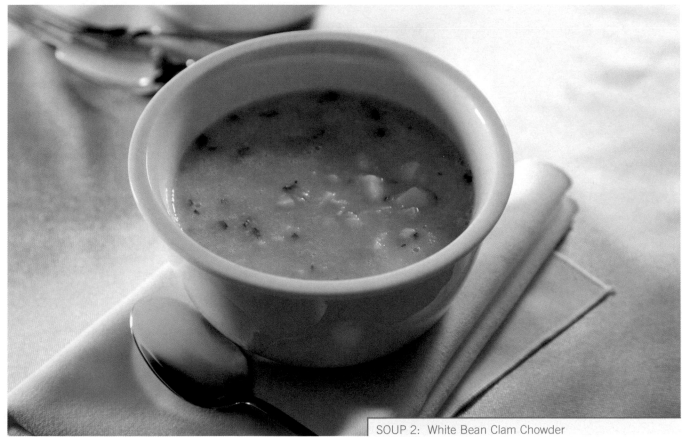

SOUP 2: White Bean Clam Chowder

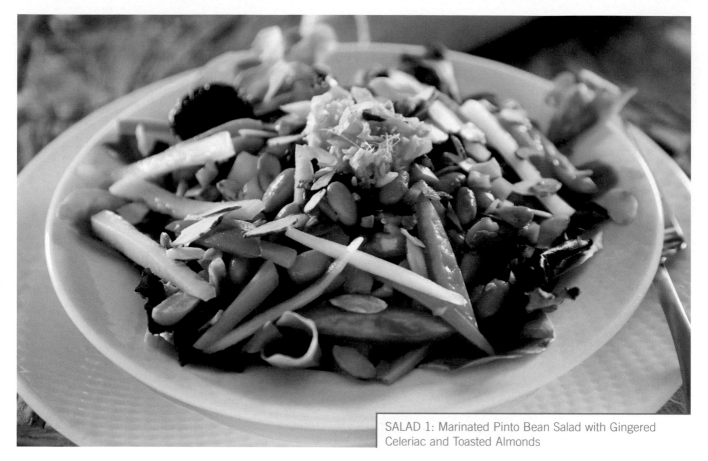

SALAD 1: Marinated Pinto Bean Salad with Gingered Celeriac and Toasted Almonds

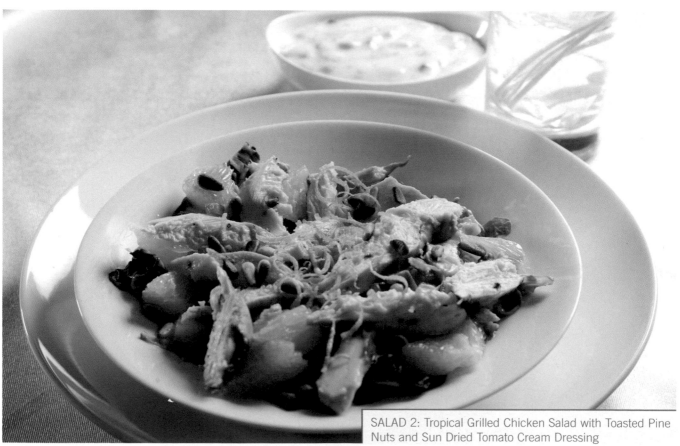

SALAD 2: Tropical Grilled Chicken Salad with Toasted Pine Nuts and Sun Dried Tomato Cream Dressing

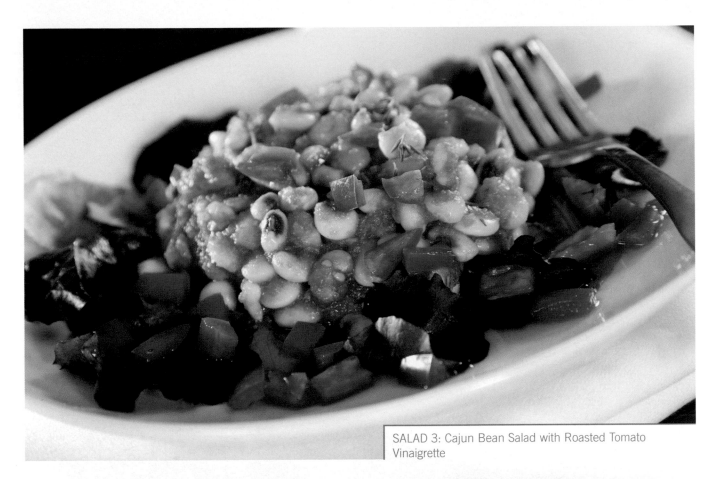

SALAD 3: Cajun Bean Salad with Roasted Tomato Vinaigrette

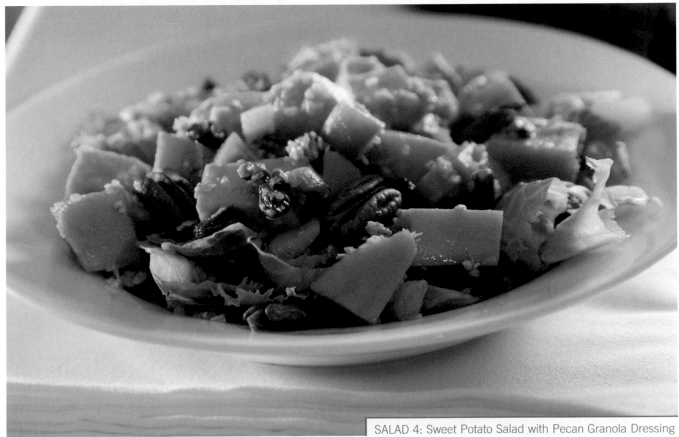

SALAD 4: Sweet Potato Salad with Pecan Granola Dressing

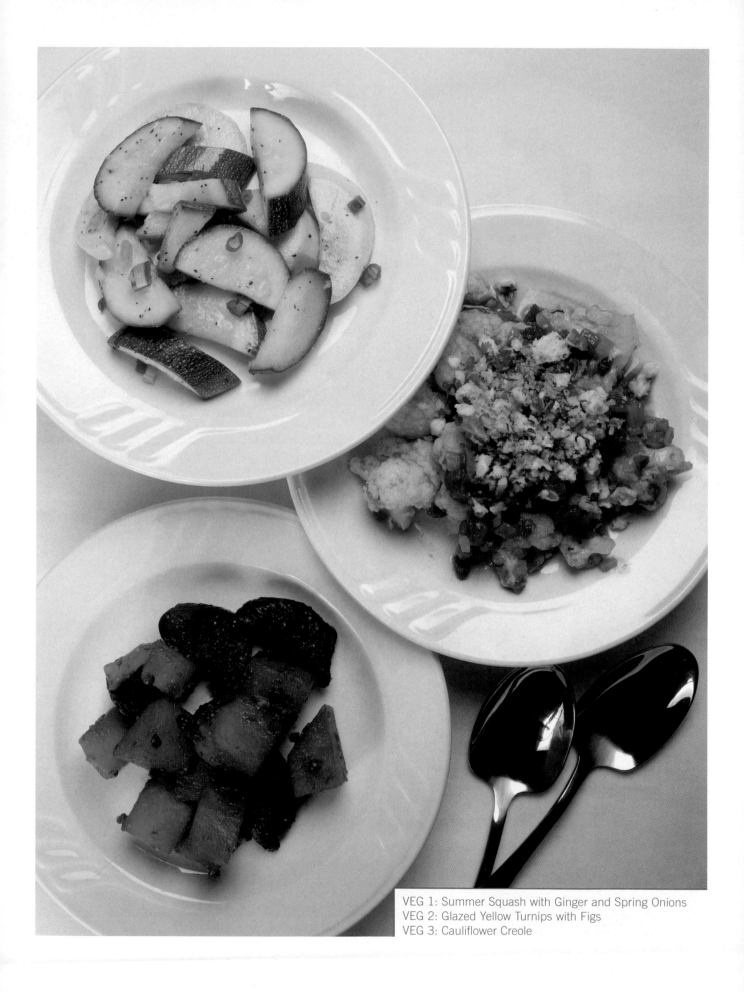

VEG 1: Summer Squash with Ginger and Spring Onions
VEG 2: Glazed Yellow Turnips with Figs
VEG 3: Cauliflower Creole

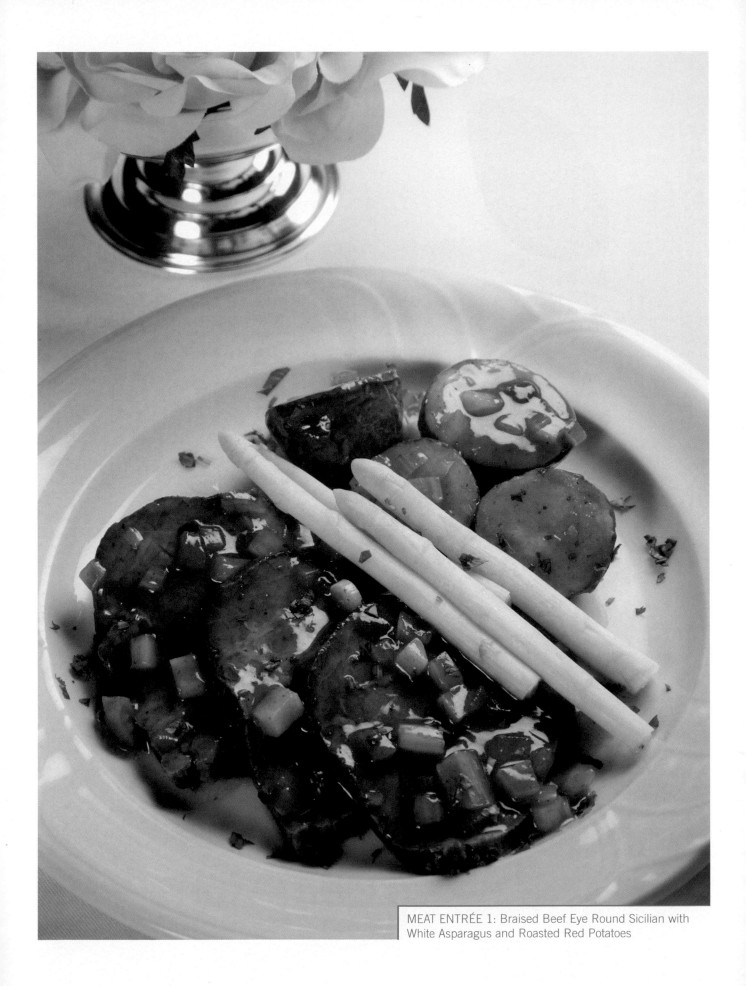

MEAT ENTRÉE 1: Braised Beef Eye Round Sicilian with White Asparagus and Roasted Red Potatoes

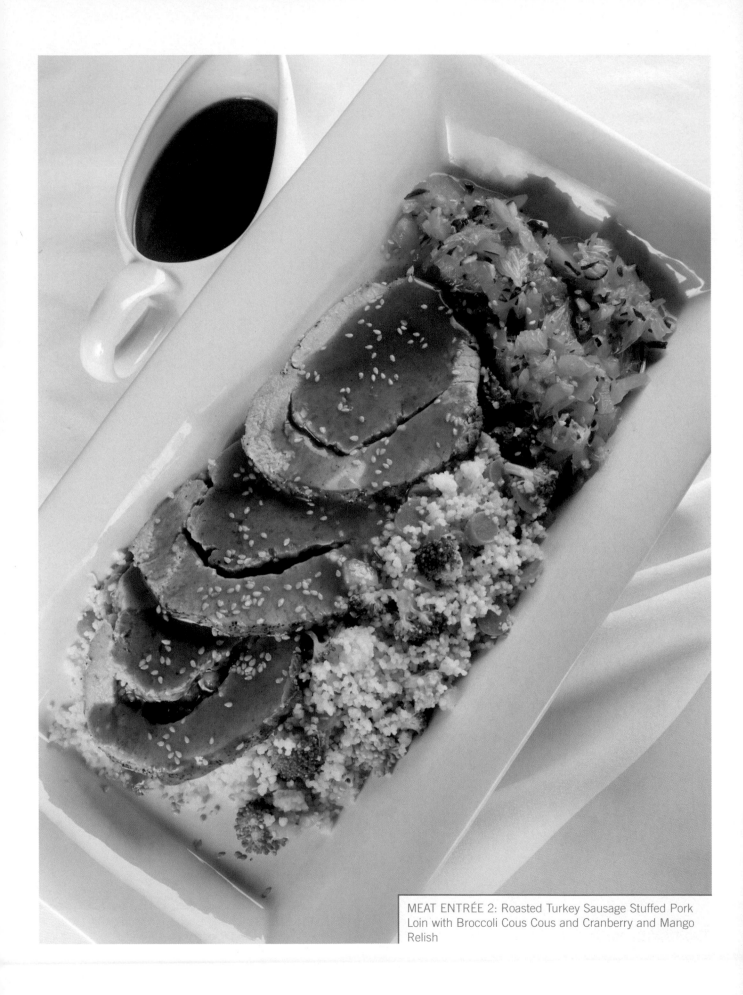

MEAT ENTRÉE 2: Roasted Turkey Sausage Stuffed Pork Loin with Broccoli Cous Cous and Cranberry and Mango Relish

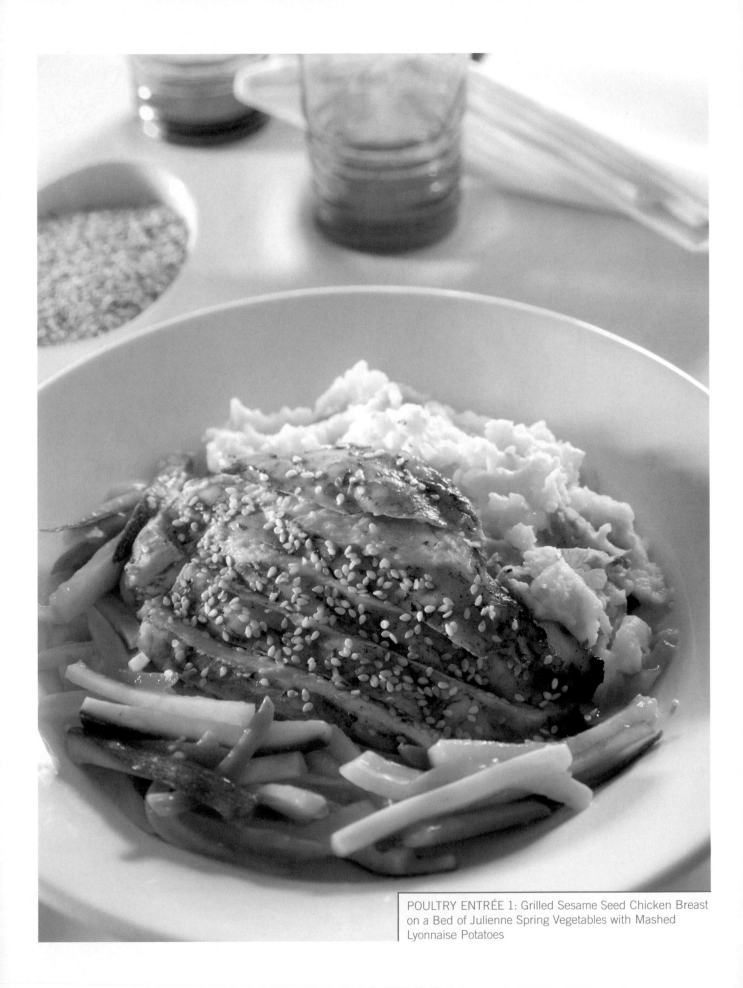

POULTRY ENTRÉE 1: Grilled Sesame Seed Chicken Breast on a Bed of Julienne Spring Vegetables with Mashed Lyonnaise Potatoes

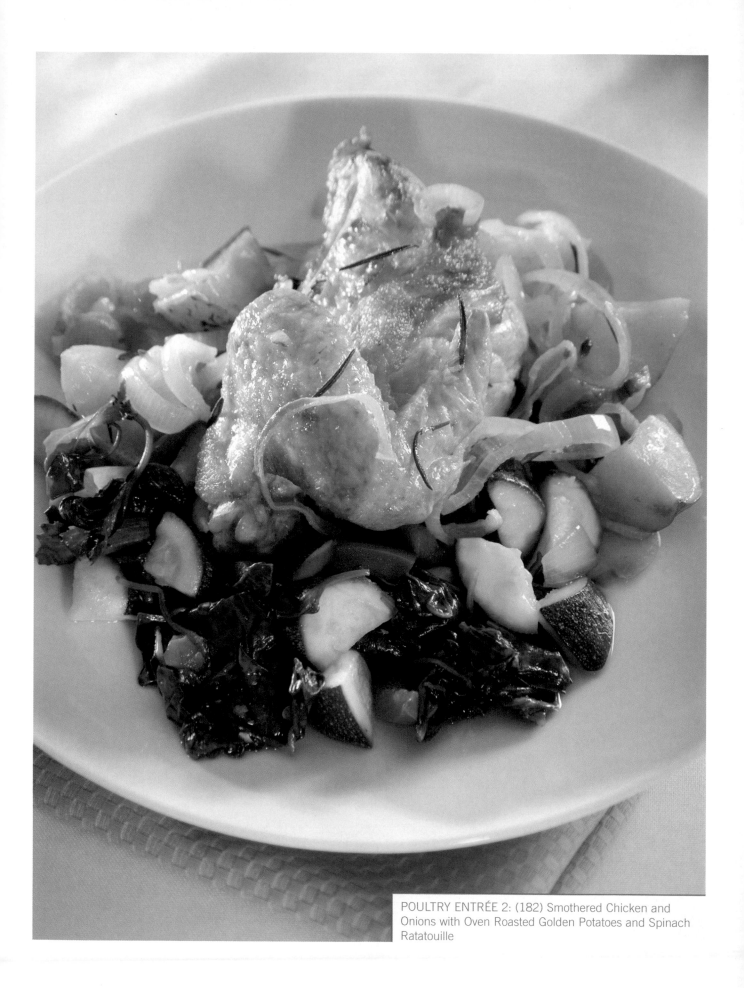

POULTRY ENTRÉE 2: (182) Smothered Chicken and Onions with Oven Roasted Golden Potatoes and Spinach Ratatouille

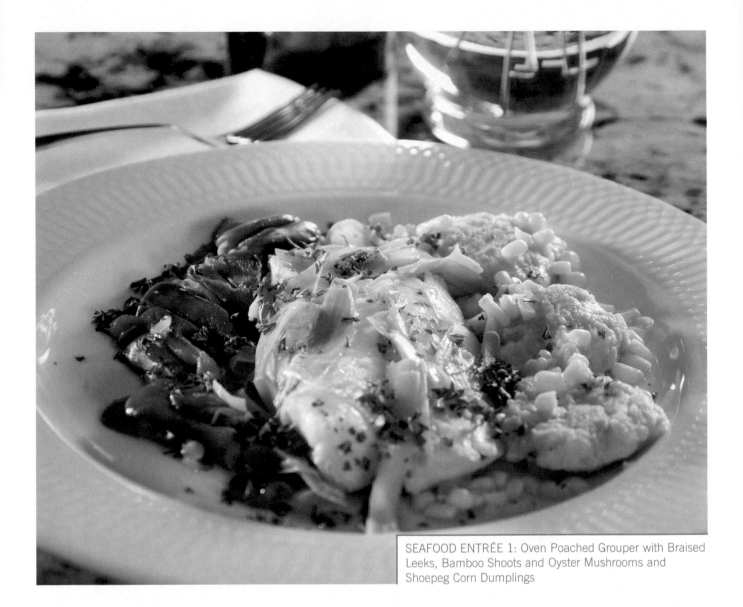

SEAFOOD ENTRÉE 1: Oven Poached Grouper with Braised Leeks, Bamboo Shoots and Oyster Mushrooms and Shoepeg Corn Dumplings

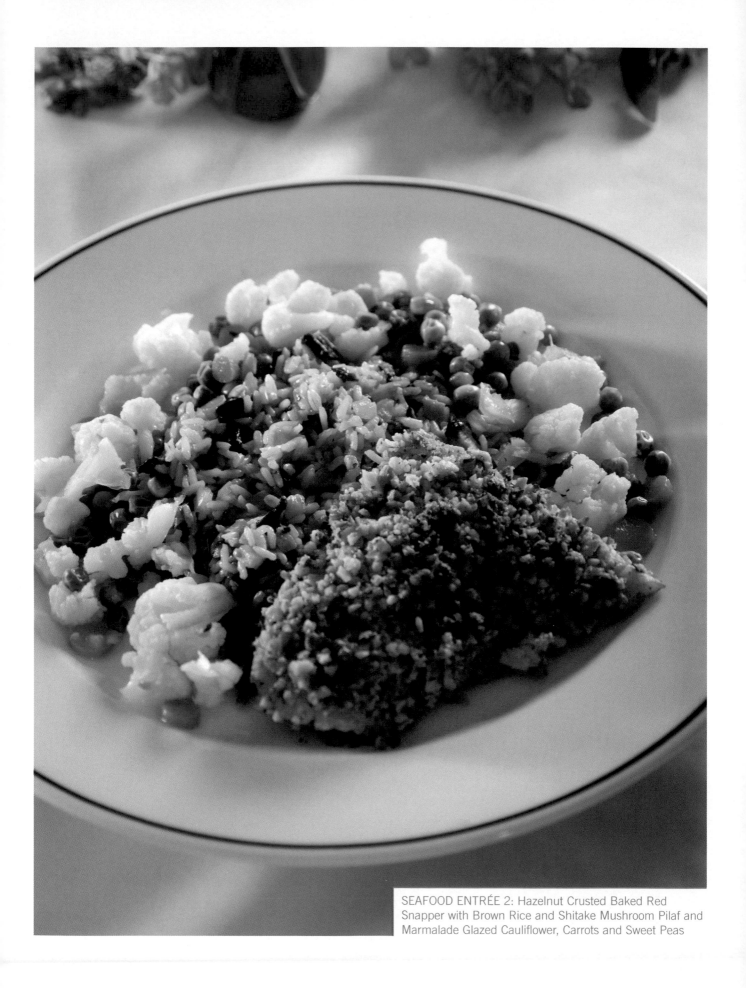

SEAFOOD ENTRÉE 2: Hazelnut Crusted Baked Red Snapper with Brown Rice and Shitake Mushroom Pilaf and Marmalade Glazed Cauliflower, Carrots and Sweet Peas

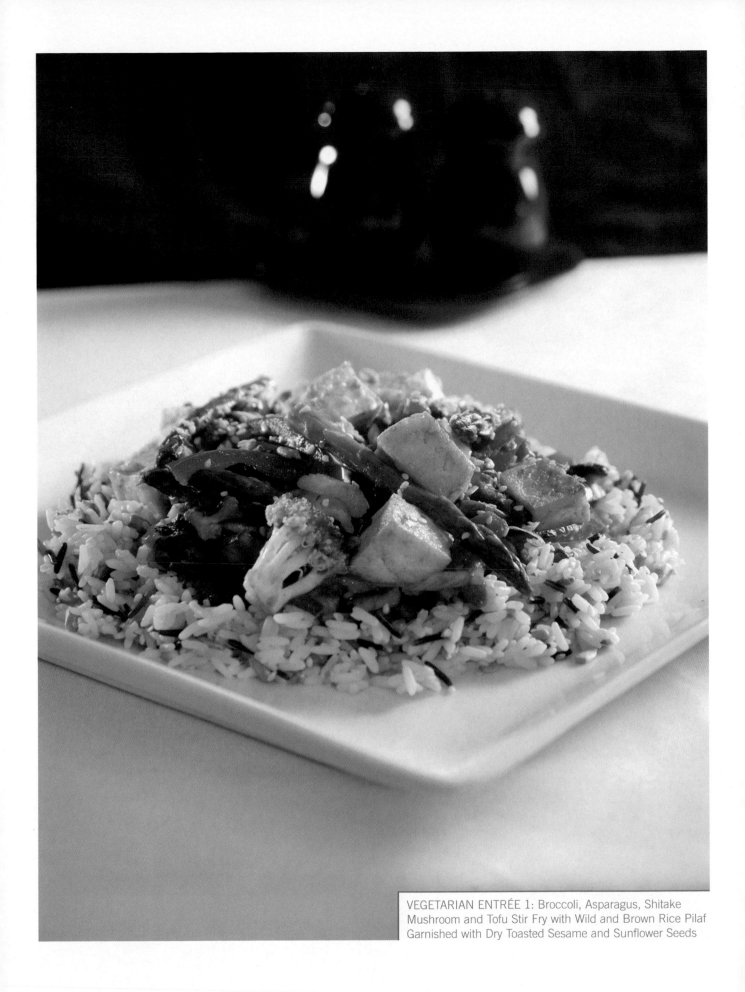

VEGETARIAN ENTRÉE 1: Broccoli, Asparagus, Shitake Mushroom and Tofu Stir Fry with Wild and Brown Rice Pilaf Garnished with Dry Toasted Sesame and Sunflower Seeds

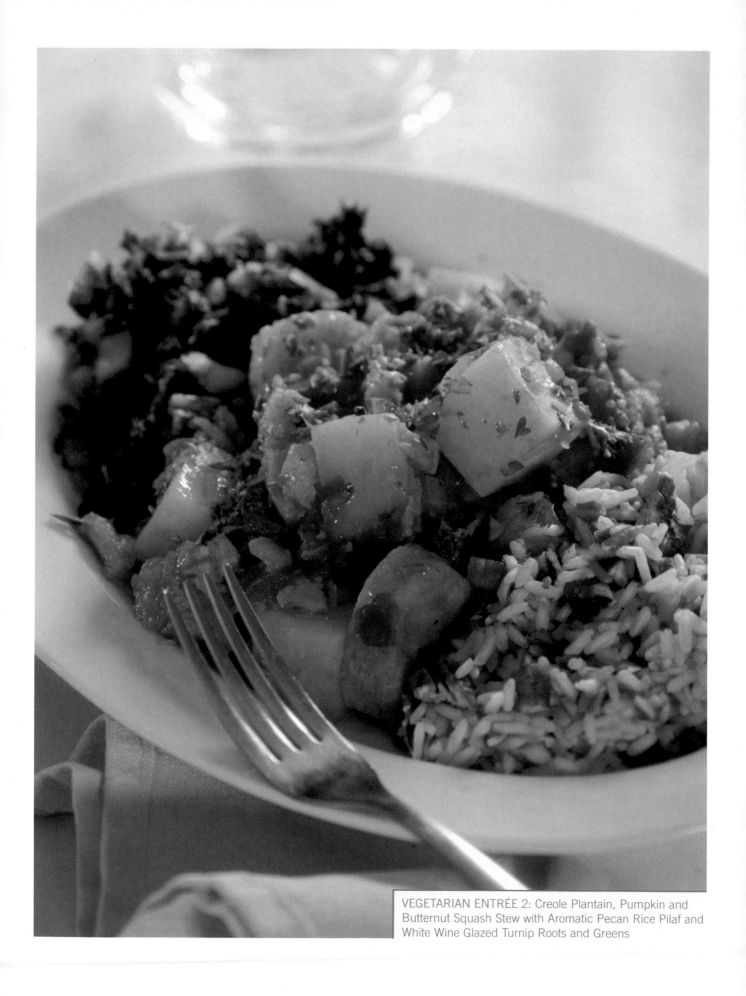

VEGETARIAN ENTRÉE 2: Creole Plantain, Pumpkin and Butternut Squash Stew with Aromatic Pecan Rice Pilaf and White Wine Glazed Turnip Roots and Greens

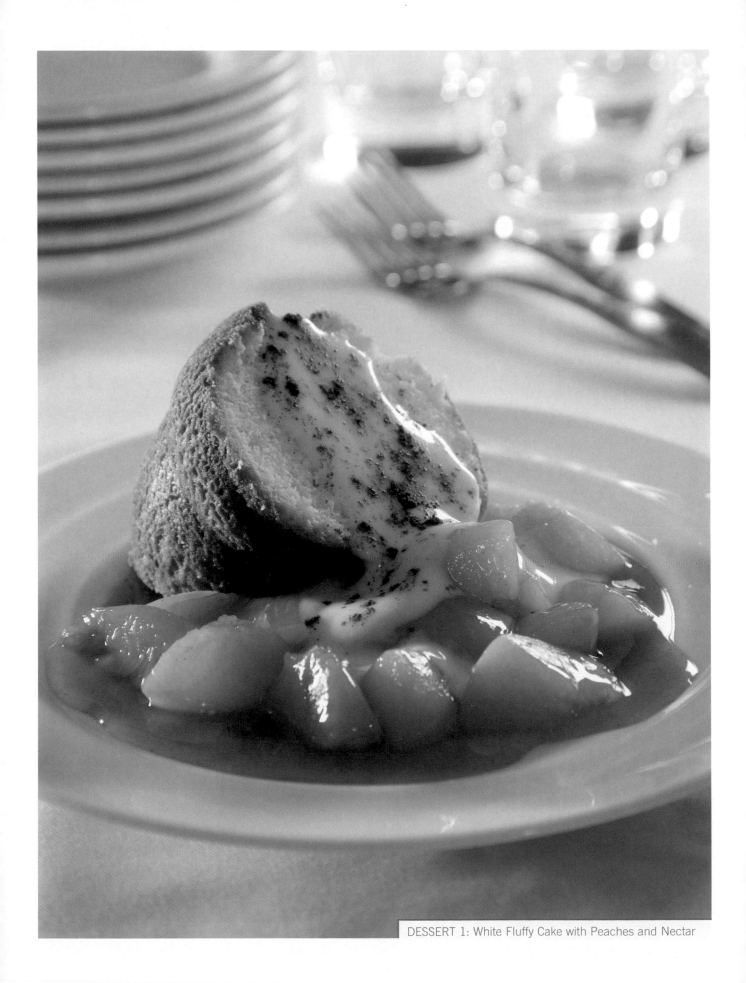

DESSERT 1: White Fluffy Cake with Peaches and Nectar

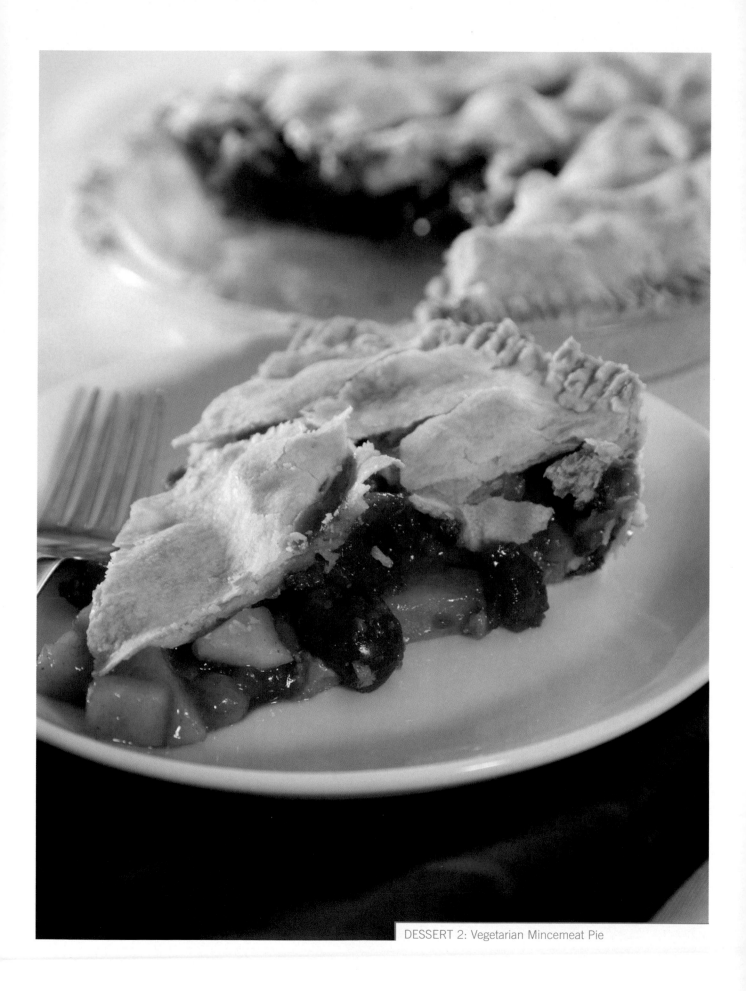

DESSERT 2: Vegetarian Mincemeat Pie

What does Adrianna have to do to keep her customers happy, knowing that the breading for the shrimp had not changed since the low-carb fad first appeared and was unlikely to change regardless of its carbohydrate content? *The resolution for this case study is presented at the end of the chapter.*

HEALTHY MENU CONSTRUCTION

Except in specialty restaurants (for example, Italian restaurants), a well-constructed menu is one that offers a variety of menu items for the adventurous, for the traditionalist, and for the nutritionally aware customer. This variety can be achieved through the use of cooking methods, styles of cuisine, and herbs and spices to create particular taste and flavor combinations. The following rules should help achieve this goal:

- Provide nutritious menu items, produced by a variety of healthy cooking styles, that are low in salt and saturated fat but do not need to be labeled as low-fat, dietary, or heart healthy.

- Well-written menu descriptions can lead consumers to make informed decisions about what foods they need or would like to eat for their own balanced diets.

- South Indian cuisine, Mexican cuisine, Spanish cuisine, American Indian cuisine, and Asian cuisine generally prepare foods simply and naturally, with an emphasis on taste and substance. Not all foods from these cuisines are low in fat, but most have low amounts of animal and saturated fats. Therefore they contain little or no cholesterol, and use vegetables and whole grains more often than do other cuisines.

- Not all menu items have to embody nutritional guidelines. For example, thin, healthy consommés, broths, or vegetable soups are not to everybody's taste. Hearty, thick soups also have their place in a nutritionally balanced menu. Moreover, customers who follow strict diets during the day may want to splurge a little at dinner, especially with dessert; other customers may eat freely during the day, cutting back on calories and fat only at dinner.

- Menu selections should accommodate customers who are on restricted diets and those who are not and offer a range of food choices. Low-carb menu items may be popular, but some people will still want their bread and potatoes, choosing to lose weight in other ways.

- Utilize as many cooking methods as possible in each menu category: appetizers, soups, salads, entrees, and desserts. Menus that feature only fried appetizers or broiled and sautéed entrees are too restrictive for the average customer. Although not all of the cooking methods will be used in each category, variety is still the key to success.

- Commercially prepared low-fat dressings come in all flavors, including the popular ranch, blue cheese, and Caesar, and should be made available to customers. Menus should state that these low-fat substitutes are available and be promoted by the waitstaff.

- Low-fat salad dressings can be made in-house as well. To create a large list of choices, the cook must first recognize the purpose of the dressing and then create reasonable substitutes that provide the same characteristics as the traditional oil-and-vinegar salad dressings.

- Nonfat salad dressing alternatives like honey mixed with a little mustard and lemon, for example, should also be available by customer request. Oil and vinegar served on the side can also allow customers to construct their own dressing with as little or as much oil as they want.

- Entrees should include grilled or broiled meats as well as roasted meats.
- Lean cuts of meats that require little or no fat to cook and fast cooking techniques should be incorporated into the menu as often as possible.
- Broiling meats releases more of the fat in the muscle than roasting does and allows the fat to drip away into the fire or grease pan; therefore, roasted Prime Rib has more fat on the plate than a similar portion of broiled rib eye steak (the same piece of beef).
- Entree choices should include some combination dinners like fettuccini and grilled chicken with wild mushroom sauce or tenderloin tips over wild and brown rice pilaf to provide the customer full meals without heavy meat portions.
- Vegetarian entrees should also be considered as daily menu items, especially if quality vegetable and starch accompaniments to entrees are already planned for the menu.

Another way to provide variety in healthy cooking is to provide vegetables and starches that accompany or are served on the side of main menu items. Many chefs over-simplify the preparation of these accompaniments and give them only marginal credit for the total enjoyment of the dish. Common accompaniments include buttered carrots, cauliflower Mornay, broccoli with hollandaise, and rice pilaf, but these are so common that they no longer entice customers to eat them. Diners then have no choice but to depend on the main item for their sustenance.

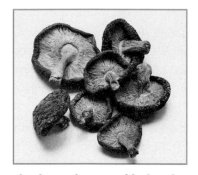

Shitake mushrooms add a lot of flavor and exotic appeal to simple and complex preparations.
David Murray © Dorling Kindersley

With some creative planning, vegetable and starch accompaniments can become an integral part of the overall impressions of a well-executed meal. A few examples include Braised Mixed Cabbages with Honey Glazed Root Vegetables, Oven Roasted Sweet Potato Home Fries with Pecans and Mint, and Teriyaki Peanut Pasta with Broccoli and Shitake Mushrooms.

To create exciting, healthier menus for customers—especially repeat customers, who are always looking for different experiences—chefs should always make taste the number one priority. Taste may be dictated by the herbs and spices used in a dish. Chefs should avoid using dominant flavors more than once in the same meal plan. For example, serving marinated basil chicken kabobs for an appetizer, basil vinaigrette for a salad, pesto for fettuccini, and wild mushroom sauce with basil for broiled flounder would be redundant. The main ingredients—chicken, lettuce, fettuccini, and flounder—are only part of the taste sensations. The taste of the basil will dominate after the first two choices. Taste is the collection of different flavors and must have balance as well as complexity. Taste is also dictated by the other flavoring ingredients used. Chefs need to be careful, for example, that everything does not end up tasting like olive oil, garlic, or bell peppers.

For desserts, the key is balance, not elimination. Not all desserts need to be on the heavy side. A good selection of sherbet, yogurt, sponge cakes, and fresh fruit cups should be offered along with heavier, more traditional choices.

CHOOSING ALTERNATIVE BREAKFAST ITEMS

American breakfast habits alternate between eating no breakfast at all and eating high-fat, cholesterol-packed meals such as bacon and eggs and sausage and biscuits. People are in too much of a hurry to eat breakfast, too groggy to cook it, or rely too heavily on fast-food breakfasts. With a little planning and foresight, however, healthy breakfast preparations can be made easily and with as much creativity as any other meal.

As just mentioned, some people skip breakfast as a form of dieting. This is a self-defeating practice, however, because people who don't eat breakfast are usually ravenous by lunchtime and tend to overeat at that meal.

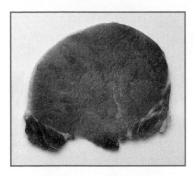

Canadian bacon is healthier than normal bacon because it is made from the lean pork loin instead of the fatty belly.

Philip Dowell © Dorling Kindersley

The human body needs a regular supply of energy foods and nutrients throughout the day. The first meal of the day is the most important meal because it helps the body recover from its repose and fasting. Other meals taken at intervals of four to five hours help the body balance its energy needs with its energy consumption. (Some researchers attest to the benefits of eating healthy snacks between meals to stave off the urge to overeat at the next meal. Healthy snacks include raw vegetables, fruits, and other nonfattening foods.)

People who eat breakfast away from home need nutritional choices for breakfast, just as they do for any other meal. Without such choices, people will either eat high-fat foods or eat elsewhere. It's not difficult to offer nutritional choices; what is needed is just another way of practicing the art of nutritional cooking.

Here are some simple strategies that will help transform traditional breakfast meals into healthy choices:

- In place of regular bacon, which is full of fat, use Canadian bacon, which is lean meat.
- In place of ham or Canadian bacon, use smoked turkey breast or grilled chicken as breakfast meats.
- In place of pork sausage, use turkey, seafood, or vegetable/soybean-based sausage.
- Poach eggs instead of frying them, and serve one egg with steamed, seasoned vegetables in place of home fries or hash brown potatoes.
- When making omelets or scrambled eggs, add one extra egg white for every whole egg used, and reduce the amount of egg yolk per portion.
- Add fruit to pancake and waffle mixes; the added moisture and flavor will reduce the need for a large amount of calorie-laden syrup.
- Add whole-wheat, buckwheat, or soy flour or a combination of flours, oats, and grains to traditional pancake and waffle mixes to increase fiber, vitamins, and minerals.
- Make your own fruit syrups with reduced calories and great natural flavor.

CREATING HEALTHY APPETIZERS

Well-planned appetizers play an integral part in the overall enjoyment of the dining experience. When properly designed, appetizers can act as a bridge between hunger and the main course and set the tone for the entire meal.

Appetizers need to be distinctive in flavors and textures but not overpowering in style or presentation. They should encompass a wide variety of flavors, cooking techniques, and portion sizes to satisfy a wide range of customers. Customers who regularly order appetizers are usually looking for value, variety, and nutritional choices.

Value-minded customers may select appetizers that are neither complicated nor expensive. They are looking to round out their meal with tasty, bite-size portions of foods, and they don't want to become overly full with the first course. Appetizers should be large enough to satisfy customers' initial hunger, but not large enough to ruin their appetite.

Customers want a variety of foods, flavors, and cooking techniques to choose from. Offer appetizers in all categories of foods, vegetables, proteins, grains, fruits, and dairy and prepared using as many cooking methods as is practical. Fried appetizers may be acceptable, but also offer grilled, poached, baked, and cold preparations to allow customers to choose the appetizer that best complements the rest of the meal.

Plan appetizers with flavors and ingredients that complement the flavors of the entrees yet do not duplicate them. The practice of offering smaller portions of entrees as appetizers or turning appetizers into entrees by adding side dishes should be avoided. Be creative with all menu sections, and offer your customers the greatest choices of flavors possible.

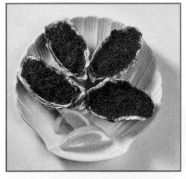

Offer a variety of appetizers to satisfy health-conscious consumers. These Oysters Rockefeller are loaded with vitamins and minerals.

David Murray and Jules Seimes © Dorling Kindersley

Using the techniques outlined in this text, it is easy to plan and construct appetizers that meet the aforementioned requirements yet maintain a high level of nutrition. Flavors do not have to be dominated by fat or sodium. Exciting flavors can be added using herbs, spices, and other ingredients.

Some traditional high-fat appetizers can be balanced with no-fat or low-fat accompaniments to lower the meal's total fat content to recommended standards. For example, the batter-fried popcorn shrimp recipe discussed in Chapter 13, which could contain as much as 32% fat, can be served with a small portion of brunoise salad on a piece of leaf lettuce (21% fat) as an accompaniment to lower the total plate fat percentage to 30%. Adding sliced fresh vegetables like tomatoes, celery, and carrots; small portions of other low-fat salad recipes; or sliced fruits and berries will also reduce the overall plate fat content.

The Wild Rice Corn Fritters with Sour Cream Cinnamon sauce recipe has been created utilizing the information contained in this book. The combination of foods on the plate make the whole dish a healthy menu item with less than 30% calories coming from fats, only 8 milligrams of cholesterol, plus a variety of vitamins, minerals, and other nutrients.

NUTRIENT-RICH, LOW-FAT SOUPS

In cultures and cuisines around the world, soups have long supplied healthy and satisfying meals. Soup making was a versatile cooking method that allowed cooks to hydrate dried meat and beans; dilute the salty taste from preserved meats; and combine vegetables, herbs, spices, and meats to form a complete meal in a single dish.

Soups continue to play an important part in various world cuisines. For some, soups supply complete meals; for others, soup is only one of many courses in a single meal. Soups can be pedestrian in design or sophisticated works of culinary art, depending on the culture in which it is prepared, the ingredients used, and the soup's place in the meal.

In the art of nutritional cooking, soups can be designed to supply all essential parts of a healthy meal in a single, satisfying dish. Proteins, carbohydrates, fats (easily kept within the recommended 30% of daily calorie intake), vitamins, and minerals come together in one pot or kettle, satisfying the most ravenous appetites, and the most restrictive diets.

Thin soups and purée soups supply the most nutrition without the fat. Cream soups can be made less fatty by using low-fat dairy products. Soups can be thickened with cornstarch or puréed vegetables; enriched with protein from herbs, tofu, or legumes; and flavored with spices and other natural flavorings to enhance the finished product.

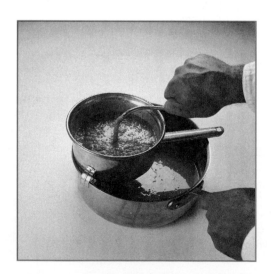

Puréed soups are often good healthy choices because they do not depend on roux for thickening. This puréed split pea soup was made without any fat, including from salt pork; it is flavored with smoked turkey necks.
Pearson Education/PH College

WILD RICE CORN FRITTERS
WITH SOUR CREAM CINNAMON SAUCE

- *Wild rice is the seed of a type of marsh grass. It naturally contains a higher level of insoluble fiber than typical grain foods, including brown and white rice. The kernels should still be slightly firm when fully cooked, giving a nice texture to the final dish.*
- *One cup of raw wild rice has 22.6 grams of protein, 120.5 grams of carbohydrate, and a slight amount of fat. It has more than twice the iron of brown rice.*
- *The buckwheat flour in this recipe is also known by the names* beechnut *(because the seeds resemble beechnuts) and* saracen *(because of its dark color). Buckwheat is rich in minerals and B vitamins and has a lower caloric value than any of the cereal grains.*
- *The corn oil in this recipe helps reduce the overall amount of saturated fat in the recipe, although there is still some fat in the low-fat sour cream.*
- *The recipe contains less than 25 milligrams of cholesterol.*

MAKES 20 2-OUNCE FRITTERS

INGREDIENTS	WEIGHT/VOLUME
wild rice	4 ounces
water	1 1/2 cups
whole kernel corn	6 ounces
celery, peeled and finely diced	2 ounces
buckwheat flour	5 ounces
baking powder	1 tablespoon
white pepper, ground	1/4 teaspoon
allspice, ground	1/2 teaspoon
egg whites	2 each
corn oil	1 tablespoon
vanilla extract	1/4 teaspoon
1% milk	1/2 cup
low-fat sour cream	1 1/2 cups
cinnamon, ground	1 tablespoon

1. Cook the wild rice in the water until tender.
2. Sift together the buckwheat flour, baking powder, white pepper, and allspice.
3. Whip together the egg whites, oil, and vanilla until well mixed, and add the mixture to the dry ingredients.
4. Add milk and stir well.
5. Add corn, celery, and rice to the mixture, and stir to incorporate all the ingredients.
6. Measure 2 ounces of the batter for each fritter, and cook them on a lightly oiled griddle.
7. Cook the fritters on one side until the batter begins to bubble; flip them over gently and cook the other side until firm.
8. Mix the sour cream and cinnamon, and spoon the mixture over each serving of fritters.

Approximate values per serving: Calories 164, carbohydrates (grams) 25.7, protein (grams) 4.6, fat (grams) 5.5, cholesterol (milligrams) 8. Carbohydrates = 60% calories, protein = 11% calories, fat = 29% calories.

If a soup is to be a complete meal, it should contain vegetable, starch, and protein. A recipe with 1 cup of vegetable; 1/2 cup of grains like rice, barley, or corn; and 2 to 3 ounces of protein could provide a complete meal depending on individual calorie requirements. A Louisiana-style gumbo, seafood chowder, or Vietnamese noodle soup could all fit into this category. Chicken noodle, cream of broccoli, or vichyssoise contain only one or two of the vegetable, starch, and protein categories and would not provide a complete, balanced meal.

To transform traditional soups into healthful meals that provide fiber and contain 30% or less total fat, follow these eight guidelines:

1. Sweat vegetables in stock instead of fat.
2. Caramelize vegetables for color and flavor in a nonstick pan or a well-seasoned griddle or grill, without the fat.
3. If using fat, substitute a vegetable oil like olive, canola, peanut, or corn oil for butter, margarine, or other animal fats.
4. Thicken soups with cornstarch, arrowroot, or puréed vegetables in place of a roux.
5. Include a variety of fiber-rich vegetables, especially leafy green vegetables and legumes.
6. Use herbs and spices to increase flavors, replacing the flavors lost through no-fat and low-sodium cooking.
7. Replace cream with low-fat plain yogurt or low-fat sour cream. The added tartness from yogurt or sour cream helps add flavor to the finished soup.
8. Decrease the overall percentage of fat calories by adding grains, potatoes, noodles, and vegetables. These supply great nutrition with little or no added fat.

The Vegetable Barley Soup recipe is an example of the sort of healthy soup that can be created when special care goes into the selection of the ingredients and the procedures for putting them together.

MAKING HEALTHY SALADS AND ENTREMETS

Salads have served many functions in the dining experience over the centuries. Depending on culture, dining practices, and health concerns, salads have been a part of meals to one extent or another.

A salad can be loosely defined as any combination of vegetables, fruits, cheeses, or protein foods bound together by a single dressing. Salads can accompany a meal, or be a meal in themselves with the proper amounts of vegetable, grain, and protein foods in a single serving. Health-conscious diners choose salads as a way of eating a balance of foods, usually low in fat and cholesterol, that have great amounts of flavor and substance.

An entremet is a small course served between large or main courses on a classic menu. Entremets were designed to be light, tasty, and easy to prepare, so guests would not be kept waiting between courses. Originally, vegetables, fruits, and pastas made up the majority of entremets served. Some culinary history connoisseurs suggest that the modern salad was a type of entremet; it was easily prepared and could be served quickly between courses that took longer to cook and serve. In this way guests would have some food in front of them at all times during the meal.

No matter what their place in the menu, salads and entremets can both meet dietary guidelines and give guests a variety of food choices and presentations.

Lettuces today are available in many different shapes, sizes, and tastes. The old standby iceberg lettuce has given way to romaine, mâche, red oak leaf, arugula, and about a dozen other

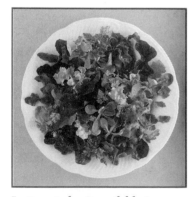

Lettuce today is available in many different shapes and sizes, as seen in this salad mix, which is marketed as spring mix.
© *Dorling Kindersley*

VEGETABLE BARLEY SOUP

- *Carrots are a known source of beta-carotene, a precursor for vitamin A.*
- *Vitamin A is needed for growth, night vision, and healthy skin. It also helps us resist infections of the respiratory tract by keeping the respiratory tract tissues moist.*
- *Barley is a good source of dietary fiber, which helps to lower cholesterol by binding to the bile acids that contain cholesterol. (The cholesterol then is eliminated through digestion and excretion processes.)*
- *The mushrooms in this recipe are a good source of chromium. Other good sources of chromium include whole-wheat breads, meats, and vegetables.*

MAKES 10 10-OUNCE PORTIONS

INGREDIENTS	WEIGHT/VOLUME
carrots, julienned	16 ounces
onions, julienned	8 ounces
bell peppers, julienned	8 ounces
vegetable stock	3 quarts
tomatoes, peeled, seeded, and diced	32 ounces
dried barley	5 ounces
rosemary leaves	1 tablespoon
thyme leaves, chopped	1 tablespoon
celery seed	1 teaspoon
black pepper, coarsely ground	1/2 teaspoon
white pepper, ground	1/4 teaspoon
salt	1/2 teaspoon
shitake mushrooms, chopped	12 ounces

1. Place the carrots, onions, bell peppers, vegetable stock, and tomatoes in a stockpot and bring to a quick boil.
2. Make a cheesecloth sachet to enclose the rosemary leaves, thyme, and celery seeds and tie it together with a string. Place the bag of spices in the simmering stockpot.
3. Add the barley, black pepper, white pepper, and salt, and reduce the soup to a simmer.
4. When the barley is cooked (about 15 minutes), add the mushrooms.
5. Allow the soup to simmer for an additional 15 to 20 minutes to cook the mushrooms through and blend the flavors together.

Approximate values per serving: Calories 332, carbohydrates (grams) 63.2, protein (grams) 8.2, fat (grams) 5.1, cholesterol (milligrams) 0. Carbohydrates = 76% calories, protein = 10% calories, fat = 14% calories.

specialty lettuces and flavorful green leafy vegetables. Some of these lettuce blends are commercially sold as mesclun or spring mix. Combining various types of lettuces in mixed salads is a simple way of balancing colors, textures, flavors, and nutrients for the entire plated salad.

Salad dressings are typically high in fat and calories and low in overall nutrition. Salads by themselves, mixed vegetable creations, are healthy choices, but the choice and amount of dressing used can transform a healthy creation into a fatty menu item.

Dressings add moisture and flavor components to the salad that either complement or contrast with the flavors of the main ingredients. The more complex and contrasting the flavors of the main salad, the less that dressing is needed to satisfy the guests' flavor palate.

Commercial nonfat salad dressings are available that give the operator a variety of products with little extra work. Depending on the size of the operation, commercial low-fat and nonfat salad dressings are a great way of creating healthier salads. Samples of these should be on hand for customers who request them, and the inventory should be replenished as demand dictates. Oil and vinegar should also be available for those who want oil-based dressings but want to control the amount of oil that is used. A high-quality olive oil and red wine vinegar are the best choices.

Low-fat or nonfat salad dressings can also be made in the kitchen. Here are four different styles of low-fat and nonfat dressings. Change the main ingredients, flavoring spices, and liquids to make hundreds of healthy recipes.

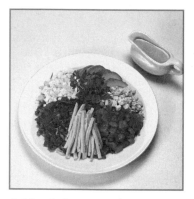

Cobb salads are popular entree-type salads, as are chicken Caesar salads and chef salads.
Pearson Education/PH College

1. Fruit juice dressings thickened with cornstarch or arrowroot
2. Lean chicken, beef, and vegetable stocks thickened with cornstarch or arrowroot
3. Fruit jellies and preserves thinned with lemon juice, vinegar, or soy sauce
4. Low-fat dressings made from standard dressing recipes by substituting low-fat sour cream or plain low-fat yogurt for mayonnaise

Salad entrees have become a popular menu choice in the last few decades. They combine a larger quantity of lettuce greens, vegetables, and protein ingredients than the typical salad course. The traditional chef salad, with julienne turkey, ham, and Swiss cheese on a bed of lettuce greens, was one of the forerunners of the grilled chicken Caesar and Cobb salads of today.

Salad as a main course should contain at least two servings of vegetables (2 cups of raw leafy vegetables or a combination of raw, cooked, and chopped vegetables); 2 to 3 ounces of a protein food (meat, chicken, fish, legumes, or tofu); and a serving of grains (rice, corn, or pasta), fruit, or dairy.

Lettuces, in general, do not have high calorie counts. Therefore, salads made primarily from lettuce or endive greens and dressed with a simple vinaigrette will contain a high percentage of fat calories overall. To offset this high fat percentage, add low-fat protein items (grilled chicken, fish, shrimp, or tofu) or other vegetables to increase nonfat calories, texture, eye appeal, and substance. In this way a plain salad, normally high in fat calories, can become a more substantial balanced menu item with appropriate fat content and rich in nutrients.

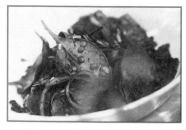

Fresh spinach makes a healthy salad green.
Ian O'Leary © Dorling Kindersley

Fresh spinach is a healthy lettuce substitute that contains enough calories to offset high fat percentages in salads. However, the traditional hot bacon dressing often served with spinach salads defeats the benefits of eating the healthy vegetable. Plenty of low- and no-fat salad dressings are more appropriate to fresh spinach salad than bacon and bacon fat–based hot dressings. Low-fat ranch or arrowroot-thickened citrus dressing make great accompaniments to this tasty vegetable. Spinach can be used by itself or in combination with other nutrient-rich salad greens to reduce overall fat percentages and add extra color, textures, vitamins, and minerals to the final preparation.

The Marinated Pinto Bean Salad with Gingered Celeriac and Toasted Almonds recipe is full of protein, carbohydrates, and other valuable nutrients. It combines multiple flavors and textures to satisfy the most discriminating customer.

MARINATED PINTO BEAN SALAD WITH GINGERED CELERIAC AND TOASTED ALMONDS

- *The olive oil used in the recipe for flavor and mouth feel is known to help reduce LDL (bad cholesterol) without affecting HDL (good cholesterol). Olive oil is low in saturated fat and contains a large amount of essential fatty acids.*
- *Pinto beans, as all legumes, contain a high amount of fiber and the essential amino acids needed for good health, and they are relatively low in fat.*
- *When eaten raw, bell peppers are one of the best sources of vitamin C, a water-soluble vitamin that must be replenished daily.*
- *Dried dates are rich in iron, which is needed to form hemoglobin, and natural sugars, which add sweetness to the finished salad.*
- *Almonds contain a better-quality protein than that found in almost any other plant.*
- *Peppers, beans, dates, and nuts are also good nutritional choices because of their fiber.*
- *The gingered celeriac provides great flavor, texture, and corresponding tastes that both complement and contrast with other flavors in the dish.*
- *When this salad is served on a bed of green lettuce, it becomes a complete meal. The combination of beans and nuts contains complete protein and could substitute for meat.*

MAKES 10 5-OUNCE PORTIONS

INGREDIENTS	WEIGHT/VOLUME
pinto beans, cooked	2 1/2 pounds
red wine vinegar	4 ounces
lemon juice, fresh	2 ounces
virgin olive oil	2 ounces
green bell peppers, small diced	16 ounces
dried dates, chopped	6 ounces
cumin, ground	1/2 tablespoon
fresh basil, chopped	2 tablespoons
black pepper, coarsely ground	1/2 teaspoon
red pepper, crushed	1/8 teaspoon
almonds, sliced and dry toasted	2 ounces
mixed lettuces (mesclun, spring mix, or house blend of varietal lettuces)	1 pound

GINGERED CELERIAC

celeriac, peeled and shredded	1 pound
fresh ginger root, grated	2 ounces
muscatel (sweet wine)	2 ounces
cardamom seeds, crushed	1 tablespoon
black peppercorns, cracked	1 teaspoon

1. Mix all the ingredients together except the almonds. Allow the mixture to rest for at least 1 hour.
2. Mix in the toasted almonds just before service.
3. To make gingered celeriac, place the shredded celeriac, grated ginger, wine, and sachet (cheesecloth spice bag) containing the cracked cardamom seeds and black peppercorns into the sauce pot. Bring the pot to a quick boil and allow it to simmer until the wine and natural juices have reduced to a syrupy consistency.
4. Remove th0e sachet, and refrigerate the gingered celeriac until quite chilled.
5. Plate a 3-ounce portion of bean and almond salad on a bed of mixed lettuces, and crown it with a 2-ounce portion of gingered celeriac.
6. Serve with other vegetable garnishes such as celery, radishes, and tomatoes.

Approximate values per serving: Calories 349, carbohydrates (grams) 53, protein (grams) 12.6, fat (grams) 9.7, cholesterol (milligrams) 0. Carbohydrates = 61% calories, protein = 14.4% calories, fat = 25% calories.

DEVELOPING HEALTHY MEAT ENTREES

There are several things to know about meat when deciding on a cut or cooking method. The composition of the muscle(s), the amount of exterior fat, the amount of marbling (interior fat), and tenderness are all critical issues in the nutritional cooking of meat products.

Composition of muscles refers to their shape and size and the direction of the grain (protein strands). Sub-primal cuts of meat may contain two or more different muscle types (bottom round roast, for example) and could be broken down into single-muscle cuts to obtain the most flexibility in cooking styles. The following points are also important in evaluating muscle composition:

- The shape of the muscle (flank steak versus top round, for example) plays a part in determining the cooking method and serving suggestions.
- The size of the muscle determines the type of cooking method that works best. Larger pieces are roasted or braised, and smaller pieces are grilled or broiled.
- The direction of the grain becomes a factor when two or more muscles are connected (such as in the bottom round of beef and veal) or in a thin muscle like the flank; cooking and cutting of these muscles require specific care.

All exterior fat on meat should be removed and not consumed. These fats can be trimmed before or after cooking. (Fat contains concentrated animal flavors because of the natural juices locked inside the fat. During cooking, these juices are released and can add flavor to slow-roasted meats.)

Nutritionists are studying the relationship between cholesterol content and the effect of removing exterior fat and the skin from chicken or turkey before cooking versus after the item is cooked. Results are not yet conclusive, but they show that the amount of cholesterol consumed differs little whether or not the meats are roasted with the skin and excess fats (which contain flavorful juices and fat-soluble vitamins but are discarded before serving the foods). The main health issue is not to directly consume these fats together with the meat; the main culinary issue is to make foods taste good without the fats. The practice of roasting meats and poultry first with fat and then trimming them for service may be a good compromise.

All meat contains a certain amount of interior fat. In beef it is called *marbling*, and it is often easy to see against the meat's natural red color. But this fat is not always visible to the eye and can be removed only by the cooking process. Broiling, grilling, rotisserie cooking, or roasting on a rack are good ways of making sure that these fats, when they melt during cooking, fall away from the meat and are not consumed.

In response to public concern, meat, including pork, is leaner today than ever before. This means that the amounts of exterior and interior fats are decreasing. Because fat is

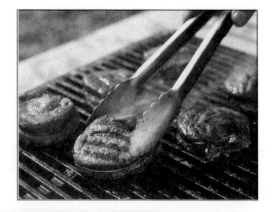

Grilling helps to reduce the amount of exterior and interior fat.
Ian O'Leary © Dorling Kindersley

controlled mostly by diet (although genetics is also involved), livestock are now fed special diets to ensure more muscle growth and less fat growth. The results are less fatty animal products in the stores and on the table.

The USDA grading of meat, veal, and lamb evaluates fat content as one of the primary factors. Prime meat contains the most fat; Choice meat contains the second most; Select meat (for beef) and Good meat (for veal and lamb) contain the least. Therefore, in selecting meats for nutritional cooking, choose Select or Good grades first, when possible, and Choice grades next; avoid Prime meats.

Meat cuts that are naturally leaner than others include the following:

Beef: Flank, top round, eye round, top sirloin, strip loins, tenderloins, first-cut brisket

Veal: Practically all cuts

Pork: Boneless loin roast, center cut loin chops, sirloin roast, tenderloin

Lamb: Sirloin roast, leg roasts, blade chops, foreshank

Venison: Practically all cuts

Despite all the health concerns regarding meat (especially red meats), beef, lamb, pork, and veal are substantially healthy foods. All of these meats contain the eight essential amino acids and adequate amounts of vitamins and minerals (particularly the amino acids, vitamins, and minerals not easily found in vegetables). Vegetarians and people who greatly reduce their meat consumption must make sure they get these vitamins and amino acids through other sources. People who eat a moderate amount of lean meat will have a less difficult time meeting their daily nutritional needs.

One of the more difficult health concerns in relation to meat consumption is portion sizes. In America, where large steaks and large roasts are standard dinner fare, the 3- or 4-ounce portions recommended by dietitians may be met with resistance. Hearty appetites must be satisfied while reducing portion sizes. There are two ways to accomplish this. First, prepare meat dishes that are full of flavor. A simple grilled steak doesn't have enough flavor contrasts or complexities to give the diner a sense of satisfaction when served in smaller portions. Instead, serve beef that has strong and distinct flavors, like tenderloin braised in citrus juice with cloves and cinnamon or sirloin steak marinated in teriyaki sauce. Second, serve smaller meat portions together with potato, rice, pasta, or vegetable dishes; a stir-fry is a good example of how this can be accomplished. The bulk of the dinner comprises several accompaniments and does not depend on the size of any one item.

The Braised Beef Eye Round Sicilian with White Asparagus and Roasted Red Potatoes is a nutritional meat entree recipe made even healthier by accompaniments chosen for their own particular nutrients, colors, or textural attributes.

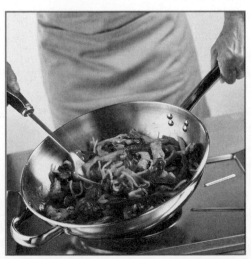

Stir-fried meals are a good way to serve proper protein portions and still satisfy your guests' appetite.
Edward Allwright © Dorling Kindersley

BRAISED BEEF EYE ROUND SICILIAN WITH WHITE ASPARAGUS AND ROASTED RED POTATOES

- *Beef eye round is a beef muscle with little internal fat. Much like the tenderloin, the outer layer of fat can be easily removed from eye round. What remains is a relatively lean piece of meat.*
- *The eye round is one of the three muscles that make up the bottom round of the hind quarter. Eye rounds can be cut from veal, venison, and lamb legs for a variety of menu choices.*
- *Because eye rounds come from the inner thigh muscle of the animal, they are not as tender as less used muscles. Braising is one of the preferred methods to tenderize the meat. All the vitamins and minerals from the vegetables, herbs, and spices remain in the braising liquid, which becomes a part of the final dish.*
- *The use of Chianti wine as a flavor enhancer reduces the need for salt to stimulate taste.*
- *Fennel is a perennial herb and vegetable relative of the carrot family and contains large amounts of vitamin C, dietary fiber, potassium, phosphorus, folate, magnesium, and calcium.*
- *Asparagus is low in calories, only 20 calories per 5.3-ounce serving (less than 4 calories per spear), and contains no fat or cholesterol. Asparagus is a good source of potassium, fiber (3 grams per 5.3-ounce serving), folate, thiamin, vitamin B_6, and rutin, a natural drug that strengthens capillary walls.*

MAKES 10 PORTIONS

INGREDIENTS	WEIGHT/VOLUME
onions, medium diced	8 ounces
celery, medium diced	8 ounces
parsnips, lightly peeled and medium diced	8 ounces
garlic, chopped	2 teaspoons
fresh basil, chopped	1 tablespoon
fresh oregano, chopped	2 teaspoons
black pepper, coarsely ground	1/2 teaspoon
Chianti wine	16 ounces
tomatoes, peeled, seeded, and diced	24 ounces
beef eye round, trimmed and cut into 1/2-inch steaks	3 to 4 pounds
lean beef stock	64 ounces
fennel bulbs, trimmed and cut into wedges	2 each
olive oil	3 tablespoons
salt	1/4 teaspoon
black pepper, coarse ground	1/2 teaspoon
red potatoes (small)	1 pound
fresh white asparagus	1 1/2 pounds
white vegetable stock	32 ounces
arrowroot	6 tablespoons

1. Mix first 9 ingredients together to make a marinade. Bring the mixture to a quick boil.
2. Immediately remove the marinade from the heat, and allow it to cool.
3. Add the steaks to the cooled marinade, and marinate for a minimum of 3 hours.
4. Remove the steaks from the marinade and pat them dry.
5. Grill the steaks just long enough to color the outsides.
6. Add the marinade and the beef stock to a straight-sided pan (rondo).
7. Bring to a quick boil.
8. Add the grilled steaks and cut fennel. Cover the pan and cook in a 350°F oven for 1 1/2 hours or until tender.
9. Mix together the olive oil, salt, pepper, and chopped garlic.
10. Add the potatoes to the dressing and stir.
11. Place the potatoes on the roasting pan, and add them to the beef in the oven for the last 45 minutes of cooking.
12. Trim the asparagus stems, and poach the asparagus in simmering vegetable stock.
13. Time the cooking of the asparagus so that it is done when the meat is ready to be served.
14. Remove the steaks and fennel when cooked and set them aside.
15. Thicken the sauce with 3 tablespoons of arrowroot per pint of strained liquid. Simmer the sauce for 10 minutes and strain.
16. Serve each steak with braised fennel, poached asparagus spears, roasted red potatoes, and sauce.

Approximate values per serving: Calories 541, carbohydrates (grams) 56.4, protein (grams) 44.6, fat (grams) 15.4, cholesterol (milligrams) 95. Carbohydrates = 42% calories, protein = 33% calories, fat = 25.6% calories.

DEVELOPING HEALTHY POULTRY ENTREES

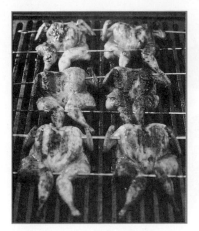

Quail are now available from most major food purveyors.
Ian O'Leary © Dorling Kindersley

Poultry has gained popularity over the past 20 years among people who are concerned about health and diet. Poultry is generally leaner and, consequently, contains less fat and cholesterol than other meats. It has long been considered a healthy alternative to red- and pink-fleshed meats.

Different species of poultry, from chickens to quail, partridge, and pheasants, are now available throughout the year. Cooks and chefs can purchase specific types and parts of almost every kind of commercially raised poultry. For example, turkey, pigeon, and pheasant are commonly available as breasts, leg and thigh quarters, wings, and ground meat. This availability allows full utilization of the products as determined by recipe specifications.

Poultry contributes protein, vitamin A, thiamin, riboflavin, niacin, phosphorus, potassium, sodium, calcium, and trace amounts of other vitamins and minerals to the human diet. All forms of poultry are generally lower in calories, total fat, and saturated fat than are red meats.

Most of the fat in poultry is found just beneath the skin. Removing the skin, before or after cooking, decreases the overall amount of fat by as much as 60% in breasts and 40% in legs and thighs.

According to the USDA, uncooked white chicken meat, with skin, contains only 65 milligrams of sodium per 3.5-ounce edible portion. The same amount of uncooked dark meat, with skin, contains slightly more, at 73 milligrams for the same size portion.

Chicken, turkey, game hen, and other lean birds lend themselves to almost any recipe or cooking procedure known to the modern cook or chef. Whether it's poaching, braising, grilling, or roasting, all healthy cooking processes can be used on poultry with great success.

Poultry (especially chicken and turkey) does present some safety and health issues. Chicken and turkey are naturally susceptible to salmonella contamination. Strict handling, preparation, and cooking guidelines must be followed to protect the health of consumers:

- Thaw frozen poultry properly (under refrigeration, under cold running water, or during the cooking process, never at room temperature).
- Always wash poultry thoroughly before preparation.

Removing the skin from poultry can reduce the amount of fat by 60%.
Pearson Education/PH College

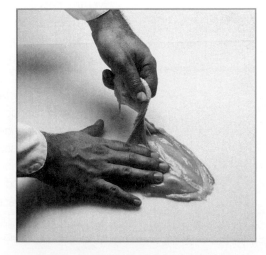

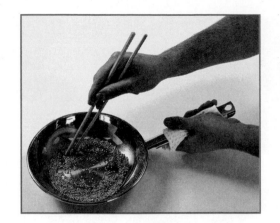

Sesame seeds are a rich source
of protein and fiber.
David Murray and Jules Selmes
© Dorling Kindersley

- Clean and sanitize knives and cutting boards after preparing poultry and before preparing any other ingredients.
- Never store raw poultry above other ingredients in the refrigerator.
- Cook poultry thoroughly, to a minimum internal temperature of 165°F.
- Cook poultry from beginning to end. Partially cooking poultry to finish at a later time can have hazardous results.
- To serve already cooked poultry hot, reheat it to an internal temperature of 165°F as quickly as possible.

Poultry is a healthy and safe food when properly prepared. It is easy to achieve variety in menus by offering more types and forms of poultry together with hundreds of different accompanying sauces and vegetables. The Grilled Sesame Seed Chicken Breast on a Bed of Julienne Spring Vegetables with Mashed Lyonnaise Potatoes is an example of a poultry entree that provides adequate protein in the chicken breast yet is a completely balanced meal when eaten together with the selected side dishes. The colors and textures of the vegetables contrast with the pale toasted color of the sesame chicken breast; all of this contrasts with the mashed red skin lyonnaise potatoes.

DEVELOPING HEALTHY SEAFOOD ENTREES

Over the past 15 to 20 years, the popularity of seafood has risen to record heights in the United States. Concerns about the negative effects of red meat consumption led to the popularity of poultry and then seafood, both of which are now vying for a greater share of American eating choices—and winning.

From meager, almost obligatory offerings on restaurant menus to spotlighted specials, seafood now appears in interesting and stylistic ways on menus across the nation. From grilled flounder on breakfast menus to tuna carpaccio on luncheon menus, seafood has found a permanent place in American cuisine.

Continued research proves that seafood can be one of the healthiest protein items in human diets. Its generally low-fat, high-protein content is the perfect combination for proper nutrition. All seafood contains omega-3 fatty acids, which appear to aid in the prevention of coronary heart disease and other ailments caused by too much saturated fats and cholesterol.

Seafood has become such a popular menu item that new harvesting and raising techniques continue to be perfected. Farm-raised seafood is now seen as a viable resource

GRILLED SESAME SEED CHICKEN BREAST ON A BED OF JULIENNE SPRING VEGETABLES WITH MASHED LYONNAISE POTATOES

- *In this recipe, sesame is used both as an oil to impart flavor and provide proper cooking lubrication and as a flavorful seed garnish.*
- *Sesame seeds are a good nutritional choice. They are 25% protein and especially rich in methionine and tryptophan; many other plant proteins lack these amino acids in adequate quantities.*
- *Natural sesame seeds (unhulled) contain 5 grams of protein, 3.1 grams fiber, and 14 grams of total fat per ounce. When toasted they offer 4.8 grams of protein, 4.0 grams fiber, and 13.8 grams of total fat.*
- *Although relatively high in fat, sesame oil is 38% monounsaturated and 44% polyunsaturated, which equals 82% unsaturated fatty acids.*
- *Marinades are used to impart flavor, so oils and other fats are unnecessary. Strong flavored ingredients thinned by vegetable stock make an excellent marinade for many lean pieces of meat, poultry, and fish with little or no extra fat added.*
- *Cooking the vegetables in the same stock that is used to make the sauce retains all the water-soluble vitamins for the final dish.*

MAKES 10 PORTIONS

INGREDIENTS	WEIGHT/VOLUME
chicken breasts, 4 to 6 ounces, boneless and skinless	10 each
sesame oil	1/2 ounce
onions, finely chopped	8 ounces
garlic, chopped	1 tablespoon
lemon juice	2 tablespoons
black pepper, coarsely ground	1/2 teaspoon
low-sodium soy sauce	2 tablespoons
white vegetable stock	12 ounces
dry white wine	8 ounces
lean chicken stock	32 ounces
carrots, julienned	10 ounces
parsnips, julienned	10 ounces
zucchini, julienned	10 ounces
yellow squash, julienned	10 ounces
arrowroot	4 ounces
sesame seeds, dry roasted	1 ounce
MASHED LYONNAISE POTATOES	
red bliss potatoes, skins on	2 pounds
virgin olive oil	2 tablespoons
onions, small diced	1 pound
garlic, chopped	1 tablespoon
low-fat sour cream	12 ounces
white pepper, ground	1/2 teaspoon

1. Whisk together the sesame oil, onions, garlic, lemon juice, pepper, soy sauce, white vegetable stock, and white wine.
2. Place the chicken into this marinade, and refrigerate it for a minimum of 1 hour.
3. Bring the chicken stock to a full boil, and add julienned carrots and parsnips. Reduce to a simmer for 15 minutes.
4. Add the julienned zucchini and yellow squash. Cook for 5 additional minutes.
5. Dissolve the arrowroot in the vegetable stock, and add it to the cooking vegetables. Simmer until lightly thickened.
6. Remove the chicken breasts from the marinade, and grill them until they are well marked and cooked through.
7. To make the mashed lyonnaise potatoes, boil the potatoes in their skins in lightly salted water.
8. Heat the virgin olive oil in a sauté pan, and cook the diced onions until they are lightly browned.
9. Add the garlic to the sauté pan, and continue to cook over medium heat for 5 more minutes.
10. Drain the cooked potatoes from the water, and place them in a large bowl with the skins still attached.
11. Add the cooked onions, garlic, and sour cream to the bowl. Mash the foods together using a hand potato masher or a whip attachment in a mixer for a few seconds (to retain some texture).
12. Place the cooked chicken breast on a scoop of mashed lyonnaise potatoes in the center of the plate with the vegetables and sauce served on the side. Pour some sauce on top of the chicken before adding sesame seed garnish.
13. Garnish with toasted sesame seeds and serve.

Approximate values per serving: Calories 511, carbohydrates (grams) 48.6, protein (grams) 41.9, fat (grams) 16.7, cholesterol (milligrams) 94. Carbohydrates = 38% calories, protein = 33% calories, fat = 29% calories.

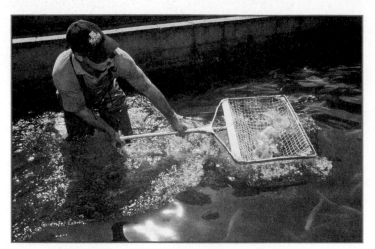

Farm-raised seafood is now seen as a viable resource.
Photo Researchers, Inc.

to ensure a good supply of seafood and shellfish in the future. As natural habitats become exhausted, farm-raised species and less-known species will begin to dominate the American culinary scene.

Seafood choices used to be regionally oriented, but this is no longer true. A continually shrinking global market means that salmon is now available in Florida, conch in Seattle, Maryland crabmeat in Denver, and Maine lobsters in Kentucky. Cooks are enjoying many healthful seafood choices. There are only a few guidelines to keep in mind in selecting seafood for nutritional menus:

- Buy only the freshest seafood possible and always from a reputable dealer.
- Be flexible to allow for seafood substitutions based on availability.
- Keep fresh seafood on ice and frozen seafood frozen until ready for use.
- Fresh seafood has a short shelf life; buy only what is needed right away.
- Most varieties of seafood can be cooked using low-fat cooking techniques (poaching, grilling, baking, and *en papillote* [in paper]).

The delicate flesh of seafood, although highly perishable, is the perfect medium for various taste and flavor combinations. Even fatty fish with stronger fish flavors like salmon, mackerel, and bluefish blend well with many herbs, spices, and other natural flavoring agents.

The Oven-Poached Grouper with Braised Leeks, Bamboo Shoots, Oyster Mushrooms, and Shoepeg Corn Dumplings is an example of a seafood entree that contributes proportionately to the overall nutritional value of the foods served while preserving the healthy benefits of the main seafood items.

OFFERING HEALTHY DESSERTS

Does the notion of healthy desserts seem like an illusion? We are so used to the mousse, cakes, and cheesecakes that fill pastry carts that it is hard to imagine that low-fat and low-calorie desserts could taste as good as traditional desserts. Most people do not believe that nutritionally prepared desserts can satisfy cravings or provide dining pleasure.

It may be asking too much of bakers to make low-fat, low-calorie, high-fiber mirror images of traditional desserts. Is a pound cake without eggs, butter, refined flour, or milk still a pound cake? Or should it be called something different?

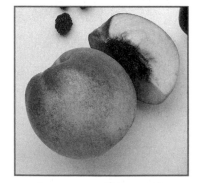

Peaches are a good source of B vitamins, folic acid, vitamin C, calcium, fiber, potassium, and beta-carotene, with a small amount of zinc.
Dave King © Dorling Kindersley

OVEN-POACHED GROUPER WITH BRAISED LEEKS, BAMBOO SHOOTS, OYSTER MUSHROOMS, AND SHOEPEG CORN DUMPLINGS

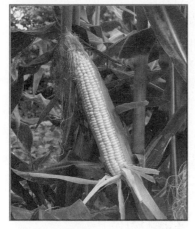

Shoepeg corn is a small white sweet corn.

Photo Researchers, Inc.

- *Grouper is low in saturated fat and sodium. It is also a good source of vitamin B_6, phosphorus, and potassium and a very good source of protein.*
- *Poaching protects the delicate flesh of the grouper and allows the flavors of the vegetables to mix and blend with the favors of the fish. Served in a shallow bowl, this dish offers great nutritional value.*
- *Bamboo shoots add texture and flavor to the dish and are a good source of soluble and insoluble fiber. One cup contains a scant 14 calories and half a gram of fat.*
- *Bamboo shoots are also a good source of potassium, phytochemicals, and phenolic acid, a potent antioxidant.*
- *Cornbread dumplings are a fiber-rich, low-fat starch accompaniment.*
- *Shoepeg corn is a small white sweet corn that holds its texture well when cooked. Corn in general is low in fat and calories and provides almost 3 grams of dietary fiber and protein per ear. Corn also contains moderate amounts of folate and vitamin C, with lots of magnesium and potassium.*

MAKES 10 PORTIONS

INGREDIENTS	WEIGHT/VOLUME
bay leaf	1 each
cardamom seeds, crushed	1 teaspoon
fennel seeds, crushed	1 teaspoon
white peppercorns, crushed	1/2 teaspoon
lean fish stock, preferably grouper	32 ounces
Sauvignon Blanc	8 ounces
shallots, finely diced	1 tablespoon
leeks, batonnet, white only	16 ounces
bamboo shoots, 1/4-inch slices	12 ounces
oyster mushrooms, sliced thin	12 ounces
grouper fillet, cut into 4- to 6-ounce portions	10 pieces
SHOEPEG CORN DUMPLINGS	
yellow cornmeal	10 ounces
flour	6 ounces
baking powder	2 teaspoons
sugar, granulated	1 tablespoon
salt	1/2 teaspoon
shoepeg corn (canned or frozen)	6 ounces
egg whites	2 each
low-fat milk	12 ounces
white vegetable stock	32 ounces

1. Using a piece of cheesecloth and butcher's twine, make a sachet of spices with the bay leaf, cardamom seeds, fennel seeds, and white peppercorns.
2. Mix together the fish stock, wine, and sachet in a sauce pot, and bring to a full boil.
3. Add the shallots, leeks, bamboo shoots, and sliced oyster mushrooms. Simmer for a few minutes.
4. Pour the mixture into a shallow roasting pan, and place the cut grouper fillets on top.
5. Cover the pan first with parchment paper and then with aluminum foil or a metal lid.
6. Bake in a 350°F oven for 40 minutes or until the fish is done.
7. To make the shoepeg corn dumplings, mix together the cornmeal, flour, baking powder, sugar, and salt.
8. In a separate bowl, whip the egg whites lightly with milk. Add them to the dry mix and blend together by hand. (Do not overmix if using a machine.)
9. Stir the shoepeg corn into the batter. (Drain the corn if canned.)
10. Bring the vegetable stock to a boil in a shallow pan, and reduce to a simmer.
11. Drop the dumpling mixture into simmering stock, using a large spoon to form elongated dumplings. Cover the pan and reduce to a low simmer. The dumplings will be cooked through in 5 minutes.
12. Serve the grouper with sauce and vegetables in the center of the plate. Garnish with two shoepeg dumplings each.

Approximate values per serving: Calories 411, carbohydrates (grams) 51.2, protein (grams) 37.9, fat (grams) 4.6, cholesterol (milligrams) 80. Carbohydrates = 50% calories, protein = 37% calories, fat = 10% calories.

When creating menu choices in the dessert category, consider the following tips:

- Decrease the amount of sugar required by one-fourth or one-half in either volume or weight (depending on how it is measured).
- Instead of using whole butter, use light butter, or a combination of butter and canola oil (low in saturated fat).
- Replace a portion of the sugar required in a recipe with fruit, fruit juice, or ground nuts.
- Some nuts and fruit are high in calories. Use half the amount in the standard recipe and chop the nuts or fruit very fine to distribute them evenly throughout the item.
- Use extracts, liqueurs, and spices to reduce salt and fats by enhancing other flavors.
- Vanilla, almond, and lemon extracts; nutmeg; allspice; mace; cinnamon; and ginger add flavor when fat and salts are reduced or eliminated.

The White Fluffy Cake with Peaches and Nectar is a dessert recipe that can be a healthy substitute for many high-fat, high-calorie dessert choices and still satisfy a hungry sweet tooth.

VEGETARIAN MENUS

Not everyone who chooses vegetarian entrees is a practicing vegetarian. Many people just like to experiment with new and exciting dishes. Others believe the low-fat mystique surrounding vegetarian cooking and occasionally choose vegetarian entrees as part of an overall controlled diet plan. Still others may try a well-prepared and satisfying vegetarian entree at the recommendation of vegetarian friends and family. Whatever the reason, the prevalence of vegetarian selections on restaurant menus continues to increase.

Vegetarian entrees go far beyond mere plates of vegetables and grain-rich foods. A plate of broccoli and green beans with a side of rice would not excite many appetites. Why would a vegetarian choose such an entree? Cooks must be ingenious in creating vegetarian entrees with taste and visual appeal.

Although the food components in a vegetarian diet come from a limited number of food groups, the numbers of choices within each group are astounding. Technological advances in horticulture and farming continue to expand these choices.

A well-planned and well-executed vegetarian entree should include a variety of items from the acceptable food groups: vegetables, fruits, nuts, seeds, legumes, and grain-rich foods for all vegetarians and vegans; dairy for lacto vegetarians; and eggs for lacto-ovo vegetarians. Three to five major ingredients, including two or three vegetables, one grain product, one seed or nut product, and a choice of legumes, can supply balanced nutrition, good visual and taste appeal, and a controlled calorie count.

Strict vegans have to take extra steps to guarantee proper protein intake in their diets. Other vegetarians can obtain adequate protein from the dairy products and eggs that they consume. Vegans, who do not eat dairy or eggs, have a greater risk of protein deficiency (particularly in the essential amino acids) than any other group of people.

Soybeans contain proteins that are the closest to animal proteins in the vegetable kingdom. Asians have long taken advantage of the healthy properties and versatility of soybeans in their cuisine. Recently, in light of increased interest in vegetarian foods, soybean consumption has spread across the globe.

Soybeans are legumes but are the only ones known to contain all essential amino acids. They are also naturally rich in fiber, calcium, iron, folate, and potassium. Soybeans are lower in starch than are many other legumes; they are also cholesterol-free and low in saturated fat and sodium.

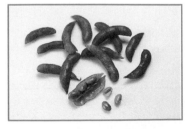

Soybeans are legumes that contain all the essential amino acids.
Pearson Education/PH College

WHITE FLUFFY CAKE WITH PEACHES AND NECTAR

- *This reduced-fat cake formula achieves only part of its rise from the small amount of creamed butter and sugar; the rest of the rise, in baking, comes from the whipped egg whites.*
- *The sliced peaches, nectar, and brandy serve as an icing to replace the more traditional buttercream icing.*
- *Other fruits, fruit juices, and fruit-flavored brandies can be substituted for the peaches to create more varieties of the same dessert.*
- *Peaches are a good source of B vitamins, folic acid, vitamin C, calcium, fiber, potassium, and beta-carotene, with a small amount of zinc.*

MAKES ONE 12-INCH TUBE CAKE, OR 12 PORTIONS

INGREDIENTS	WEIGHT/VOLUME
butter	2 ounces
sugar, granulated	3 ounces
skim milk	8 ounces
pure vanilla extract	1 teaspoon
almond extract	1/2 teaspoon
flour, sifted	12 ounces
baking powder	1 tablespoon
egg whites	4 ounces
sugar, finely granulated	2 ounces
cling free peaches, peeled and thinly sliced	32 ounces
peach nectar	8 ounces
peach brandy	2 ounces

1. Cream the butter and sugar together until very light and fluffy.
2. Mix together all the wet ingredients, and stir them into the mix.
3. Sift together all the dry ingredients and fold them into combined mixture.
4. Beat the egg whites until light and fluffy. Add the finely granulated sugar slowly while continuing to whip until soft peaks form. Fold gently into the mix.
5. Pour the mixture into a lightly greased tube cake pan, and bake at 350°F for 45 to 60 minutes. (The cake is done when the sides pull away from the pan and the cake springs back when pressed with a finger.)
6. In a sauté pan, heat the peaches with the nectar and simmer them together for 10 minutes.
7. Remove the peaches from the heat and add brandy. Cool the sauce.
8. The sauce can be served cold or warm over the sliced cake. Sorbet or low-fat yogurt could also be served with the cake.

Approximate values per serving: Calories 218, carbohydrates (grams) 40.6, protein (grams) 5.1, fat (grams) 4.2, cholesterol (milligrams) 10.1. Carbohydrates = 73% calories, protein = 9% calories, fat = 17% calories.

Soybeans are also versatile. They can be eaten as a vegetable, turned into milk and cheese substitutes, fermented into a rich sauce (soy sauce), and mashed or ground into many other marketable forms.

A vegetarian diet is not necessarily low in fat. Care must be taken not to fill vegetarian entrees with fatty beans, nuts, and seeds or overuse vegetable oils in frying, baking, dressing, and marinating foods. A vegetable kabob that has been marinated in an oil-rich dressing and served with a peanut, almond, or walnut sauce is not a low-fat item. Stir-fried vegetables are not necessarily low-fat items either. Care must be taken to measure only the proper amount of oil required to do the cooking and cut the vegetables into thin, small pieces to ensure fast cooking.

Offer vegetarian entrees that embody the healthy properties of nonmeat items, using the guidelines of counting the calorie content of fats and mixing vegetables, grains, and vegetable protein foods to ensure a balance of vitamins and minerals.

SUMMARY

Designer Nutrition

Except in specialty restaurants (Italian restaurants, for example), a well-constructed menu is one that offers a variety of menu items for the adventurous, the traditionalist, and the nutritionally aware customer. This variety can be achieved by using different cooking methods, styles of cuisine, and herbs and spices to create particular taste and flavor combinations.

The human body needs a regular supply of energy foods and nutrients throughout the day. The first meal of the day is the most important, because it helps the body recover from its repose and fasting. Other meals taken at intervals of four to five hours help the body balance its energy needs with its energy consumption.

All menu categories can be designed to offer customers better choices for planning their own meals. One main way to achieve this is to offer menu items prepared in a variety of ways (frying versus broiling/grilling or sautéing) and to select items as much for their nutritional values as for their flavor and eye appeal. Appetizers, salads, soups, entrees, and desserts can satisfy both hunger and nutritional needs when planned and executed properly, with the emphasis on health, diet, and taste.

CASE RESOLUTION

The discussion of low-carb versus healthy eating is continuing well into the twenty-first century. Adrianna's job is to serve and not educate, so she would be advised not to enter into a discussion of the value or dangers of low-carb diets.

The best thing that Adrianna could do is to review the items on the menu that do not contain any breading at all (such as broiled, steamed, or sautéed food items) and suggest the healthier preparations to her customers. She might also suggest that they substitute an additional healthy appetizer or salad for the breads or rolls that are normally served with meals.

REFERENCES

Hartbarger, J. C., and N. J. Hartbarger. 1983. *Eating for the eighties: A complete guide to vegetarian nutrition.* New York: Berkley Publication Group.

Hillman, H. 1981. *Kitchen science.* Boston: Houghton Mifflin.

Hunter, B. T. 1972. *The natural foods primer.* New York: Simon and Schuster.

McCormick and Co. 1984. *Spices of the world cookbook.* New York: McGraw-Hill.

1. How can a variety of cooking methods and seasonings enhance the dining experience for health conscious diners?

2. Are there any world cultures that practice healthy eating concepts as a way of life?

3. What are some characteristics of a nutritionally prepared appetizer?

4. What are some characteristics of a nutritionally prepared lunch or dinner entree?

5. What are some characteristics of a nutritionally prepared dessert?

APPENDIX I

WINES FOR COOKING

France, Italy, Germany, Spain, Portugal, Australia, and the United States all produce excellent wines—from the common table wines to the sophisticated varietal and sparkling wines. The only way to learn the proper use of these different wines is to taste them and cook with them.

FRANCE

The French winemakers have worked diligently to develop an excellent wine-making tradition. It is wise to investigate the different French wines when choosing the right wine for the kitchen.

All of France's six main wine-producing regions—Bordeaux, Champagne, Burgundy, Alsace, Rhône, and Loire—offer a variety of excellent wines. Each region is further divided into distinct districts that produce their own types and qualities of wine. Bordeaux, for example, is subdivided into nine districts where specific wines are produced: Médoc, Graves, Saint Émilion, Pomeral, Sauternes, Premières Côtes de Bordeaux, Côtes de Bourg, Côtes de Blay, and Entre-Deux-Mers. Wines produced in each of these regions and subdistricts have distinct characteristics, which make the task of choosing the right wine difficult but enjoyable.

Although complex, the task of choosing the right French wine can also be educational and fun. It may be best to start with the Bordeaux region, which is well known for its red wines from Médoc and Saint Émilion. Burgundy is known for its world-famous whites, especially from the Chablis and Mâconnais districts.

A sweeter wine, such as one of the whites from Sauternes, would be appropriate to mellow the bitter taste of turnips and endive. These wines are produced from overly ripe grapes that are almost raisins. In these grapes, the juices have partially evaporated, which leaves behind a high concentration of sugars, increases the glycerin, and thus reduces the acids. The resulting wines will be fruitier and sweeter than most other varieties.

Champagnes, when used in cooking, give a light body to many sauces, especially berry and other fruit sauces served with duck, lamb, or pork. Although the effervescence of champagne is lost during cooking, the character of the excellent wines used in the making of champagne remains on the palate. When Dom Perignon, the seventeenth-century Benedictine monk associated with the invention of champagne, invented the bubbly wine, he insisted on using only the finest white wines for the base. The true champagne producers of today still insist on this tradition.

ITALY

An excursion through Italy's wine regions would be equally exciting and educational. Perhaps because of the great influence and financial support of the Catholic Church in the production and distribution of wines, Italy can boast of having one of the finest array of wines in the world. The Catholic monks who raised vineyards to produce their sacrificial wines took great pains to produce the finest wines in the world.

Wines are produced almost everywhere in Italy, from the Piedmont, one of the northernmost regions, to Sicily, the southern island that is the home of the Marsala wines.

Some of the best Italian red wines come from the northern Piedmont. The noble grape of this region is called the *nebbiolo*. Barbera and grignolino grapes are also important in the Piedmont and Lombardy regions for producing a wide range of reds. These wines are excellent cooking wines whose character withstands longer cooking methods like braising and stewing.

The white grape trebbiano, also grown in the north, is the base grape for Soave, one of Italy's most popular white wines. Soave is excellent for use in poultry dishes, seafood sauces, and stews.

From Tuscany come the popular Chianti and Chianti Classico wines. Although it is among the most famous Italian wines in the United States because of its straw-wrapped bottle, Chianti Governato has few culinary attributes. This particular Chianti is intended to be drunk while quite young and is sold in the popular straw fiasco more for decoration than for any other purpose. Because of its youth, however, Chianti Governato cannot contribute a full-bodied character to sauces or stews. Many chefs believe, therefore, that Chianti does not make a good cooking wine. The other varieties—Chianti Vecchio and Chianti Classico Riserva—are excellent cooking wines. These wines are aged from two to three years and acquire a more developed character suitable for cooking and for marinades. Chianti Classico Riserva is the perfect flavoring liquid for braising rabbit and quail and for shellfish ragouts and sauces.

From Sicily come some great wines used in kitchens around the globe. Mount Etna, the volcano on the eastern end of Sicily, has contributed a fertile volcanic ash to much of the island. This ash is a perfect grape vine fertilizer. The best wines are produced from grapes grown directly on the volcano's slopes and bear its name: Etna bianco, Etna rosso, and Etna rossato.

Perhaps the most famous Sicilian wine is Marsala, a fortified wine, which means that brandy was added to raise alcohol content in the bottle after the fermentation had ceased. The volcanic soil in which the wine's grapes are grown gives Marsala an acid undertone that withstands the highest cooking temperatures, as in sautéing techniques. Marsala is popular not only for cooking but also for drinking. The sweet Marsala makes an excellent dessert wine; the dry Marsala is generally used for cooking.

GERMANY

Germany is also divided into several wine-growing regions. The three that are most famous are the Rheingau, Rheinhessen, and Rheinpfalz.

From Rheingau come some of the most famous wines in the world. Johannisberg, Hallgarten, and Rauenthal are a few of the most popular. This region's wines have excellent body, flavor, and character and are among the longest lived of any German wines. They are generally fruity in nature and can add great depth to sauces, marinades, and desserts.

From the region of Rheinhessen come the most popular liebfraumilchs. Liebfraumilch is neither a district nor a vineyard but is rather a blending of wines. Liebfraumilch is an excellent drinking wine that may be used as an aperitif (before-dinner cocktail), as a beverage consumed with the meal, or as an after-dinner wine. Liebfraumilch's consistent flavor makes it a great cooking wine for soups, stews, and sauces.

Rheinpfalz is Germany's largest wine-producing region. Although much of this region's product is consumed by Germans, its excellent white and red table wines make good cooking wines when available in the United States. Table wines are usually blended from multiple varieties of grapes and usually have less distinctive characteristics than varietals; in Rheinpfalz, this is not the case.

SPAIN

Spain's southernmost wine region, Andalucía, is the home of the country's most prized viniculture possession, sherry wine. The lands that produce the finest of these wines are situated between the Guadalquivir and the Guadalete rivers. Jerez de la Frontera is the primary shipping port for sherry.

The sherry we know today is the product of soil, fruit, and the intricate solera system. Solera is a controlled blending system that takes seven to ten years to complete. Sherries are also fortified with brandy.

The best sherries for cooking are the finos, which range from the very dry manzanilla to the pale dry amontillado, which also has a slightly nutty flavor. The sweet sherry wines, oloroso, cream, and tawny, may be used in dessert sauces and fillings.

PORTUGAL

Of all the wines produced in Portugal, the fortified port wine is the most prized in the culinary arena. Port is fortified before fermentation has completely ceased, which leaves some of the unused sugars behind. Port is, therefore, always a sweet wine. Port's significant character gives distinction to sauces and stews.

Port comes in three types: vintage, ruby, and tawny. Each of these wines is excellent for drinking and as a flavoring liquid for cooking.

Vintage port is produced only during exceptional years, when nature has cooperated fully with the winegrowers. If rain, sun, and the soil work together through the entire growing season, an exceptional wine full of character, bouquet, and flavor can be achieved. These conditions usually occur about every three to four years. Vintage ports need several years to mature fully in the bottle and may be too costly for regular kitchen use. For the special occasion or feast, however, there can be no substitute.

Ruby and tawny ports are aged in wooden casks, which give character to these otherwise young, fruity wines. They are usually blended wines, which ensures a consistency in style and quality similar to that achieved in the sherry solera system. Tawny ports that are blended and well wooded (aged) are generally more consistent and thus better for culinary use than are younger ports.

Another Portuguese wine is the popular Madeira, which takes its name from the island on which the grapes are grown. The name Madeira means the "wooded isle." The island of Madeira was discovered by Portuguese sailors on their way south around Africa in search of the spice islands. Captain Joso Goncalves of the Portuguese navy was given the task of settling the island and establishing it as a resting place for other ships. Finding it to be completely covered by a dense forest, and being short of manpower and time, Goncalves decided to burn the trees as a quick means of clearing the land.

Captain Goncalves was later rewarded for his deed. The volcanic island covered by a thousands of years of decaying organic matter was completely covered by several feet of freshly produced potash as a result of Goncalves's actions. Captain Goncalves accidentally made Madeira one of the most fertile wine-producing islands in the world. This combination of volcanic soil, organic debris, and potash was perfect for the cultivation of grape vines and, later, sugarcane. One of the oldest domesticated grape varieties, the malvasia candiae, was transplanted from Crete to this new lush home. Before long Portugal had a thriving wine-producing colony.

There are four types of Madeira: sercial, verdelho, bual, and malmsey. Sercial is the driest and is suitable in most culinary applications. Verdelho is less dry. Bual is almost sweet. Malmsey is the sweetest and is almost liqueur-like in consistency and taste.

APPENDIX II

AN ANTHOLOGY OF THE MOST GENERALLY USED HERBS AND SPICES

Allspice was a relatively new spice to the Europeans who settled America, although it is one of the only spices native to the Americas. Found abundantly in the Caribbean islands, it is the fruit of a tropical evergreen of the myrtle family. Often referred to as the Jamaican pepper, the berries are picked green and allowed to sun dry. This transforms them into a form resembling plump peppercorns, without the hot bite. Allspice gets its common name because of its resemblance in flavor to a blend of other spices, such as cloves, cinnamon, and nutmeg. It can be bought in dried berry form, which is preferable to crushed or ground, and is easily crushed under a rolling pin before being added to a variety of dishes. Allspice is excellent in flavoring meat, poultry, and seafood stews and sauces, especially those with venison, rabbit, duck, turkey, shrimp, and mussels. Although tradition prefers the use of allspice in pies and puddings, it is also excellent in vegetable dishes, including the family of winter squashes, greens, and root vegetables.

Anise is an old spice known throughout the Mediterranean region. It has been used to flavor everything from alcohol (anisette) to curries. Combined with mace, allspice, ginger, coriander, and cumin, anise adds character to many vegetarian dishes, which are the mainstay of southern Indian cuisine. Anise can be bought as an extract, which is distilled with alcohol, and it is excellent for flavoring cream sauces and puddings. Its seeds can be easily ground and used to flavor many stews and fricassees or left whole as desired. It is excellent in salad marinades in combination with dill and sweet peppers, or just by itself with cucumbers and sour cream.

Basil is one of the Mediterranean's most widely used herbs. It grows easily in most climates, and its seeds are successfully stored for replanting the following growing season. Because of the ease of growing basil in hothouses, it is available fresh year-round. Basil is part of the mint family and has a slightly mint taste when first eaten. In dried leaf form that minty taste is almost lost, but basil's characteristic sweet flavor remains. Besides its popular use in Italian tomato sauce and salad dressings, basil is also a good seasoning to use for roasting meats, poultry, and fish. It is an excellent blending herb when used in combination with some of the more powerful-tasting herbs like cumin and tarragon. Fresh basil leaves may also be chopped and mixed with salad greens or marinated eggplant for excitement and character. There are at least four related basils for the modern cook to use: lemon basil, cinnamon basil, red basil, and Israeli basil (lemon and cinnamon because of the related flavors they impart; red basil for its color; and Israeli basil for its hardiness).

Bay, or laurel leaves, as they are sometimes called, come from an evergreen whose cultivation dates back to ancient history. In Greece and imperial Rome bay leaves were used as a symbol of wisdom and glory; they were often tied into a crown worn by emperors and kings (bay leaves are also a symbol for scholarship; the word baccalaureate means "laurel berries"). As a gardening shrub, laurels add a robust aroma to gardens throughout Europe. Bay is well known for its contributions to stews and meat pies. It gained this reputation because of its year-round availability: In the cold winters, when herbs were unavailable and imported spices costly, farmers would merely pick a few bay leaves from their gardens to lend spice to their soups and stews. Along with the game they hunted and the dried beans that were stored for the winter, they could easily make great-tasting meals with the addition of a few bay leaves. Bay has a very strong flavor when fresh, and only a few leaves are needed. To impart its flavor in sautéed dishes, bay leaves can be fried in hot oil and then removed from the dish, leaving behind their aroma.

Caraway is known to most Americans only as the seeds found in rye breads. This is unfortunate because the flavor is an excellent enhancer for many other dishes as well. Germans and Austrians know about the benefits of caraway, and this seed finds its way into many of their dishes. Goulash is a stew with caraway and paprika as the main flavors. Sauerbraten and sauerkraut both complement the taste of caraway. Caraway is an excellent spice for strong-flavored dishes like these and others made with lamb or venison. It is also an excellent accompanying spice with flavors like sesame, sage, or sweet potato.

Cardamom is an underestimated spice today. It is found rarely in some bakery items and sausage recipes, but it is generally forgotten. At one time, however, it was so popular that its rich fragrance was used as the essence in some of the more valuable perfumes and oils of ancient Rome. Cardamom is the second most expensive spice (saffron comes first), because the pods containing the seeds are cut from the plant by hand, for a crop yield of only 250 pounds per acre. It is native to India, although modern sources also include Guatemala. Cardamom comes in seed form and is easily crushed or ground as needed. It is excellent when used in dishes that need a subtle yet distinguishing taste (rice pilaf or creamed onions), but it can also be used in combination flavors (curries and meat pies). Cardamom was one of the original curry spices and rightfully has a reputation of being one of the great blending spices.

Cassia is similar in taste to cinnamon but a little more pungent. It also comes from the bark of an evergreen, and it is harvested and dried in the same way as cinnamon.

Cayenne pepper was one of the "spices" discovered by Christopher Columbus when his ships reached the Caribbean islands. One of the varieties of the genus *Capsicum*, cayenne is related to sweet bell peppers, jalapeños, and chilies. Cayenne pepper pods grow 3 to 4 inches long, are narrow and taper to a point, and are red. The pods are first dried and then crushed (leaving the whole seeds and similar size pieces) or ground very fine. Like all spices, cayenne will eventually lose its potency in ground form; however, this fact is not generally known because when freshly ground, cayenne pepper's potency is extreme. Cayenne is also used to produce liquid hot sauces used as flavoring spices for soups and stews.

Celery seed, because of its close resemblance in taste to its mother plant, is used frequently as a spice in various food preparations. It is a small seed that does not have to be crushed or ground to release its flavor. Its concentrated celery flavor is quickly detected in almost any dish it is used in, and it is excellent in cold food preparations and hot food recipes. Celery seed offers a unique blending taste that can smooth out otherwise pungent tastes or enhance some of the most delicate flavors.

Chervil has long been considered one of the essential herbs in French and other Mediterranean cuisines. It shares a place with tarragon and parsley as one of the three fines herbes used in many French dishes and soups. In dried form it has almost no taste, just as dried parsley has no distinguishing taste, and therefore it has not gained much popularity in American cooking. Now that it is available in fresh form throughout the world, its popularity is sure to rise. Chervil can be used in meat and vegetable dishes and has a clean and refreshing taste. Its flavors are easily extracted when sautéed in oil or steeped in stock or sauces. It should never be added too early in the cooking process; in fact, it should only be added to the dish or soup just before removing it from the heat source because its delicate flavor dissipates quickly.

Cinnamon has had one of the most romantic and adventurous histories of all the spices. The Arabs, who transported cinnamon from the East into Europe, were determined not to share in the trade of this valuable spice and created unbelievable stories about its collection and transport to scare off anyone even thinking of competing. A story recorded by Herodotus tells of a great bird in the Far East who builds its nest out of sticks of cinnamon high in the rocky peaks of great mountains. According to Herodotus, to collect the spice, traders must climb these peaks and risk their lives. Naturally, stories like these also kept the price of cinnamon very high.

Actually, cinnamon comes from the bark of a laurel-like evergreen found in Ceylon. It was not until the Portuguese captain Vasco da Gama reached India by sea in 1498 that the myths about cinnamon were finally put to rest. Modern traditions dictate that cinnamon can be used only in bakery items. In truth, cinnamon has as much flexibility as any other spice. It is excellent for sautéed potatoes and for June peas, carrots, sweet potatoes, and even brussels sprouts. Cinnamon has long been used in cream sauces for famous dishes like Greek moussaka and in meat pies and stuffing for turkey, quail, pheasant, and duck. It is also good for seafood stuffing for flounder or for making deviled crab. Cinnamon should be bought and used in stick form whenever possible; the stick can be used to flavor a stock or sauce and then removed and used over again. When the stick form cannot be used, fresh ground cinnamon is adequate. Like any preground spice, cinnamon's potency is lost quickly with age.

Cloves are dried, unopened blossoms of a tall evergreen nearly 30 feet high. The tree's crimson buds are picked before they open and dried on palm leaf mats (in the drying process, the buds turn reddish brown). Cloves can be purchased either whole (which are easily crushed) or ground (ground cloves are potent when fresh). Cloves, and especially their oil, have been used throughout the centuries as a cure for many ailments. The use of clove oil as a pain reliever is well documented. Clove oil is used in medicinal teas to aid in digestion and to reduce fevers. Cloves are traditionally used to flavor hams and spice cakes. Their distinctive taste, however, could be used to flavor a variety of dishes (vegetable dishes and savory pies and fillings, for example). Cloves are also one of the great blending spices; they blend well not only with cinnamon, nutmeg, and allspice but with sage, fennel, caraway, anise, and bay leaves.

Coriander has a marked place in history. In the Bible (Exodus 16:31) there is a description of the life-saving bread called *manna*, which fell from the sky to help feed the Israelites in the desert: "The bread from heaven tasted of coriander seed and honey." Coriander blends well with the taste of whole grains, which have a similarly nutty taste when roasted. Coriander seeds are small round spheres, light brown, with a thin shell easily ground or crushed with a rolling pin. Coriander is excellent in sausage recipes and savory dishes of all descriptions. Coriander is used in some of the world's best chutneys, and it blends well with most varieties of fish and shellfish.

Cumin has long been recognized as one of the world's most widely used spices. It is native to Egypt (which gives it one of the oldest histories of any spice used in cooking) and is predominant in foods of the Near East and Latin America. It comes in seed and ground form and is the characteristic flavor of chorizo, the famous Spanish sausage. Cumin is the main flavor in two very different spice blends, chili powder and curry powder. Cumin has a fairly dominant flavor that blends well with sage, thyme, garlic, or ginger; it gives exciting flavor to rice, beans, potatoes, vegetables, meat dishes, fish, and poultry. Freshly ground cumin seeds can also be used to flavor biscuits or wafers; cumin lends a certain Mediterranean flair to such foods.

Dill can be used either for its leaves or its seeds, although its seeds are more pungent than its leaves. Dill is not a true perennial, but it will grow back every year from seeds that fall on the ground. Dill is the characteristic flavor of the world-famous dill pickle, and dill seems to do extremely well with other marinated preparations as well. Dill has an intense flavor and should be used with other dominant flavors (with sour cream and in vinegar dressings, for example).

Fennel, or finocchio, as it is called by the Italians, has a flavor similar to anise yet is a little more delicate. Fennel's flavor blends well in many cooking and baking preparations. Fennel may be used for its leaves (like dill), for its seeds, or as a vegetable. Fennel produces a stalklike plant similar in texture to pascal celery with a slightly rounder bulb at the root. Fennel, as a vegetable, can be braised, simmered, or sautéed; it can also be used as a flavoring vegetable for stews and soups and a variety of other dishes. Fennel is the characteristic flavor in Italian sausage and has gained world popularity for its use in tomato sauces, soups, and stews. It is used to flavor many European-style hearth breads and is a popular ingredient in foccacia and sandwich rolls.

Garlic, which originally came from Asia, enjoys as intriguing a history as any of the other herbs and spices. Its medicinal properties, though only scientifically evidenced in the twentieth century, have long been associated with warding off evil spirits (in medieval times sickness was perceived as the work of an evil spirit) and with promoting lasting youth. Modern research suggests that garlic can help lower cholesterol and strengthen the immune system, but these findings are still speculative. Garlic is a bulbous plant made of several smaller cloves. It is generally used fresh and is preferred in this form. Because of its popularity, garlic can also be found in several dried forms, from chopped and minced to flakes and powder. The juice from garlic can be processed and used in its liquid form to flavor sauces and stews. Garlic's flavor changes dramatically when roasted or fried, producing a milder and a sweeter version, respectively.

Ginger is one the oldest spices used in cooking. Centuries ago, Chinese sailors carried potted ginger on long journeys so they could enjoy its fine flavor and benefit from its medicinal properties. Today ginger is used frequently in Asian and Pacific Island cuisine. Ginger has a peppery flavor and gives curry powder its spicy hot characteristic. The fresh ginger root can be easily shredded, chopped, or grated and is available year-round. Ground dried ginger loses most of its characteristics and should be avoided. Ginger is excellent with summer and winter squash, celery, rutabaga, and turnips; it is also good with savory poultry and meat dishes and seafood stews.

Horseradish is a root that is native to Eastern Europe. Today it is grown around the world wherever other root crops are grown. The roots are first washed thoroughly and then ground with their skins (the skins give horseradish its characteristic tang). A small amount of water is added during the grinding process to provide a smooth consistency. Horseradish should be refrigerated to help retain its highly volatile properties. Grinding fresh horseradish releases vapors 10 times more potent than the vapors released from opening a jar of horseradish; these vapors may be too powerful for the average person to bear. Buy fresh ground horseradish from a reputable vendor and you will be guaranteed a consistent product ready for use in your recipes.

Horseradish is used mainly in cold sauces like cocktail, barbecue, and mustard. Because of its potency, it is generally used as a condiment spice.

Juniper is a berry that is widely known for its use in the flavoring of some English gins. Its sweet aromatic taste has been used for many years as an essential ingredient in game stews like venison or rabbit, but juniper can also be used to flavor vegetable dishes like cabbage, broccoli, and onion. Juniper has a strong but sweet taste that can blend well with other characteristic tastes without being lost.

Mace is the aril, or thin skin, around the nut of the nutmeg that is removed and then dried and ground. Its taste, therefore, resembles the nutmeg but is somewhat milder. Mace is much more versatile than nutmeg because its sweet taste is easily blended with other tastes without overpowering them, as is sometimes the case with nutmeg. Mace is more expensive than nutmeg because it is only a small part of the whole nut, yet its delicate fragrance can enhance the most subtle of flavors. Mace can also be used to stimulate vibrant flavors because its sweet taste lingers in the mouth and in the nostrils.

Marjoram, which is sometimes called *sweet oregano*, is one of the most popular herbs of the southern Mediterranean region. It grows wild almost everywhere dirt and sun are found and is a hardy perennial. Marjoram is similar in taste to thyme but not as pungent and can therefore blend well with thyme and oregano. Whenever a dish calls for a subtle flavor of fresh herbs, marjoram is an excellent choice.

Mint has a sweet and slightly peppery taste. It, too, is a hardy perennial that renews itself every spring for fresh cuttings. Mint has a strong characteristic flavor that should be used in moderation in cooking. A little mint can enhance the flavor of green peas; too much mint can dominate the delicate flavor of some vegetables. As a replacement for salt in vegetable cooking, a touch of mint gives both sweetness and a peppery spice to many foods.

Mustard is related to the cabbage family and is used for its green broad leaves, which are high in vitamin A, magnesium, potassium, iron, and fiber, and for its dried pungent seeds. Mustard seeds produce the characteristic spicy taste of prepared mustard. Mustard has been used in cooking for thousands of years. Its leaves can be cooked and served like a vegetable, and its seeds can be ground into a spicy condiment. The ground seeds are mixed with water and allowed to rest for 10 to 15 minutes; the water stimulates enzyme growth, resulting in a hot and volatile flavor. Mustard seeds are very small and can be easily crushed, or they can be used whole to develop their taste through longer cooking processes. In creating recipes, however, it is difficult to judge how much mustard to use because the flavor is not released until late in the cooking process. Recipes using mustard should be tested thoroughly and adjustments made until a satisfactory amount of mustard is identified. Generally, too little mustard is used to give any value to the taste, or too much is used and overpowers the taste.

Nutmeg is the nut, or kernel, of a large fruit that resembles a yellow plum. Nutmeg grows on a large evergreen and is allowed to ripen and dry on the tree. When the fruits are dry they split open, revealing a bright red aril, the mace, with the nutmeg in the center. Nutmeg has a strong characteristic taste that can easily overpower other more subtle tastes. A few specks of nutmeg can beautifully enhance the flavor of greens and potatoes, whereas a half teaspoon of nutmeg can overwhelm other flavors. Nutmeg is excellent when used with some of the stronger flavors like venison, lamb, sweet potatoes, and cabbage, but in small amounts nutmeg can be used in almost all preparations. Nutmeg blends extremely well with cinnamon, mace, and allspice (an American spice blend commonly referred to as pumpkin pie spice) and can be used for other fruit, squash, or potato pies.

Oregano, commonly referred to as the "pizza pie spice," is related to marjoram yet has a much more pungent flavor. Oregano is a perennial that grows wild throughout the southern Mediterranean, and it has been used in all types of recipes from meat stews and pies to fish soups and shellfish chowders. Oregano's potency holds up well when dried; however, fresh leaves are preferred.

Paprika is the dried ground flesh of a red capsicum pepper called *Capsicum annum*. Until the nineteenth century, paprika was always hot, and then Hungarian spice millers developed a process to remove the seeds and hot membrane inside. Paprika takes its name from a Hungarian word meaning "Turkish pepper." Although Christopher Columbus was the first to bring paprika peppers back to Spain, paprika's full introduction as a dried spice did not come until much later. Today there are both Spanish and Hungarian paprikas. The Spanish variety is less pungent. Paprika is one of the main flavoring ingredients in Hungarian goulash and is often used in spice mixes like chili powder, Old Bay, and Caribbean jerk.

Parsley has been underrated as an herb and overrated as a garnish. Because of its ease in growing, parsley is available fresh year-round. It has a sweet slightly minty taste when eaten fresh, but it loses its flavor quickly when dried. Fresh chopped parsley can be stored for several days by following this simple procedure: Place the chopped parsley in a cheesecloth bag and rinse it thoroughly with cold water. Then, using the bag, squeeze the parsley until no more water comes out. Remove the parsley from the cheesecloth, and place it in a closed container with a few pieces of stale bread. The bread will help remove all the excess moisture and keep the parsley in a semidried state. Parsley is one of the better edible garnishes. When eaten fresh, it acts like a breath freshener and leaves the palate clean and fresh.

Pepper has long been one of the most prized of all the world's spices. It adds excitement to almost every dish and is identifiable in any combination. Green, white, and black peppercorns are all the same berry. Green peppercorns are picked green, cured in brine, or freeze-dried. Black peppercorns are picked green and dried in the sun, which turns their outer skin black. White peppercorns are ripened on the tree and have a slightly crimson color. Their outer skin is removed, leaving behind the white peppercorn.

Black peppercorns are the most pungent and green the least pungent. Black and white peppercorns are usually cracked with the flat blade of a knife or ground in a pepper mill for the most flavor. Because of the prevalence of pepper in recipes, the practice of cracking or grinding your own pepper may be too cumbersome. In this case it is better to buy cracked or restaurant-grind (coarse) peppercorns for a rich peppery taste. Finely ground pepper should be avoided unless a recipe specifically calls for its use. Ground white pepper is usually used to season white or blonde sauces because black pepper will leave behind small specks in the sauces. Red pepper should not be confused with the other peppers. Red pepper is of the capsicum family called *cayenne* and is related to chili peppers and bell peppers.

Peppercress has bright light green leaves with parsley-like foliage. Its peppery flavor gives it its characteristic name. It can be used in whole leaf form as a salad green, or it can be chopped and used as an herb.

Rosemary is most popular in the eastern Mediterranean. Its leaves come from an evergreen that grows on the rocky coasts of Italy, Greece, and Turkey. Rosemary has a distinct flavor that is excellent in any number of savory dishes. Fresh rosemary is available year-round because it comes from an evergreen. The fresh leaves can be chopped finely and left in the preparation; if the dried form is used the leaves are tough and should be removed from the dish before serving. A sachet may be needed to remove the leaves easily when the cooking is complete.

Saffron is the dried stigmas from the flower of the saffron crocus, which grows throughout the Mediterranean region. The tiny stigmas must be picked by hand. An estimated

750,000 plants are needed for 1 pound of saffron, so the price of this flavorful spice has always been extremely high. Saffron has a flavor that is worth the price. It is one of the primary spices used in the world-famous French seafood stew called *bouillabaisse*, and it is used to flavor many Spanish dishes, like paella. The beauty of saffron is that only a small amount is needed to give a recipe a unique signature taste.

Sage is another of those spices for which, in America, tradition has dictated only a few culinary applications (turkey with sage dressing, country breakfast sausages). In other areas of the world, sage is used more for its medicinal properties than for cooking. The people of the Mediterranean believe that a tea made from the leaves of fresh sage can relieve almost every kind of digestive or intestinal problem. Sage has a very distinctive taste, which makes it more versatile than other delicately flavored herbs and spices. Its flavor can enhance stews, pies, stuffings, and sausages. Sage is also good on its own as a flavoring for potato dishes, corn, carrots, celery, turnips, and vegetable greens. Purple sage is also available; its taste is the same as regular sage.

Savory is an herb whose taste most closely resembles that of thyme, yet it is not as pungent. Savory can be used in a variety of savory dishes or as the primary seasoning for beans, peas, rice, leeks, and potatoes.

Sesame is a spice that has lost its allure over the centuries. At one time in history, sesame was so favored that it was believed to possess supernatural powers. The Arabian prince Ali Baba, in searching for a city's hidden treasure, commanded the secret passage door to open by chanting the words, "Open sesame." Sesame seeds contain 60% oil. This extracted oil was once used to light lamps and has been used in Asian cooking for thousands of years. Today, a common use for the toasted seeds is to flavor and garnish hamburger buns and other breads. Sesame deserves a more vibrant place among the world's seasonings: Its flavor is unique, especially when roasted before use. Sesame can be used to highlight the flavors of any stuffing or breading or to flavor salad dressings and marinades. Sesame oil can be used alone or as part of other frying mediums in many sautéed dishes. Sesame oil is great in oriental stir-fries, where it is commonly used, and also in sautéed lamb, venison, chicken, and veal dishes.

Tarragon has earned a high place among the world's seasonings for its unique taste and versatility. Tarragon is not as easily grown as some of the other herbs, yet the demand for this herb has created a world market for its fresh leaves as well as for tarragon leaves preserved in brine. Dried tarragon should be avoided because it tends to have a very "grassy" taste. Tarragon gained world recognition for its use in béarnaise sauces and in cream sauces for poached fish and shellfish. A simple dish of a toasted English muffin with Gruyère cheese and crabmeat becomes an excellent luncheon item or appetizer when topped with fresh béarnaise sauce. Tarragon oil and vinegar are used commonly in salad making and in vegetable and meat marinades.

Thyme is a popular spice. Not only does it provide good-character tastes by itself, as in Cajun jambalaya, but it is excellent in blending with other spices. Thyme has small leaves that dry well, but the dried herb has a more pronounced flavor than fresh thyme and can overpower delicate tastes. Fresh thyme has a distinctive flavor, yet it enhances other flavors rather than hiding them. Thyme can be used in almost any type of dish, including as a flavoring in biscuits, rolls, and muffins. Lemon thyme has just a hint of lemon flavor. Israeli thyme is a little more pungent with slightly larger leaves.

Turmeric is a spice with little flavor of its own and is generally used as a coloring spice in curries, soups, and rice dishes. Turmeric is sometimes used in place of saffron in paella and other dishes because of its low cost; however, the taste is sacrificed.

Vanilla is not usually thought of as a spice, yet it fits both the botanical and culinary definitions of spices. Vanilla is the pod of a climbing orchid grown in tropical America. The pod is dried slowly in the sun, on top of palm leaves, and turned many times during the drying process. Vanilla is most readily available as an extract, which has been distilled with alcohol, yet its dried pods are superior. The pods can be infused for their flavor in stocks or sauces and then rinsed off and stored for later use. One single vanilla bean can last through several applications. Tradition dictates that vanilla is used primarily in dessert applications. Its versatility is much greater than that, however. Vanilla is great with fish and seafood, chowders, and savory meat dishes; its slight sweetness can enhance an otherwise unexciting flavor. Only a small amount of vanilla is needed to turn the taste completely around to one that is unique and pleasant.

Wasabi is an Asian spice that is gaining in popularity in Western cuisine. It is the root of *Wasabia japonica* and is ground into either a dry powder or a wet paste. The character flavor of wasabi resembles a combination of mustard and horseradish. Wasabi can be found in most Asian food stores and is available from specialty food vendors.

FOOD WEIGHTS AND MEASURES

Food	Weight	Measure (approximately)
Allspice	1 oz.	4 1/4 Tbsp.
Almonds (chopped)	1 lb.	3 1/4 cups
Apples (fresh)	1 lb.	3 medium or 4 small
(sliced)	1 lb.	2 1/2 cups
(diced)	1 lb.	2 3/4 cups
Apricots (fresh)	1 lb.	5–7 large
Asparagus (fresh)	1 lb.	15–20 stalks
Avocado	1 lb.	2 medium (3 small)
Bacon (cooked)	1 lb.	80–90 slices
(cooked; diced)	1 lb.	15–20 slices
(raw)	1 lb.	2 cups
Baking powder	1 oz.	2 1/4 Tbsp.
Baking soda	1 oz.	2 1/4 Tbsp.
Bananas (fresh)	1 lb.	2 1/2–3 medium (4 small)
(mashed)	1 lb.	2 1/2 cups
Barbecue sauce	1 lb.	2 cups
Barley, pearl (uncooked)	1 lb.	2 1/2 cups
Basil (dried)	1 oz.	1 1/2 cups
(fresh)	1 oz.	1 cup (50 medium leaves)
Bay leaves	1 oz.	1 3/4 cups
Beans, green (fresh; cooked)	1 lb.	3 1/2 cups
Beans, lima (fresh)	1 lb.	3 1/2 cups
Beef (diced; cooked)	1 lb.	3 1/4 cups
Beef (ground; uncooked)	1 lb.	2 1/4 cups
Beets (diced; cooked)	1 lb.	2–3 1/2 cups
(fresh)	1 lb.	3–4 medium
Blackberries (fresh)	1 lb.	3–4 cups
Blueberries (fresh)	1 lb.	2–3 cups
Bran flakes	1 oz.	1 cup
Bread (fresh; dry crumbs)	1 lb.	9 1/2 oz.
(loaf; fresh)	1 lb.	15–18 slices (1/2 inch thick)
(crumbs; dry)	1 lb.	4 cups
Broccoli (florets)	1 lb.	3 3/4 cups
(head)	1 lb.	1 medium
Brussels sprout (fresh)	1 lb.	4 cups
Butter	1 lb.	4 4-oz. sticks (2 cups)
Buttermilk (fresh)	1 quart	4 cups
Cabbage (raw; fresh)	1 lb.	1/2 small head
(shredded; lightly packed)	1 lb.	4 cups
(cooked)	1 lb.	2 cups
Cake mix (standard; boxed)	18.25 oz. (1 lb. 2 1/4 oz.)	4 cups
Cantaloupe	3 lb.	1 medium
Caraway seeds	1 oz.	4 Tbsp.
Carrots (fresh; whole; raw)	1 lb.	4–6 medium
(diced)	1 lb.	3–3 1/2 cups
Catsup (bottle)	2 lb. 4 oz.	36 oz.
Cauliflower (florets)	1 lb.	3 3/4–4 cups
(head)	1 lb.	1 medium

Food	Weight	Measure (approximately)
Cayenne pepper	1 oz.	4 1/2 Tbsp.
Celery (chopped)	1 lb.	3–3 1/4 cups
(diced)	1 lb.	4 cups
Celery salt	1 oz.	2 1/2 Tbsp.
Celery seed	1 oz.	4 Tbsp.
Cheese, cheddar/Swiss	1 lb.	4–4 1/4 cups
Cheese, cottage	1 lb.	2–2 1/2 cups
Cheese, cream	1 lb.	2 cups (4 8 oz. pkgs)
Cheese, mozzarella (shredded)	1 lb.	3–3 1/2 cups
Cheese, Parmesan/Romano (commercially grated)	1 lb.	3–3 1/2 cups
(freshly grated)	1 lb.	7 1/2–8 cups
Cheese, Slices (commercial)	1 lb.	16–19 slices
Cherries, maraschino (drained)	1 lb.	50–60
Cherries (fresh)	1 lb.	40–45
Chicken (cooked)	1 lb.	3–3 1/2 cups
Chili powder	1 oz.	4 Tbsp.
Chives	1 oz.	3 1/4 cups
Chocolate, baking	1 lb.	16 squares
Chocolate (grated)	1 lb.	2 cups
(melted)	1 lb.	3 1/2 cups
Chocolate chips (all regular size chips)	1 lb.	2 1/2 cups
Cilantro (fresh)	1 oz.	1 cup (scant)
Cinnamon (ground)	1 oz.	3 3/4 Tbsp.
(sticks)	1 oz.	6–8 pieces
Cloves (ground)	1 oz.	4 Tbsp.
(whole)	1 oz.	4 3/4 Tbsp.
Cocoa	1 lb.	4 cups
Coconut (shredded/flaked)	1 lb.	4 1/2 cups
Coffee (coarsely ground)	1 lb.	5 cups
Coffee, instant	1 oz.	1/2 cup
Coriander seed (whole)	1 oz.	6 Tbsp. (scant)
(ground)	1 oz.	5 Tbsp. (scant)
Corn, whole kernel (canned;drained)	1 lb.	2 1/2–3 cups
Cornflake crumbs	1 lb.	4 1/4 cups
Cornmeal (coarse)	1 lb.	3 cups
Cornstarch	1 lb.	3 1/2 Tbsp.
Corn syrup	1 lb.	1 1/2 cups
Crabmeat flaked	1 lb.	3 cups
Cracker crumbs	1 lb.	5 1/2–6 cups
Crackers, graham (whole)	1 lb.	63–65
(crumbs)	1 lb.	3 1/2–4 cups
Cranberries (cooked)	1 lb.	1 1/2 cups
(raw)	1 lb.	4 cups
Cranberry sauce (jellied)	1 lb.	2 cups
Cream of tartar	1 oz.	3 Tbsp.
Cream, sour	1 lb.	2 cups
Cream, whipping	1 pt.	4–5 cups
Cucumbers	1 lb.	2–3 large
Cumin	1 oz.	4 Tbsp.
Curry powder	1 oz.	4 1/2 Tbsp.
Dates (pitted)	1 lb.	2–2 1/2 cups
Dill	1 oz.	3/4 cup
Eggplant	1 lb.	7–8 slices
Eggs (hard-cooked, chopped)	1 lb.	2 1/2 cups
(hard-cooked, chopped)	1 dozen	3 cups
(whole in shell)	1 lb.	8–10 large

Food	Weight	Measure (approximately)
Flour, all-purpose, bread	1 lb.	4–4 1/2 cups
Flour, cake/pastry	1 lb.	3–3 1/2 cups
Flour, whole wheat	1 lb.	3 3/4–4 cups
Garlic (fresh; cloves)	1 oz.	5–6 large
(fresh; minced)	1 oz.	2 1/2–3 Tbsp.
Garlic powder	1 oz.	3 Tbsp.
Garlic salt	1 oz.	2 Tbsp.
Gelatin, unflavored (granulated)	1 oz.	3 Tbsp.
Ginger (ground)	1 oz.	4 Tbsp.
Grapefruit sections	1 lb.	2 1/2 cups
Grapes (seedless; fresh)	1 lb.	3–3 1/2 cups
Ham (cooked; diced)	1 lb.	3–3 1/2 cups
(ground)	1 lb.	2–2 1/2 cups
Honey	1 lb.	1 1/2 cups
Horseradish (prepared)	1 oz.	2 Tbsp. (scant)
Ice cream	5–6 lb.	1 gallon
Jam/jelly	1 lb.	1–1 1/2 cups
Kiwi	1 lb.	5–6 small
Lemon juice	1 lb.	2 cups (8–10 lemons)
Lemon peel (dried)	1 oz.	4 Tbsp.
(fresh)	1 oz.	4 Tbsp.
(fresh)	1 lemon	2 Tbsp.
Lettuce	2 lb.	1 head
(chopped/shredded)	1 lb.	6–7 cups
Limes (fresh)	1 lb.	4–5
Macaroni (cooked)	1 lb.	3–3 1/2 cups
(dry)	1 lb.	4 cups
Mace	1 oz.	4 Tbsp.
Mango	1 lb.	2 small; 1 large plus 1 medium
Margarine	1 lb.	2 cups
(whipped)	1 lb.	2 1/2 cups
Marjoram (leaves; dried)	1 lb.	1 cup
Marshmallows (large)	1 lb.	85–90
(miniatures)	1 lb.	7 1/2–8 cups
Mayonnaise	1 lb.	2 cups
Meat, any (cooked; chopped)	1 lb.	2–2 1/2 cups
Milk, evaporated	1 lb.	1 3/4 cups
Milk, whole/2%/skim	1 lb.	2 cups
Milk, nonfat (dry)	1 oz.	6 Tbsp.
Milk, sweetened (condensed)	1 lb.	1 1/2 cups
Monosodium glutamate (Accent)	1 oz.	2 Tbsp.
Mushrooms (canned; bits and pieces)	1 lb.	2 cups
(cooked)	1 lb.	1 1/2 cups
(fresh; sliced)	1 lb.	4 1/2–5 cups
(whole)	1 lb.	80 small
		40 medium
		20–25 Large
Mustard (ground)	1 oz.	5 Tbsp.
(prepared)	1 oz.	2 Tbsp.
Mustard seed	1 oz.	2 1/2 Tbsp.
Noodles (cooked)	1 lb.	2 1/2–3 cups
Nutmeats	1 lb.	4 cups

Food	Weight	Measure (approximately)
Nutmeg	1 oz.	3 1/2 Tbsp.
Oats, quick cooking (as purchased)	1 lb.	5 cups
Oil, vegetable	1 lb.	2 cups
Olives (ripe; sliced)	1 lb.	3 1/2 cups
(ripe; drained)	1 lb.	140 small
Onions (dehydrated; chopped)	1 oz.	5 Tbsp.
(fresh)	1 lb.	2 1/2–3 cups
(mature, as purchased)	1 lb.	4–5 medium
Onions, green (sliced)	1 lb.	2– 2 1/2 cups
Onion powder	1 oz.	3 Tbsp.
Onion salt	1 oz.	2 1/2 Tbsp.
Orange	1 lb.	4–5 medium
Orange juice (frozen; reconstituted)	6 oz.	3 cups,
Oregano (ground)	1 oz.	5 Tbsp.
(leaf)	1 oz.	3/4 cup
Oysters (stretched)	1 lb.	2 cups
Paprika (ground)	11 oz.	4 Tbsp.
Parsley (chopped)	1 oz.	3/4–1 cup
(flakes; dry)	1 oz.	1 1/3 cups
(fresh)	1 oz.	3/4–1 cup
Pasta; different varieties (cooked)	1 lb.	2–3 cups
Peaches (canned, sliced, drained)	1 lb.	2–2 1/2 cups
(fresh, as purchased)	1 lb.	3–4 medium
(sliced; frozen)	1 lb.	2–2 1/2 cups
Peanut butter	1 lb.	2 cups
Peanuts (shelled)	1 lb.	3 cups
Pears (canned; drained; diced)	1 lb.	2 1/4 –2 1/2 cups
(fresh, as purchased)	1 lb.	3–4 medium
Peas (cooked; drained)	1 lb.	2–2 1/2 cups
Pecans (chopped)	1 lb.	4– 4 1/2 cups
(shelled; pieces)	1 lb.	4–4 1/2 cups
Pepper, cayenne	1 oz.	5 Tbsp.
Pepper black or white (ground)	1 oz.	4 Tbsp.
Pepper, red (crushed)	1 oz.	6–6 1/2 Tbsp.
Peppercorns	1 oz.	6 Tbsp.
Peppers, green	1 lb.	2–3 medium
(chopped)	1 lb.	3– 3 1/2 cups
Peppers, jalapeno	1 lb.	14–16 medium
Pickle (chopped)	1 lb.	3 cups
(relish)	1 lb.	2–21/2 cups
Pimento (chopped)	1 oz.	1 Tbsp.
(canned; drained; chunks)	1 lb.	2–3 cups
Pineapple (crushed; drained)	1 lb.	1 3/4 cups
(crushed; undrained)	1 lb.	2–2 1/2 cups
(fresh)	3 lb.	1 pineapple
(slices; canned; drained)	1 lb.	8–12 slices
Plums	1 lb.	5–6 medium
Poppy seeds	1 oz.	3 Tbsp.
Potato chips (crushed)	1 lb.	2–2 1/4 qts.
Potatoes, white (fresh, as purchased)	1 lb.	2–4 medium
(cooked)	1 lb.	2–3 cups
Potatoes, sweet	1 lb.	2–4 medium
Poultry seasoning (ground)	1 oz.	6 Tbsp.
Prunes (pitted, cooked)	1 lb.	3 cups
Pudding mix (instant)	1 lb.	2 1/2 cups
Pudding (regular)	1 lb.	2 1/4 cups
Pumpkin (cooked)	1 lb.	2–2 1/2 cups
Radishes (fresh) whole	1 lb.	40–50 cups
Raisins (as purchased)	1 lb.	3–3 1/4 cups
Raspberries (fresh; frozen)	1 lb.	3–3 1/4 cups

Food	Weight	Measure (approximately)
Red hots candy	1 lb.	2– 2 1/2 cups
Rhubarb (fresh; chopped)	1 lb.	2 1/2–2 3/4 cups
Rice, aborio	1 lb.	2 1/2 cups
Rice, brown	1 lb.	2 1/2 cups
Rice, cereal (crisp)	1 lb.	4 qts. or 16 cups
Rice (converted)	1 lb.	2 1/2 cups
(cooked)	1 lb.	2 1/2 cups
Rice, wild	1 lb.	2 1/2 cups
(cooked)	1 lb.	5 cups
Rosemary leaves	1 oz.	9–10 Tbsp.
Sage (ground)	1 oz.	1/2 cup
(rubbed)	1 oz.	1/2 cup
Salmon (canned)	1 lb.	2 cups
Salt, table	1 oz.	1 1/2 Tbsp.
Sausage (bulk)	1 lb.	2 cups
Sesame seed	1 oz.	3 Tbsp.
Shortening	1 lb.	2 1/2 cups
Shrimp (cooked; peeled)	1 lb.	3 1/2 cups
Soda, baking	1 oz.	2 1/2 Tbsp.
Spaghetti (cooked)	1 lb.	2 1/2 cups
(canned; tightly packed)	1 lb.	2–3 cups
Spinach (canned; frozen)	1 lb.	5–6 qts
Squash (slender)	1 lb.	3 1/2–4 cups
Strawberries (fresh; frozen)	1 lb.	3 –3 1/2 cups
(sliced; with syrup; frozen)	1 lb.	2–2 1/2 cups
Sugar, brown (solid pack)	1 lb.	2 cups
Sugar, corn/maple	1 lb.	1 1/2 cups
Sugar, granulated	1 lb.	2 1/4 cups
Sugar, powdered	1 lb.	3 1/2 cups
Tapioca (after cooking)	1 lb.	7 cups
Tarragon leaf	1 oz.	1 cups
Tea (instant)	1 oz.	1/2 cup
Thyme (ground)	1 oz.	6 Tbsp.
(leaves)	1 oz.	3/4 cup
Tomatoes (diced)	1 lb.	2 1/2 cups
(fresh)	1 lb.	2–3 medium
(undrained; canned)	1 lb.	2 cups
Tomato paste	1 lb.	2 cups
Tuna (canned)	1 lb.	2 cups
Turmeric (ground)	1 oz.	4 Tbsp.
Vanilla and all other extracts	1 oz.	2 Tbsp.
Vinegar	1 lb.	2 cups
Walnuts (shelled)	1 lb.	3 1/2 –4 cups
Whipping cream	1 lb.	2 cups
Yeast (dry)	1/4 oz.	1 envelope
Yogurt	1 lb.	2 cups
Zucchini (fresh; shredded)	1 lb.	3 1/2 cups

GLOSSARY

absorption Process of moving smaller nutrients from the intestines into blood for transport throughout the body.

acid/base balance A state of equilibrium in the blood between compounds that give off hydrogen and ones that receive hydrogen.

adrenaline A stress hormone secreted by the adrenal glands.

alpha-linolenic acid An omega-3 fatty acid; examples include canola oil and flaxseed.

antibodies Proteins produced to fight off intruders called *antigens*.

antioxidants A chemical substance that protects body cells from damage.

arachidonic acid An omega-6 fatty acid; precursor to prostaglandins, substances that activate platelet aggregation, vasoconstriction, and clotting.

ascorbic acid Vitamin C.

atherosclerosis Hardening and thickening of arterial walls.

beriberi A deficiency of thiamin, a B vitamin; this disorder is manifested by weakness, poor appetite, nerve damage, and fluid retention.

beta-carotene The most abundant carotenoid; precursor to vitamin A.

bile A fat emulsifier; made in the liver and stored in the gallbladder.

calcitriol Fully activated hormone form of vitamin D.

carotenoids Any of various pigments (as carotenes)—usually yellow to red—found widely in plants and animals.

catalyze Facilitate or speed up chemical reactions. Enzymes act as catalysts.

celiac disease Inability to metabolize gluten; leads to nutrient deficiencies.

cheilosis An abnormal condition of the lips characterized by scaling of the mouth's surface and fissure formation in the corners.

cholecalciferol Inactive dietary form of vitamin D.

chylomicrons A lipoprotein unit, containing triglycerides and cholesterol, transported from the intestines ultimately to the blood.

chyme Liquefied mass of food moving from the stomach to the duodenum.

chymotrypsin A digestive enzyme from the pancreas.

coenzyme A molecule that attaches to an enzyme to activate or enhance the enzyme's function.

cofactor A chemical that activates and works with an enzyme.

collagen Protein substance of connective tissues.

complementary protein Combination of two protein sources to achieve a better amino acid balance.

complete protein A protein containing all essential amino acids.

culinary art Taking food beyond what is required for sustenance into a realm of appreciation and discrimination.

dextrose Another name for glucose.

dietary fiber Edible, indigestible fiber naturally found in plants.

dietitian Someone who received specialized education in college or graduate school along with a dietetic internship. Dietitians often take a national examination to become registered dietitians (RDs).

digestion A process where food undergoes conversion into substances small enough for absorption.

dipeptide Contains two amino acids linked together.

disaccharides Sugars comprising two monosaccharides, for example, maltose, sucrose, and lactose.

DNA (deoxyribonucleic acid) and RNA (ribonucleic acid) Carriers of genetic information.

duodenal Referring to the duodenum or the beginning of the small intestine.

duodenum The first part of the small intestine.

edema Excessive fluid buildup.

eicosanoid Hormone-like substance that regulates body functions, including inflammation, vasodilation, platelet aggregation, and immune response.

elastin A protein substance that works with collagen to provide elasticity.

emulsifier An agent that forms a stable mixture of two immiscible liquids.

enzyme A molecule necessary for a chemical reaction to occur but is not used up in the reaction.

epithelial tissue Tissue that lines the body—the skin on the outside and the mucous membrane on the inside.

ergocalciferol Synthesized plant form of vitamin D.

essential nutrients A nutrient we must consume in the diet.

exchange system Foods grouped together based on similar nutrient content.

fatty acid An organic acid found in animal and plant materials. Three fatty acids combine with glycerol to create a triglyceride.

fermentation A chemical reaction converting carbohydrate into its constituents, specifically, carbon dioxide and alcohol.

fructose Fruit sugar; the sweetest monosaccharide.

functional fiber Isolated, extracted, or synthetic fiber.

galactose A simple sugar found in milk; constituent of lactose.

galactosemia Inability to metabolize galactose that could lead to mental retardation if untreated.

gastric lipase An enzyme in the stomach that digests fat.

gastrin A hormone that stimulates production of gastric hydrochloric acid.

gelatinase An enzyme that breaks down gelatin.

glucagon A hormone that raises blood sugar.

glucose A simple sugar and major energy source for humans.

gluten A plant protein found in wheat, rye, and barley.

glycogenesis Metabolic process of converting glucose into glycogen for energy storage.

guild A group of professional tradesmen tied together by a single craft.

hemoglobin An iron-containing pigment made of protein that transports oxygen in the blood.

homocysteine Amino acid by-product of protein metabolism that may increase risk of cardiovascular disease.

hormone Substance produced in one part of the body with action elsewhere in the body.

hydrochloric acid Acid that activates pepsinogen.

hydrolysis Chemical reaction involving water.

hypercholesterolemia Raised blood cholesterol, which is a risk factor for heart disease.

hyperkeratosis Thickening of the skin's stratum corneum layer.

hypoglycemia Low levels of blood sugar.

incomplete protein A protein lacking all essential amino acids.

insulin A hormone made of protein in the pancreas that facilitates the uptake of glucose, or sugar, from the blood into cells.

intestinal lipase An enzyme that hydrolyzes fat into fatty acids and glycerol.

intrinsic factor Gastric protein required for vitamin B_{12} absorption.

kwashiorkor Severe protein malnutrition often seen in children from developing countries; potbelly is one characteristic.

lacto-ovo vegetarian Vegetarian who consumes milk, dairy products, and eggs.

lactose Milk sugar.

lacto vegetarian Vegetarian who consumes milk and dairy products.

lingual lipase An enzyme formed in salivary glands; digests minimal amounts of fat in the mouth.

linoleic acid An omega-6 fatty acid; examples include corn and soybean oils.

lipid A variety of substances soluble in fat but not in water.

lipoproteins A fat unit containing protein on the outermost layer to transport it through water.

macronutrients Nutrients needed in larger quantity; refers to the calorie-containing nutrients, carbohydrate, protein, and fat.

malnutrition A condition resulting from dietary consumption that was either inadequate or excessive.

malt A type of grain that produces alcohol.

maltose Malt sugar produced during fermentation.

marasmus Severe protein and calorie malnutrition.

menadione Synthetic vitamin K soluble in water.

menaquinone Vitamin K_2; synthesized by intestinal bacterial flora.

microorganisms A life-form so tiny it requires a microscope to see it.

monoglyceride Glycerol with only one fatty acid.

monosaccharides Simple sugars, such as glucose, fructose, and galactose.

monounsaturated Fatty acid with a single double bond in its carbon chain.

mouth feel The sensory evaluation of food in the mouth.

niacin equivalents (NE) Denotes tryptophan and natural niacin intake combine to provide total niacin intake.

nonessential nutrients A nutrient that can be made from other nutrients. We do not have to eat nonessential nutrients.

non-heme iron Major component of dietary iron, but poorly absorbed.

nutritional science The study of food and nutrients and their application to health.

nutritionist Someone who may have undergone specialized training in nutrition to apply science to dietary practice.

oligosaccharides Chain of three to nine monosaccharides.

omega-3 fat An essential fatty acid most Americans consume too little of. The first double bond is located on the third carbon from the omega end.

omega-6 fat An essential fatty acid consumed abundantly. The first double bond is on the sixth carbon from the omega end.

osteomalacia Adult vitamin D deficiency disease; softening of the bones.

oxidize Combine with oxygen.

pancreatic Pertaining to the pancreas, a gland involved in digestion.

pancreatic amylase Enzyme from the pancreas that digests carbohydrate.

pancreatic lipase An enzyme made in the pancreas and released in the intestine to digest fat into free fatty acids.

pasteurization A process of heating food to a high enough temperature to render disease-causing microorganisms impotent.

pepsin An enzyme found in the digestive process that breaks down protein into polypeptides.

pepsinogen A precursor to pepsin.

pesco vegetarian Vegetarian who consumes fish.

phylloquinone Vitamin K_1; major form of vitamin K found in plant foods.

physiological property A property having to deal with the functioning of the human body.

phytochemicals A substance in plants involved in protecting human health.

polypeptides Long chains of amino acids.

polysaccharides Several monosaccharides joined together.

polyunsaturated fat Fatty acid with more than one double bond in its carbon chain.

probiotic Substance that promotes healthful microorganism growth.

protein Chemical compounds of carbon, hydrogen, oxygen, and nitrogen.

provitamin A A substance requiring conversion to vitamin A before the body can use it.

Recommended Dietary Allowance Established daily recommendations for intake of nutrients to meet requirements for most healthy people.

rennin An enzyme that coagulates, or curdles, milk.

retinal Form of vitamin A used to convert light into nerve impulses for sight.

retinoic acid Derivative of vitamin A.

retinoids Class or group of the different forms of vitamin A; includes retinal, retinol, retinoic acid.

retinol Form of vitamin A in foods of animal origin. Also called *preformed vitamin A.*

retinol activity equivalent Unit of measurement for vitamin A.

rickets Childhood vitamin D deficiency; softening of the bones.

salivary amylase Enzyme secreted in the mouth required to convert starch to sugar.

saturated As in saturated fat; indicates the chain of carbons in fat's chemical structure can hold no more hydrogen atoms.

scurvy A deficiency disease resulting from inadequate vitamin C intake, characterized by bleeding gums.

smelt Melting or fusing ores to separate metallic components.

stomatitis Inflammatory mouth disease resulting from riboflavin deficiency.

sucrose Table sugar.

tocopherols Group name for different forms of vitamin E.

toxicity Quality or condition of being toxic.

transit time The time required to eliminate ingested food from the body.

triglyceride The most abundant form of fat found in foods and in the body; composed of glycerol and fatty acids.

tripeptide Contains three amino acids linked together.

trypsin A digestive enzyme from the pancreas.

tubers Underground plant; potato.

vegan Strict vegetarian who eats only plant products.

vitamins Compounds the body requires in very small amounts to maintain life. Examples include vitamin C and niacin.

water balance The relationship of water made in the body and water lost or given off.

Wernicke's encephalopathy Acute brain disease caused by thiamin deficiency; seen in alcohol abusers. Sufferers lack muscle coordination and experience confusion.

xerophthalmia Dryness of the conjunctiva and cornea due to vitamin A deficiency.

INDEX

A

acids
  alpha-linolenic, 89, 92, 97, 100
  arachidonic, 89, 100
  erucic, 92
  linoleic, 89, 90, 92, 95, 100
  oleic, 92
adenosine triphosphate (ATP), 142
adequate intake, *see* AI
Administration on Aging (AoA), 167
adrenaline, 51, 72
Africa, 154, 179–80, 231
AI (adequate intake), 17, 30, 32, 63, 84, 95,
    103, 109, 114, 121, 127, 133–34,
    139, 144, 148–49, 153, 157–59
ALA (alpha-linolenic acid), 89, 91–92, 95,
    97, 100
alcohol, 8, 21–22, 24, 51, 70, 116, 123, 230,
    244–45, 247, 249, 265
alcoholic beverages, 21–22, 79, 229,
    244–45, 276
alkali, 115, 133–34
alkaloids, 221
allergic, 14, 84–85, 155, 276
alpha-linolenic acid, *see* ALA
aluminum, 162
American Cancer Society, 170, 175, 215
American Dietetic Association, 42, 44, 67–68,
    135–36, 182, 191, 195
American Heart Association, 90, 169–70,
    174–75, 178, 182, 194
American Journal of Clinical Nutrition, 53,
    67–68, 100–01, 175
amino acids, 50, 68, 70, 72–73, 79, 85, 101,
    122–23, 125, 143, 159, 199, 245,
    261, 289, 293
  limiting, 73, 75
  nonessential, 72, 75
amylase, 46–48
amylopectin, 46–48
anosmia, 223, 227
antibiotics, 114, 128
antibody, 72
antioxidants, 8, 84, 101, 106–07, 111–12,
    129, 136, 156, 165, 169–71,
    175, 184, 210
Apicius, 4, 234
appetizers, 70, 223, 256, 277, 279–82, 298
apples, 8, 46, 58, 61, 63, 67, 82, 111, 201,
    220, 246–47
Arachidonic Acid (AA), 89, 100
aromatics, 212, 231, 233–34
  vegetable, 233, 248
aromatized wines, 245
arrowroot, 265–66, 284, 286, 290, 293
arsenic, 138, 162
ascorbic acid, 16, 97, 200
asparagus, 119, 125–26, 211, 290
atherosclerosis, 39, 92, 101, 169
Atkins, 177, 182–84, 194
avocado, 122–25, 129

B

bacteria, 105, 113–14, 133
  vitamin-K-producing, 114
baking, 45, 59, 62, 92, 204, 212, 229, 234,
    237, 244–47, 268–69, 274, 294,
    297–98
baking soda, 115, 130
balance of foods, 263, 284
bamboo shoots, 295
bananas, 123–25, 133
barley, 8, 47, 53, 58, 62, 67, 73,
    284–85
Basal Metabolic Rate (BMR), 154,
    191–92
basic tastes, 221
basil, 222, 225, 234–35, 239, 280
beans, 44, 47, 52, 55, 59–61, 64, 70, 73–74,
    76–77, 79, 85, 95, 203, 212,
    266–67, 287
beef, 4, 73, 77, 95, 143, 153, 170, 204, 243,
    253, 258–60, 266, 272, 280, 286,
    288–90
beers, 8, 79, 159, 226, 229, 244–47, 276
beriberi, 8, 9, 104, 115–16, 134
berries, 2, 4, 56, 59, 160, 207, 225,
    246–47, 282
beta-carotene, 97, 105–07, 169–70, 200, 204,
    208, 239, 285, 294, 297
beverages, 1, 5, 21–22, 40, 83–84, 142, 180,
    219, 225–26, 233, 247
bile, 93
  acids, 61, 65, 285
biotin, 19, 29, 41, 115–16, 127–29, 135,
    201, 211
  toxicity, 128
blood, 28, 50–52, 64, 72, 79, 89, 90, 94, 96,
    142–43, 146, 148, 150, 161, 163,
    169–70, 172
  calcium levels, 139
  cholesterol, 93, 95
  clotting, 91, 139
  glucose, 183
  pressure, 148–49, 172, 174, 181
  sugar, 43, 50–52, 64, 168, 182
BMI (body mass index), 16, 178–79, 185
body mass index, *see* BMI
bone loss, 167
bones, 70–71, 77, 81, 85, 139–43, 157–58,
    160, 167, 195, 204, 266, 269
boron, 138, 160, 167
brain, 106, 123
bran, 121, 123
breads, 23–24, 26, 36, 44–45, 47, 51–52,
    59, 64, 71, 74, 76, 78–79, 83, 98,
    143, 146
breakfast, 51, 61, 78, 99, 280–81
Brillat-Savarin, Jean Anthelme, 5, 11, 206,
    216, 218, 222, 227
broccoli, 113–14, 119, 122, 131, 134
brown sauces, 266
buckwheat, 73, 75, 275, 281, 283

butter, 3, 27–28, 82, 87–89, 96–100, 140,
    213, 242–43, 264–65, 267–70,
    275, 284, 294, 296–97
  clarified, 267–68

C

cadmium, 138, 155, 162
cakes, 46, 59, 62, 187, 268–69, 274, 278, 297
calcitonin, 139
calcium, 15–16, 29–31, 33–34, 41, 54, 60,
    82–84, 109–10, 137–43, 157, 160,
    163–64, 167–68, 173, 200,
    290–91, 296–97
  absorption, 54, 63, 139–40, 142, 165
  deficiencies, 139, 144
  supplements, 141–42
cancer, 10, 27, 34–35, 65, 77, 84, 131–32,
    134–35, 155, 162, 165, 169–71,
    174–75, 177, 181–82
canned fruits, 147, 173, 204
canola oil, 88–90, 92, 97, 100, 256, 268, 296
cantaloupe, 107–08, 117, 132
carbohydrates, 14–15, 21–22, 31, 37–38,
    43–45, 47–53, 55–59, 67–68,
    71–72, 77, 182–83, 208, 282–83,
    285–87, 290, 293
carbon, 43, 67, 70, 72, 85, 89
  chain, 89, 96, 100
  dioxide, 8, 43–44, 50, 150
carcinogens, 65, 160, 215
carob, 61–62
carotenoid, 105, 107, 132, 210
carrots, 11, 40, 46, 58, 67, 104–05, 107–08,
    132, 152, 173, 210, 212, 220, 225,
    235, 239, 255, 271–72, 285
catalyze, 70, 85
cauliflower, 114, 129, 132–33
celeriac, 236, 239, 287
celery, 11, 44, 59, 199, 210, 212, 220, 225,
    233, 235, 237, 239, 255–57, 264,
    270–71, 282–83
cellulose, 44, 46, 58, 64, 98
cereals, 23–24, 36, 46–47, 53, 59, 61–62, 64,
    74–75, 83, 99, 150, 153, 173, 188,
    208–09
cheese, 23, 51, 74, 83, 92, 139, 143, 146,
    259, 284
chicken breasts, 270, 292–93
chickens, 95, 143, 149, 159, 188, 205–06,
    214, 258–60, 266, 270, 272–73,
    280, 286, 288, 291, 293
  free-range, 205–06
child, 14, 80–81, 154, 187
childhood, 15, 167, 169, 187
China, 39, 40, 155, 231, 241
chloride, 29, 137–38, 144, 148–50, 163, 221
chlorophyll, 144
cholesterol, 9, 10, 21–22, 27–29, 33–34, 64,
    87, 89, 90, 92–95, 97, 100–01,
    107, 109, 112–13, 121, 257, 271,
    282–85, 287–88, 290–93, 295–97

chromium, 29, 60, 137, 150, 159, 163, 285
cinnamon, 225, 230, 232–35, 283, 289, 296
cis-retinal, 106
cobalamin, 127
coenzyme, 115, 118, 122–23, 133–34
cofactor, 104, 134, 163
coffee, 99, 206, 221, 230, 259
collagen, 81
Columbus, Christopher, 232
Committee on Diet and Health, 64, 67
compound butters, 243
convenience foods, 6, 7, 10, 99
cookies, 98–99, 187–88, 190
cooking
    foods, 211, 215
    healthy, 11, 257, 280
    low-fat, 212–13
    methods, 211, 215, 255, 257–58, 263,
        267–68, 272, 279, 281, 288, 298
        no-fat, 255, 257
    oils, 242, 257
copper, 29, 60, 79, 137, 150, 153, 156, 163
corn, 9, 47, 58, 62, 67, 69, 73–74, 89, 97,
        100, 173, 232, 268–69, 283–84,
        286, 295
    oil, 91–92, 256, 270, 283–84
    starch, 265, 267, 286
coronary heart disease, 34–35, 39, 89, 94, 292
crackers, graham, 56–57

D

Daily Reference Values, see DRVs
Daily Values, see DVs
dairy, 9, 14, 23, 40, 43, 55, 82–83, 85, 139,
        157, 275, 281, 286, 296
    foods, 23, 40
    products, 24, 37, 55, 82–85, 87, 93, 100,
        139, 144, 150, 168, 171, 296
DASH (Dietary Approaches to Stop Hyperten-
        sion), 21, 173–75
DASH diet, 174–75
Deficiency and toxicity, 140, 143–44, 148–49,
        151, 153–60
desserts, 187, 230, 239, 246, 248, 274–75,
        279–80, 297–98
    healthy, 274, 294
dextrose, 45
diabetes, 14, 50–53, 64, 159, 165–66,
        168–69, 172, 174–75, 177–78,
        181–82, 184, 193
diet
    fad, 70, 191
    healthy, 1, 28, 56, 152, 174, 184
    high-carbohydrate, 55, 183–84
    high-fiber, 56, 59, 64, 169
    higher-protein, 75, 183
    vegetarian, 82, 84, 86, 296, 298
dietary cholesterol, 64, 92–93, 95, 101
dietary fat, 10, 34, 87–89, 94–95,
        100–01, 170
dietary fiber, 58, 62–64, 67, 140, 170, 285,
        290, 295
Dietary Guidelines for Americans (DGA), 13–14,
        19, 20, 22, 25, 30, 40, 42, 63, 185,
        192, 195
Dietary Reference Intakes, see DRIs
Dietary Reference Values, see DRVs

dietitians, 9–11, 51, 148, 169, 185, 188, 289
    registered, 10, 169, 194
disaccharides, 45–46, 49, 68
disease, 8, 9, 13, 26, 30, 33–34, 41, 50, 53,
        57, 61, 80, 87, 165–66, 174–75,
        181, 195–96
    celiac, 53, 262
    protein-deficiency, 80
diverticulosis, 64–65
DNA, 44, 72, 142, 153
dried beans, 9, 58, 67, 167, 170, 212, 266
dried herbs, 234
DRIs (Dietary Reference Intakes), 13–14, 16,
        20, 22, 30–32, 40, 42, 95, 97, 150,
        157, 159
DRVs (Daily Reference Values), 28–32
DV (Daily Value), 28–33, 38, 42, 59

E

egg yolks, 92–93, 107, 121, 133, 152, 168,
        265, 281
eggplant, 132
eggs, 9, 23–24, 44, 51, 62, 70–71, 73, 76,
        81–85, 97, 111, 117, 119, 122–23,
        128–29, 169–70, 205–06, 267–68,
        271, 280–81, 296
    substitute, 108
eicosanoids, 88, 90–91
Eijkman, Christiaan, 9
elastin, 81
electrolytes, 21, 137, 144, 147, 149, 163–64
emu, 260
emulsifier, 93
endosperm, 56–57
energy, 2–4, 21, 43–44, 48–52, 55–56, 67–68,
        72, 75, 85, 95, 101, 142, 168, 170,
        173, 185
    balance, 21, 25, 184
    metabolism, 115, 127, 136
    sources, 43, 45, 50, 56, 67, 72, 85,
        142, 168
entrées, 253, 255–56, 261, 274, 279–81,
        296, 298
entremets, 284
enzymes, 104, 115–16, 122, 133
essential amino acids, 70, 72–73, 75, 85,
        261–62, 287, 289, 296
ethnic cuisines, 39, 41
Europe, 4, 9, 206, 231, 241, 246, 262
exchange list, 28
exercise, 10, 24–25, 51, 55–56, 67, 144, 165,
        168–69, 177–78, 182–84, 191–92,
        194, 272

F

fat, 1–4, 21–22, 24–35, 27–49, 31–53, 36–40,
        77, 87–101, 173, 182–83, 185–88,
        212–15, 242–43, 253–76, 279–91,
        295–98
    body, 88, 95, 100, 185–86
    calories, 3, 213, 243, 284, 286
    replacers, 98
fat-soluble vitamins, 98, 214, 288
fatty
    acid chains, 89, 90, 94, 100
    acids, 21, 41, 50, 54–55, 64, 68, 72, 83,
        85, 89–94, 97, 100–01, 287

alpha-linolenic, 92, 97
    polyunsaturated, 89, 90, 100–01
    saturated, 22, 28–29, 96, 254, 267, 269
    unsaturated, 97, 293
    fish, cold-water, 172, 204
FDA (Food and Drug Administration), 26, 28,
        32, 34, 36, 41, 73, 92, 98, 155,
        185, 193, 195
fennel, 220, 225, 233, 235, 239, 264, 290
fermentation, 8, 46, 245
fiber, 29, 33–34, 43–45, 47, 52, 56–59,
        61–65, 67–68, 82, 84, 88, 173,
        262–63, 287, 292–94, 296–97
    functional, 58
    soluble, 34, 52, 58, 61–62, 65, 67, 170
fiber-containing foods, 59
fish, 3, 4, 22–24, 69, 70, 76–77, 81–83, 85,
        91–92, 97–98, 100, 118, 120,
        122–23, 127, 133, 138–39, 143,
        162–63, 173–74, 204, 214, 286
    salted, 4
flavin adenine dinucleotide (FAD), 116
flavonoids, 8, 65, 132, 198, 210–12, 257, 266
flavor
    building, 217, 224–26
    components, 263, 286
    enhancers, 220, 242, 290
flavoring ingredients, 247, 255, 262, 266–67,
        270, 280
flavorings, 211, 229, 233, 239, 242, 249, 265,
        270
flavors, 2, 3, 11–12, 100, 147–48, 211–14,
        217–21, 223–27, 229, 232–45,
        247–48, 254–59, 262–72, 274–77,
        279–82, 284–89, 295–96
    characteristic, 100, 247
    complementary, 235, 237
    construction of, 224–26
    contrasting, 235, 274
    perception of, 217, 225–26
flesh foods, 77, 81–82, 144, 146, 150
flour, 36, 43, 52, 56, 62, 257–58, 261, 265,
        274, 281, 295, 297
    whole-grain, 56, 59
fluoride, 41, 137, 150, 157–59, 163, 167, 221
foie gras, 253
folate, 15, 17, 34, 41, 59, 60, 115–16,
        123–27, 135, 198, 209–10, 212,
        290, 296
    deficiency, 125
    dietary, 125
    fortification, 124, 126
    losses, 126
folic acid, 115, 123–26, 135
food
    labeling, 25–26, 36, 38–39, 41
    labels, 13–14, 25–34, 36–37, 39, 41–42,
        45, 59, 63, 73, 96, 197
Food and Drug Administration, see FDA
Food Guide Pyramid, 23–25, 30, 39, 42, 263
foods
    bitter, 221
    calorie-dense, 191
    cold-sensitive, 208
    fiber-free, 62
    fiber-rich, 65
    grain-rich, 296

high-potassium, 148, 174
high-protein, 80
high-sodium, 223
high-sugar, 169
higher-calorie, 148
low-sodium, 83
lower-calorie, 37
nutrient-dense, 21, 166
France, 5, 39, 40, 179–80, 206, 241
free radicals, 170
fresh herbs, 166, 229, 233–34, 236, 242,
    244, 249, 266, 275–76
fructose, 45–47, 49, 50, 52, 66, 220
fruit
    juices, 32, 144, 169, 235, 249, 275, 296–97
    purées, 268
    sauces, 204, 246
fruitarians, 81–82
fruits, 11, 21–24, 34, 44–46, 51–52, 58,
    76–77, 84–85, 98–99, 169–70,
    173–74, 183–84, 198–204,
    246–47, 281, 296–97
Funk, Casimir, 9

G

galactose, 45–46, 49, 50, 52, 68
gallbladder, 93–94, 177
game meats, 258–60
garlic, 8, 95, 235, 237–38, 242–43, 249, 264,
    270, 280, 290, 293
gastrin, 79
gelatin, 73, 80–81, 83
germ, 56–57
glands, thyroid, 139, 153–54
glucose, 44–53, 62, 66, 72, 85, 153, 168
    converting, 50, 115, 118, 121
    units, 48, 67
gluten, 53, 71, 73, 261–62, 275
glycemic index, 52–53, 175
glycerol, 89, 94, 100
glycogen, 43, 50–51, 54–55
goiter, 154–55
grain products, 23, 34, 64, 66, 173, 263, 296
grains, 8, 9, 21–23, 25, 40, 47, 59, 65–66,
    73–75, 82–85, 144–46, 152–53,
    156–57, 159–60, 173–74,
    263–64, 284
gram, 31, 98, 213
Greece, 40, 42, 61, 178–80
guar gum, 58, 64–65
gums, 46–47, 58, 64, 98

H

HDL (high-density lipoprotein), 94–95, 245, 287
health
    claims, 9, 26, 32–35, 41
    conditions, 53, 178, 181
    professionals, 13–14, 19, 27, 36, 51, 56, 61,
    73, 158, 160, 163, 169, 185, 194
heart disease, 10, 35, 64, 88, 97, 100, 161,
    165–66, 169–70, 174–75, 177–78,
    181–82, 184, 194
    risk of coronary, 34, 39, 89
heat, 6, 44, 96–97, 138, 144, 197, 199,
    201–02, 207, 210–12, 215, 221,
    234, 257, 268, 297
hemicelluloses, 46, 58, 64

hemoglobin, 72, 150, 152, 156
Henry, Prince, 231
herbs, 6, 8, 61, 99, 148, 212, 229, 232–35,
    239, 243, 245, 247–49, 255–57,
    266–67, 279–80, 282
high blood pressure, 10, 27, 34, 145–46,
    148–59, 162, 167, 169, 172–75, 193
high-density lipoprotein, see HDL
high-fiber foods, 61, 63–64
Hippocrates, 104–05
hormones, 43, 50–51, 72, 75, 79, 84, 88,
    100, 139, 142, 153, 156, 168
humidity, 158, 207–08
HVP (hydrolyzed vegetable protein), 263
hydrochloric acid, 79, 149
hydrogen, 43, 54, 67, 70, 72, 85, 89, 96
hydrogenation, 28, 87, 96–97
hydrolyzed vegetable protein, see HVP
hypercholesterolemia, 88, 161
hypertension, 34, 145, 150, 172, 174–75,
    178, 181
hypoglycemia, 51–52, 182

I

ice cream, 9, 10, 54, 62, 76, 83, 92, 98–99,
    178, 194
immune function, 133–34
India, 61, 231–32
indoles, 132
infants, 14, 55, 68, 77, 84, 139, 151, 154,
    156, 158
insoluble fiber, 58, 67, 283, 295
insulin, 43, 50–51, 64, 72, 153, 159, 161,
    164, 168–69, 175, 181–82
International Units, see IU
intestines, 47, 54, 56, 64–65, 79, 94, 137, 163
    small, 49, 50, 56, 64, 67, 79, 93
iodine, 18, 20, 29, 72, 137, 150, 153–55,
    163–64
    deficiency, 154
iron, 16, 18, 20, 29, 30, 33, 59, 60, 63, 72,
    130, 135, 137, 150–52, 156–57,
    163–64, 205, 245, 283, 287
    absorption, 142, 152–53, 156
    deficiency, 27, 151
    dietary, 151–52
    heme, 152
    nonheme, 152
isoflavones, 65, 262, 132
IU (International Units), 106, 108–09, 111,
    113, 133

J

jalapeños, 221, 225, 236, 240
Japan, 40, 42, 241
Jerusalem artichoke, 239
Joint National Committee on Prevention,
    172–73, 175

K

kale, 108, 114, 132
kidneys, 77, 109, 116, 121, 123, 125, 142,
    144, 148, 156, 160, 162
kilocalories, 116–17, 119
Kirschenbaum, 189–90, 194
kohlrabi, 239
kwashiorkor, 80

L

LA (linoleic acids), 91, 95, 224
labels, 14, 26–30, 32, 36–39, 41, 45, 59, 67,
    141, 168
lactase, 49, 54–55, 168
lactose, 14, 45–46, 49, 54, 66, 82, 85, 142, 168
    intolerance, 43, 54, 70, 85, 168
lamb, 199, 234, 289
lard, 89, 267, 269
LDL (low-density lipoprotein), 28, 61, 64, 87,
    89, 94–95, 181, 287
lead, 8, 9, 51, 53, 55, 65, 90, 99, 139, 142, 144,
    146, 148, 163, 169, 180–81, 219–20
lead-soldered cans, 163
leafy vegetables, 160, 210
    flavorful green, 286
lean meats, 61, 77, 85, 95, 98, 253, 259, 269,
    276, 281, 289
lecithin, 90, 93, 142
legumes, 21, 40, 46–47, 52, 64, 70, 73–76,
    82–83, 95, 139, 144, 150, 263–64,
    266–67, 286–87, 296
Liebig, Justus von, 8
lignins, 58, 62
linoleic acids (LA), 91, 95, 224
lipids, 87, 89–91, 93–95, 97, 99–101, 142
    dietary, 89, 90, 100
lipoproteins, 94, 101
    low-density, 28, 61, 87, 89, 94, 181
liqueurs, 225, 244–45, 247–58, 269,
    274–76, 296
liver, 50–51, 53, 64, 73, 79, 80, 92–95,
    104–05, 107–11, 114, 118, 121,
    123, 125–26, 129, 133–34, 136,
    138, 150–51, 156, 159–60
    oil, 107
lobster, 204–05, 243
locust bean gum, 61–62
low-density lipoprotein, see LDL
low-fat, 2, 9, 22, 26–27, 41, 73, 99, 140, 169,
    184, 237, 252–53, 255–57, 275,
    286, 294
    cooking process, 213–14

M

macrominerals, 137–38, 163–64
macronutrients, 15, 32, 37, 42, 101
magnesium, 20, 29, 41, 60, 63, 79, 137–38,
    142–45, 160, 163, 167, 173, 200,
    221, 245, 290
    deficiency, 144
malnutrition, 1, 2, 224
maltose, 45–46, 48–49, 66, 225
manganese, 29, 60, 79, 137, 150, 157, 163
marasmus, 80–81
margarine, 78, 83, 88, 96–100, 242–43,
    267–69, 284
marinades, 77, 242, 244, 247, 255–56, 262,
    269–70, 290, 293
meat substitutions, 259–60
meats, 8, 9, 22–24, 37, 69, 70, 76–77, 81–84,
    152–53, 173–74, 213–15, 226,
    234–35, 252–53, 258–59, 261,
    269–72, 285–91
    charred, 215
    flavorful, 260
    processed, 37

mena-menaquinone vitamin K2, 113
mercury, 138, 162–63, 172
Mexico, 39, 40, 179–80
microminerals, 137, 150, 163
micronutrients, 9, 32, 42, 160
microorganisms, 8, 22
milk, 21–24, 44–45, 53–55, 73–74, 80–83,
    98–99, 107–08, 110–11, 117–19,
    121–22, 125, 127–28, 133, 139,
    142–43, 146, 148–50, 156,
    167–68, 188, 258, 283, 294–95
  fat, 26, 140
  products, 21–22, 52, 54–55, 62, 70, 81,
    139, 167–68, 175
  protein, 80, 84
  sugar, 14, 46
minerals, 14–15, 29, 30, 32, 41, 56, 58–59,
    137–39, 149, 155–57, 159–61,
    163–64, 200–01, 204–12, 262–63,
    281–83, 289–91
mirepoix, 235, 249, 266
molds, 174, 198, 207, 262
molybdenum, 18, 20, 29, 60, 137, 150,
    160, 163
monoglyceride, 89, 94
monosaccharides, 45–47, 49, 68
monosodium glutamate, 146–47, 220
monounsaturated, 22, 25, 87, 89, 92, 95, 97,
    100, 263, 293
mouth feel, 3, 98, 263, 266–68, 287
mushrooms, 59, 159, 161, 221, 225, 236,
    240–41, 259, 262, 285
My Pyramid, 13–14, 22, 25, 28, 40, 42, 82,
    184, 196

N

NAD (nicotinamide adenine dinucleotide),
    118, 133
National Academies Press, 41–42, 67–68,
    85, 163
National Restaurant Association (NRA), 34, 36,
    39, 41–42
National Weight Control Registry (NWCR),
    182, 184
NE (niacin equivalent), 119, 133
nectar, 45, 297
niacin, 8, 9, 16–17, 29, 36, 41, 59, 60,
    115–16, 118–22, 135–36, 201,
    204, 291
  deficiency, 118–19
  dietary, 120
  equivalent, 119, 133
nicotinamide adenine dinucleotide, *see* NAD
nitrites, 112
nitrogen, 70, 72, 75, 85, 103
NLEA (Nutrition Labeling and Education Act),
    13–14, 26–27, 32–33, 35–36, 41,
    96, 254
NRA, *see* National Restaurant Association
nutmeg, 225, 233–35, 296
nutrient
  database, 140, 205
  deficiencies, 53
  valuable, 202–03, 210–11, 213, 286
nutrient absorption, 53, 149
Nutrient Data Laboratory, 77, 185
Nutrition Labeling and Education Act, *see* NLEA

nutritional
  cooking, 2, 11, 202, 204, 214, 217, 238,
    252–53, 263, 265–66, 275,
    281–82, 289
    guidelines, 198, 215, 264
    of meat products, 277, 288
  guidelines, 10–11, 13–15, 17, 19, 21,
    23, 25, 27, 29, 31, 33, 35, 37, 39,
    41, 243
nuts, 6, 14, 22–23, 35, 51–52, 70, 75–76,
    81–82, 84–85, 144–45, 156–57,
    159–60, 173–74, 208, 287, 296
NWCR, *see* National Weight Control Registry

O

obese, 178–79, 182, 185
obesity, 1, 4, 15–16, 36, 41, 77, 97, 165, 169,
    174, 177–84, 187–88, 194–96
  adult, 16
Occupational Safety and Health Administration,
    see OSHA
odors, 92, 97, 218, 223–24, 226
  primary, 217, 222–23, 235
oils, 22, 24–25, 39, 40, 79, 87–91, 93–95,
    97–101, 146, 173, 213–15, 234,
    242, 268–70, 279, 286, 293
  flavored, 235, 242, 249, 268
  nonflavored, 243
olestra, 98
olfactory neurons, 166, 222–23
oligosaccharides, 45–47
olive oil, 40, 52, 87–88, 92, 95, 97, 100, 242,
    268–69, 280, 287, 290
omega-3, 39, 87, 90–92, 95, 101
  fatty acids, 35, 38, 62, 83, 85, 89–92, 95, 97,
    99, 100, 169, 172, 175, 204, 292
omega-6, 90–92, 95
  fatty acids, 38, 87, 89, 91–92, 95, 97, 100
onions, 212, 225, 235–38, 257, 264, 266,
    270–71, 275–76, 285, 290, 293
oregano, 222, 225, 234–35, 239
OSHA (Occupational Safety and Health
    Administration), 161
osteomalacia, 109, 133
osteoporosis, 27, 34, 139–41, 156, 158, 160,
    165–67, 175
oxidation, 97, 111–12, 115, 156, 199, 208
oxygen, 43–44, 50, 67, 70, 72, 85, 97, 150,
    156, 170, 197, 199, 201–03,
    210–11, 215
oysters, 139, 153, 156, 159, 205, 225, 241

P

pancreas, 49–51, 72, 79, 94, 151
pantothenic acid, 29, 41, 57, 60, 115–16,
    121–22, 135
  function, 121
  loss, 121
parathyroid hormone, 139, 142
Pasteur, Louis, 8
peanuts, 14, 143, 145, 173, 268–69, 275–76,
    284, 298
pearl onions, 237–38, 272
peas, split, 145, 265–66
pectin, 46, 58, 64–65, 170
pellagra, 9, 115, 118–20
pernicious anemia, 127, 134, 136

phylloquinone, 113–14
  vitamin K1, 113
phytochemicals, 103, 131–32, 134
pepsin, 79
pepsinogen, 79
pH, 142, 197, 199, 210–11, 215
phenylalanine, 14, 72
phospholipids, 89, 90, 93, 100
phosphorus, 18, 20, 29, 41, 60, 137–38,
    142–43, 160, 163, 205, 245,
    290–91, 295
photosynthesis, 43–44, 200
physiological, 2, 3, 140, 202
phytates, 66, 152–53
phytochemicals, 65, 84, 97, 170, 295
polypeptides, 79
polysaccharides, 45–48
polyunsaturated fats, 39, 88, 90, 92, 95,
    100–01, 263
pork, 82, 95, 149, 199, 200, 254, 258–60,
    288–89
Portugal, 179–80, 231
potassium, 21–22, 29, 34, 60, 137–38, 144,
    147–49, 163–64, 173–74, 200,
    205, 245, 290–91, 294–97
potatoes, 24, 40, 43, 47, 67, 73, 148, 159,
    173, 210, 232, 260, 263–64,
    266–67, 278–79, 290
poultry, 22–24, 44, 62, 70, 76, 81–83, 85,
    173–74, 199–201, 206, 211–12, 214,
    234–35, 258–59, 269–70, 291–93
pregnancy, 77, 139, 151, 153–54
pressure, osmotic, 144, 148
Pritikin, 182–84, 195
processed protein foods, 76
protein, 104, 106, 125, 127
  animal, 55, 83–84, 261, 296
  complementary, 73, 86
  complete, 40, 73, 83, 85, 287
  deficiency, 80, 296
  digestion, 79
  quality of, 69, 70, 73, 75, 85
  synthesis, 72, 153–54
provitamin, 105–07, 133
pseudovitamins, 131
psyllium, 61
pyridoxine, 121–22
  functions, 122

Q

Qualified Health Claim, 34–35

R

RAE (retinol activity equivalent), 105–06
RDAs (Recommended Dietary Allowances),
    15–18, 29–32, 75, 138, 142–44,
    148–49, 151, 153–56, 160, 163
RDIs (Reference Daily Intakes), 28–30, 32
RDs (registered dietitians), 10, 194
Recommended Dietary Allowances, *see* RDAs
Redux, 193
Reference Daily Intakes, *see* RDIs
refined carbohydrates, 182–84
refrigerator, 2, 6, 207–08, 216, 292
registered dietitians, *see* RDs
rennin, 80
retinoids, 105

retinol, 29, 105, 133
  equivalents, 29
retinol activity equivalent, *see* RAE
riboflavin, 16, 29, 36, 41, 60, 115–19, 135,
  199, 204, 209, 291
  content, 118
  deficiency, 117
ribonucleic acid, *see* RNA
rice, 8, 23–24, 43, 47, 53, 67, 73–76, 78, 82,
  156, 170, 212, 265–67, 272, 274,
  283–84
rickets, 107, 109–10, 133
RNA, 44, 72, 142, 153
rosemary, 225, 235, 239, 285
roux, 265–66, 282, 284
Russia, 178–80, 239

S

sachet, 234, 249, 287, 295
sage, 221–22, 225, 234–35
salads, 51, 61, 82, 99, 238–39, 241, 261,
  275, 279–80, 284, 286–87, 298
salivary amylase, 48–49, 67
salmon, 111, 119–20, 124, 128–29
salt, 1–3, 10–12, 21–22, 59, 76–77, 82, 88,
  98, 146–48, 150, 155, 166, 174,
  217, 290, 295–96
  substitutes, 148
sandwiches, 11, 36, 188, 238, 241, 261–62
saturated fats, 25, 27, 31, 33, 36, 82–83, 87, 89,
  90, 95–97, 99, 100, 243, 256–58,
  267–72, 279, 291–92, 295–96
sauces, 98, 138, 211–13, 223, 234–35,
  237–39, 247–48, 251–53, 255,
  257–58, 262–67, 272, 274, 290,
  292–93, 297–98
  emulsified, 265
  thickened, 266
  traditional, 265, 267
scurvy, 8, 129–30, 134
  citrus fruit cures, 128
seafood, 3, 70, 153, 156, 159, 162, 170,
  204, 206, 212, 215, 234, 265, 269,
  292, 294
seasonings, 3, 5, 214, 223, 233, 242–43,
  270, 274
seeds, 44, 47, 73, 75, 95, 153, 169, 173, 221,
  232–33, 239–40, 245, 248, 261,
  296, 298
seitan, 261–62
selenium, 18, 20, 29, 35, 42, 60, 97, 137,
  150, 155–56, 163, 170, 200
sesame, 75, 213, 242, 269, 293
  seeds, 230, 292–93
shallots, 237–38, 266–67, 270
shrimp, 92, 204–05, 243, 255–57, 278–79, 286
  popcorn, 255–57
simplesse, 83, 98
skin, 105–06, 108–09, 117, 119–20, 124,
  129–30, 134–35
  cancer, 110
  dry, 120, 133
  flaky, 123, 134
sodium, 21–22, 27, 29, 33–34, 36, 38, 88,
  137–38, 144–50, 163–64, 204–05,
  242–43, 257, 275–76, 291, 295–96
  chloride, 146, 150, 221

soups, 53, 61, 82, 138, 166, 189, 211–12,
  234–35, 239, 246, 261–63, 266,
  274, 277, 282, 284–85
sour, 166, 217, 219–20, 224–25, 243–44, 265
  five basic tastes of, 217
soy
  products, 82, 84–85, 89, 100, 139
  protein, 34, 82
soybeans, 55, 63, 73, 95, 139, 144–45, 152,
  242, 262–63, 296, 298
Spain, 61, 179–80, 232
Spanish onions, 235, 237–38
spice route, 231
standards of identity, 26
steaks, flank, 76–77, 214, 258, 269–70, 288
steam, 211
stewing, 213–14, 269
stock, 211–12, 234–35, 237, 253, 262,
  266–67, 270, 284, 293
stomach, 49, 50, 56, 67, 70, 79, 80, 93, 137,
  142, 149, 163
sucrose, 45–46, 49, 53, 66, 84
sugar, 21–22, 24, 43–53, 59, 64, 66–68, 70,
  76–79, 84, 98–99, 142, 182–84,
  187–88, 225, 248, 295–97
  cane, 46, 84, 232
  molecules, 45
  refined, 84, 183, 257, 274–75
sulfur, 72, 137–38, 150, 163
sweet potatoes, 46, 58, 67, 152, 173, 208, 210
swordfish, 138, 205

T

tannin, 152
taste
  bitter, 218, 221, 225, 227
  buds, 218–21, 226, 235
  cells, 219–20
  hairs, 219
tempeh, 261–62
tenderloin, 81, 253, 289–90
tetany, 139
thiamin, 8, 9, 16, 29, 36, 41, 60, 115–19, 133,
  135–36, 199, 200, 210, 212, 290–91
  deficiency, 115–16
  loss, 116
thickening agent, 48, 58, 266–67
thyroxin, 153–54
tocopherols, 111
tofu, 55, 73–74, 77, 82, 85, 99, 139–40, 167,
  261–63, 282, 286
tongue, 3, 217–21, 226–27
Tournedos Rossini, 253
toxicity, 18, 32, 106, 109, 112, 114, 116–17, 119,
  121, 123, 125, 127–29, 132, 134,
  140, 143–44, 148–49, 151, 153–60
trans fats, 21, 28, 30, 87–88, 96–97,
  100–01, 169
trans-retinal, 106
triglycerides, 89, 90, 93–94, 100, 159, 181
tryptophan, 118–19
tubers, 47, 210, 239
tuna, 78, 83, 120, 122, 124, 128, 149, 188,
  204–05
turkey, 143, 212, 232, 234, 258–59, 281,
  288, 291
turnips, 200, 221, 225, 234–35, 264, 266

U

UL (Upper Level), 18, 30, 32, 139, 142, 144,
  148–49, 151, 153, 155–61
umami, 217, 220–21, 265
United States Department of Health and
  Human Services, 172–73, 175
unsaturated fats, 28, 96
Upper Level, *see* UL
U.S. Department of Agriculture, *see* USDA
USDA (U.S. Department of Agriculture), 14,
  20–27, 30, 40, 42, 63, 66, 77,
  82, 182–84, 192, 195–96, 200,
  204–05, 215–16, 254

V

vanadium, 138, 160–61
vasodilation, 88, 144
veal, 82, 239, 243, 259, 288–90
vegans, 81–82, 296
vegetable oils, 22, 96, 173, 256, 267–70,
  284, 298
vegetable protein, 272
vegetables
  fiber-rich, 284
  fruit, 264
  green, 145, 211, 220, 284
  healthy, 262
  nutrient-rich, 253
  vitamin-rich, 212
vegetarians, 30, 69, 81–84, 261, 289, 296
venison, 258–60, 289–90
vermouth, 245
very-low-density lipoprotein (VLDL), 61
Vidalia, 236–38
vinegars, 77, 93, 142, 159, 220, 225, 229, 235,
  243–44, 249, 262, 269–70, 279, 286
vitamin
  A, 28–29, 33, 174, 201, 204, 209, 285, 291
  B_1, 9, 59, 115
    functions, 115
  B_2, 116
  B_3, 115
  B_5, 121
  B_6, 29, 41, 60, 115, 122–24, 135, 201,
    290, 295
    deficiency, 123
  B_{12}, 82, 84–85, 115, 122–23, 127–28,
    135, 209
    absorption, 122, 127
    deficiency, 127
  B_{15}, 131
  B_{17}, 131
  C, 8, 16, 32–33, 42, 97, 131, 152, 160–61,
    169, 174, 184, 198, 201, 204–06,
    209–12, 257, 287
  D, 19, 28–29, 41, 66, 84–85, 93, 97, 141–42,
    163, 168, 171, 175, 199, 201
  D_1, 130
  D_2, 109, 133
  D_3, 109
    25-dihydroxy, 109
    25-hydroxy, 109
  E, 15, 29, 42, 169–70, 201
  K, 19, 29
  fat-soluble, 103, 130, 132
  water-soluble, 200, 210–2, 287, 293
VLDL, *see* very-low-density lipoprotein

W

walnuts, 35, 89, 92, 97, 100, 173, 242, 269
water balance, 72, 147
weight, 1, 23–24, 27, 37–38, 59, 65, 70, 75,
 86, 154, 165, 178, 182, 184–87,
 189, 248
 loss, 65, 148, 160, 166, 168, 178, 181–82,
 187–88, 190–91, 195–96
wheat, 47, 53, 56, 58–60, 67, 73, 75, 119–22,
 129, 134, 143, 156, 275, 281
 bran, 124, 129
 fiber, 66

germ, 116, 123, 125
 oil, 112–13
whole-grain
 breads, 51, 59, 66
 products, 21, 170
wines, 8, 40, 77, 79, 83, 159, 211, 224–25,
 229, 244–46, 252, 262, 265–67,
 269–70, 274–76, 287
women, 2, 14–15, 22, 26, 31, 63–64, 94–95,
 97, 138, 140–41, 143, 148, 151,
 153, 158–60, 167
world cuisine, 5, 6, 221, 231–32, 282

World Health Organization, 46–47, 68, 178–80,
 195

Y

yogurt, 23–24, 51, 54, 71, 82–83, 85, 139, 143,
 243, 280, 284

Z

zinc, 15, 18, 20, 29, 60, 63, 79, 137, 150,
 153–54, 163, 167, 174, 245, 294,
 297
 deficiency, 153